Making Money in
a Health Service
Business on Your
Home-Based PC

Making Money in a Health Service Business on Your Home-Based PC

Second Edition

Rick Benzel

Paul and Sarah Edwards, Series Editors

McGraw-Hill
New York   San Francisco   Washington, D.C.   Auckland   Bogotá
Caracas   Lisbon   London   Madrid   Mexico City   Milan
Montreal   New Delhi   San Juan   Singapore
Sydney   Tokyo   Toronto

Library of Congress Cataloging-in-Publication Data

Benzel, Rick.
    [Making money in a health service business on your home-based PC]
    Rick Benzel.—2nd ed.

        p.   cm.
    Formerly published under the title: Health service businesses on
your home-based PC
    Includes index.
    ISBN 0-07-913139-5 (p)
    1. Medical fees—Data processing—Vocational guidance.   2. Home-
based businesses—Vocational guidance.   3. Collecting of accounts—
Data processing—Vocational guidance.   4. Medical transcription—
Vocational guidance.   5. Insurance, Health—Adjustment of claims—
Vocational guidance.   I. Title.
R728.8.B46   1997
651'.961—dc20   96-29742
                                                                              CIP

McGraw-Hill

A Division of The **McGraw-Hill** *Companies*

Copyright © 1997, 1993 by The McGraw-Hill Companies, Inc. All rights
reserved. Printed in the United States of America. Except as permitted under the
United States Copyright Act of 1976, no part of this publication may be reproduced or distributed in any form or by any means, or stored in a data base or
retrieval system, without the prior written permission of the publisher.

        5 6 7 8 9 0   DOC/DOC   9 0 2 1 0 9

P/N 0-07-006104-1
PART OF
ISBN 0-07-913139-5

*The sponsoring editor for this book was Scott Grillo, the editing supervisor was
Penny Linskey, and the production supervisor was Pamela Pelton. It was set in
Vendome by Renee Lipton of McGraw-Hill's Professional Book Group composition unit.*

Printed and bound by Donnelley/Crawfordsville.

This book is printed on acid-free paper.

To Terry, Rebecca, and Sarah

CONTENTS

Contents

PREFACE

When I wrote the first edition of this book, I did not anticipate the enormous interest it would generate among people seeking a new career. As I followed the sales of the book over several years, however, I became both proud and less surprised by its success because I realized that it was fulfilling a tremendous need for information and advice. I salute readers of the second edition of this book—by buying this book, you are already proving that you know how to approach a business or career decision as important as the one you may now face: by getting the best information available.

This second edition reflects an extensive amount of updating. Much has changed since the first edition of this book relative to the three businesses covered. The new material falls into the following categories:

Healthcare industry trends. New trends are occurring in healthcare that affect all three businesses. The foremost of these is managed care, which has had an impact on the medical billing profession, in particular.

Statistical and factual updates. One of the underpinnings in this book is to show some of the statistical data that indicate the growth and trends in healthcare. You will find many new charts and tables that businesspeople can use to plan their future.

Technological advancements. As always, there is a constant stream of new software, enormous improvement in hardware, and many other changes that can improve life for the small or home-based business. For example, the area of digital recording is beginning to alter the medical transcription field, opening up more opportunities for the home-based business. The maturation of the Internet also creates a fertile area for updating, as many companies and associations now have Web sites that you can visit for information and advice.

Case histories. Since the first edition, I have spoken to or interviewed hundreds of people who were either seeking to get into one of the businesses in this book or who were already successful at it. This new edition contains many of the best stories I heard that can serve as meaningful inspiration for you.

Business trends. In the first edition, I made many recommendations about how to get into each business; some of that information has had to be updated. I have focused especially in the chapter on medical billing to provide better, more reliable information about which business opportunity vendors to work with if you are interested in purchasing training and support along with the specialized medical billing software required for this profession.

CD-ROM capability. As you can see, the publisher has graciously agreed to include a CD-ROM with this book. This contains software demos for medical billing software.

According to an informal survey I conducted, the majority of people who bought the first edition of this book seemed to be interested in starting a medical billing service. For this reason, I have expanded the material on medical billing and made it the largest chapter in this book. This is not to suggest that the other two professions covered are slighted; there is truly an astonishing amount of information on CAP work and medical transcription, but I have tried to answer the many questions hundreds of people have asked me about medical billing. I apologize to those who may have wanted more information on the other two businesses, but I am sure you will not be disappointed with any chapter.

I probably don't need to convince you of the benefits of working for yourself. Self-employment *is* the wave of the future. It allows you the greatest freedom of choice, flexibility, and control of your life. Working for yourself provides an opportunity to make your own decisions and reap your own rewards. Indeed, self-employment can change your entire point of view on the meaning of life.

I know, because it has changed mine. After a 15-year career in publishing, working for several companies in Boston and Los Angeles, I made a transition in 1991 into my own home business as a professional writer and editor. Since that decision, I have not regretted once working for myself. In fact, I have never been more challenged or exhilarated in my professional life as I am now.

Part of my exhilaration comes from working on this book. Although I was not very familiar with the healthcare field when I wrote the first edition, I have truly become fascinated by all three businesses included here, and I have learned a great deal about each one. As a writer who focuses largely on small and home-based businesses, I sincerely believe that the three businesses in this book are among the best you can start if you enjoy the field of healthcare and you have either a background in it or an affinity for it.

Please note, however, that none of the businesses in this book is a get-rich-quick scheme. These are all businesses in which you must work hard.

I don't want to mince words about that. These are careers that require knowledge, effort, and marketing on your part.

I hope you find the information helpful if you are trying to decide on a new career. Let me add that the health field undergoes many changes on a frequent basis. The technology of medical billing and transcription changes, federal and state government rules and regulations about Medicare and Medicaid change, the insurance companies and HMOs that underwrite health insurance policies change, and even doctors and hospitals change. In short, while I believe this book to be as accurate and up-to-date as possible at the time of its writing, please be aware that you may learn slightly different information, rules, and regulations by the time this book reaches your hand or when you get into business. This only reflects how important it is to keep up with the profession you ultimately select.

Thank you for your time.

—RICK BENZEL

ACKNOWLEDGMENTS

As is the case with nearly every book published, many people contributed to the project in some form. I would like to thank especially the following pivotal people for their special role in helping me. First, I thank my wife Terry, and my daughters Rebecca and Sarah, for being there. I thank my personal friend L.F. for her invaluable guidance in my writing career. I express my gratitude to Paul and Sarah Edwards, who introduced me to these healthcare fields and the opportunity to work on this book. To Scott Grillo, my editor, many thanks for recognizing the value of enhancing the first edition of this book.

I am especially grateful to Randi Goldsmith, Director of McGraw-Hill Computing, for her leadership in developing the CD—Rom accompanying this book, and to Barry Kaplan of Mega Space, who worked endless hours to organize and program the CD—Rom into a clean, unified presentation.

I also thank my editing supervisor, Penny Linskey, for her excellent shepherding of the manuscript through final production.

In working on this second edition, I utilized many resources, particularly the knowledge and experience of many people in these businesses. I thank everyone who agreed to an interview, whose profiles you find in this book.

Special thanks go to the following individuals for spending hours of their time with me discussing their businesses and in some cases reading portions of the manuscript: my medical billing mentor Merry Schiff of Medical Management Software; Nancie Lee Cummins of Medical Management Billing; Richard Wunneburger, Ken Fisher, Cheryl Hamilton, and everyone at InfoHealth and Synaps Corporation; Jeff Ward, Darlene Pickron, and Will Crandell of Medisoft/The Computer Place; Gary Knox of AQC Resources; Norma Border of NACAP; my dear friends Tom and Nancy Koehler of In Home Medical Claims; Pat Forbis of AAMT; Linda Campbell of HPI; Ann Jacobsen of Medicode; author Donna Avila-Weil; Bernie Magoon of Lanier; and Scott Faulkner of Dictaphone.

Notices

- **Straight Talk**®, **Digital Express**® and **MVP**® are registered trademarks of Dictaphone Corporation. **Express Writer**™ is a trademark of Dictaphone Corporation.

- **Business Plan Pro**™ is a trademark of Palo Alto Software.

- **OneClaim Plus**® is a registered trademark of Santiago SDS, Inc.

- **Lytec Systems** is a division of National Data Corporation.

All other software is protected under copyright or trademark by its owner.

1

The Booming Healthcare Business

The healthcare professions are booming. Whether you are seeking to enter a completely new career or are branching out from an allied health field, now is a great time to consider starting your own business in healthcare. Today, and for many decades into the future, healthcare will remain a growing, thriving, recession-proof, profitable field for entrepreneurs and people seeking home-based businesses. Given the demographics of America's aging population with its growing need for medical attention, along with the new baby boom and a number of other factors, you have an irrefutable fact: the healthcare professions abound with opportunity. Healthcare has already become the second largest occupational sector in the United States, after the food industry. It is estimated that there were more than 10.5 million Americans employed in the health field in 1995, and projections for growth through the year 2000 are among the highest of all industries.

The upshot of this trend is a boon for the person interested in opening a small- or home-based business. With insurance companies, hospitals, labs, doctors' offices, and ancillary health businesses all looking to save money and lower costs, many opportunities exist for the home-based sole proprietor or small business entrepreneur. Smaller businesses can operate more efficiently, cut expenses, and be more productive. In fact, small businesses represent an important key to halting or at least slowing down the inflationary 8 percent to 10 percent annual growth rate in expenditures that has marked American healthcare for the past 15 years. New technologies and new ways of working are also changing the face of health careers and providing profitable opportunities for home-based and small business entrepreneurs.

Astounding Facts and Figures

A constant stream of statistics demonstrates the enormity of the American healthcare system and its projected nonstop growth. Unfortunately, it is difficult to put together a coherent snapshot of healthcare in America, because the significant time lag in collecting data and putting the statistics together makes the numbers appear to be outdated. There are also many statistics that are constantly being revised, so it is often impossible to compare facts from one month to the next and from one source of information to another, or even to determine which fact is reliable.

However, each year the Health Insurance Institute of America compiles an excellent guide to the healthcare industry, based on data collected by various government agencies and private associations. This guide, entitled *The Source Book of Health Insurance Data*, presents an impressive array of charts, tables, and text from which you can gather an astonishing knowledge about U.S. healthcare. Consider the following facts and tables as a general barometer of our healthcare industry and its opportunities:

- In 1995, the U.S. National Health Expenditure (NHE) broke the $1 trillion mark, and in 1996 (as this book was being written) it was projected to increase to $1.08 trillion. That's an 8 percent increase in healthcare spending over one year.

- Of the $1+ trillion spent in 1995, $987 billion was spent on personal healthcare (as opposed to research, construction of health facilities, and government public health programs that are not care related). Personal healthcare includes expenses for hospitalization and physician care, dental services, home health care, drugs and medications, vision products, and nursing home care. Figure 1-1 shows the breakdown of personal healthcare dollars in 1995.

■ The NHE has been slowly eating up the American economy. In 1995, the NHE was equal to more than 14 percent of the entire Gross Domestic Product (GDP), which means that healthcare consumes nearly one-eighth of all dollars produced in the United States. Even worse, it is projected that the NHE, which has been rising at a rate of 8 percent to 11 percent per year since the 1980s, will soon compose nearly one-fifth of the entire GDP. Table 1-1 projects the estimated increases in the NHE for 1996 through 2005. As you can see, within a decade, the NHE will exceed $2 trillion, nearly 18 percent of the GDP.

■ Of the $1 trillion spent for NHE in 1995, Medicare accounted for $190 billion to provide services to nearly 38 million people. The majority of Medicare money is spent on hospital and physician services. According to the Health Care Financing Administration (HCFA, pronounced Hick-fah), the federal agency that runs Medicare and is affiliated with the Department of Health and Human Services, nearly 30 percent of Medicare expenditures pay for the care of elderly people in the last years of their lives. Look again at Table 1-1 and notice how Medicare is expected to grow over the next decade. By 2050, HCFA projects there will be nearly 70 million Americans on Medicare, if the program survives that long.

■ In 1995, Medicaid—a combined HCFA and state government program—spent an additional $140 billion to cover more than 36 million

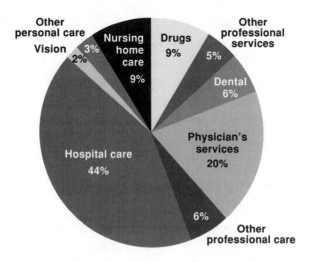

Figure 1-1
Breakdown of
personal health care
expenditures in 1995

people (some people are covered by both Medicare and Medicaid). Combining Medicare and Medicaid, government subsidized insurance paid for nearly one-third of all healthcare in the country in 1995.

In addition to these figures, consider the following interesting demographic facts about the U.S. population and our healthcare needs:

- According to the latest available *complete* and *reliable* figures from the Health Insurance Association of America, in 1993, 220 million of 260 million Americans had some type of health insurance coverage, provided generally by private insurers, employer-run group plans, or government-sponsored programs.

- In 1993, there were 5,260 community hospitals in the United States with nearly 1 million hospital beds, and an average 65 percent occupancy rate. The number of hospitals has been decreasing over the past decade because of rising costs and increased use of outpatient services.

- In a typical year in America, there are about 25 million blood pressure checks, 90 million urinalyses, and 90 million blood tests performed.

- The number of doctors in the United States is mushrooming. According to figures from the American Medical Association (AMA), in 1993, a total of 653,000 physicians were distributed among many different specialties. The largest number, more than 100,000, were in internal medicine. In addition, according to HCFA, it is estimated that by the year 2000, there will be nearly 660,000 doctors, 161,000 dentists, and 40,000 osteopaths practicing in the United States, almost double the numbers in 1970. Furthermore, there are nearly 250,000 licensed pharmacists in the country. Table 1-2 (page 6) shows a breakdown by types of physicians.

- According to the latest figures from the National Center for Health Statistics, in 1993 there were more than 1.6 billion physician contacts between doctors and patients in the United States. This figure includes all contacts in person, via telephone, or at a hospital or facility. Women averaged 6.7 visits per year, while men averaged only 5.2 contacts per year. Table 1-3 (page 7) shows a breakdown by age and sex of physician contacts.

As you can see from the data, the healthcare industry is on a rollercoaster ride up, with no major downturns expected. Why is this so? The answer lies in a number of undeniable trends.

TABLE 1-1

Projected National Health Expenditures: 1996–2005

	1996	1997	1998	1999	2000	2001	2002	2003	2004	2005
Total National Health Expenditures	$1,087.1	$1,173.5	$1,269.3	$1,372.1	$1,481.7	$1,600.4	$1,728.8	$1,866.5	$2,014.2	$2,173.7
Private	594.7	641.3	693.7	749.4	807.9	871.8	940.1	1012.5	1089.3	1171.3
Public	492.4	532.2	575.6	622.8	673.7	728.7	788.7	854.0	924.9	1002.4
Medicare	208.9	227.8	247.8	269.9	293.5	319.1	347.4	378.5	412.8	450.9
Medicaid	150.2	163.8	179.2	195.9	214.5	234.6	256.5	280.1	305.7	333.4
Other	133.3	140.6	148.6	157.0	165.7	174.9	184.8	195.3	206.4	218.1
Average % increase from previous year		7.9%	8.2%	8.1%	8.0%	8.0%	8.0%	8.0%	7.9%	7.9%
Gross Domestic Product (GDP in $billions)	$7,506.6	$7,921.3	$8,360.9	$8,822.9	$9,301.1	$9,821.5	$1,0359.2	$10,926.0	$11,524.0	$12,155.5
National Health Expenditure as a % of GDP	14.5%	14.8%	15.2%	15.6%	15.9%	16.3%	16.7%	17.1%	17.5%	17.9%
U.S. Population	275.9	278.2	280.5	282.8	285.0	287.2	289.4	291..5	293.6	295.7
Per Capita Expenditures	$3,941	$4,218	$4,525	$4,852	$5,198	$5,572	$5,975	$6,404	$6,861	$7,352

Source: Health Care Financing Administration (HCFA), Office of Actuary: Data from Office of National Health Statistics.

DEMOGRAPHIC FACTS. The U.S. population is rapidly expanding. Whereas we were 190 million in 1960, we are now more than 270 million people and growing. Of special note is the fact that the distribution of the U.S. population has a high proportion of people who need regular healthcare services: babies and new mothers, the middle aged, and the elderly. For example, in *each year* of the decade of the 1990s, nearly 4 million babies will be born. Also in each year of the 1990s, more than 20 million children will be below the age of 5, more than 4 million people will turn 45, and more than 2 million people will become 65. As you can readily imagine, these figures reflect a huge demand for healthcare services.

TABLE 1-2

Physicians
(Federal and
Nonfederal) by
Selected Specialty
and Activity, 1992

Specialty	Total Physicians	Patient Care	Office Based	Hospital Based
Anesthesiology	28,148	27,034	19,998	3,120
Cardiovascular diseases	16,478	14,709	11,460	1,407
Dermatology	7,912	7,550	6,318	371
Radiology	18,156	14,117	10,858	2,209
Emergency Medicine	15,470	14,813	9,373	3,796
Family Practice	50,969	49,269	40,479	2,555
Gastroenterology	7,964	7,121	5,724	538
General Practice	20,719	20,475	18,575	1,600
General Surgery	39,211	37,792	24,956	2,919
Internal Medicine	109,017	99,502	65,312	8,445
Neurology	9,742	8,559	6,330	917
Obstetrics/Gynecology	35,273	34,136	27,115	1,947
Pediatrics	44,881	41,482	29,110	3,851
Pathology	17,005	13,910	7,948	3,154
Ophthalmology	16,433	15,970	13,752	675
Orthopaedic surgery	20,640	20,244	15,832	1,277
Nuclear Medicine	1,372	1,181	736	307
Urology	9,452	9,214	7,688	573
Psychiatry	36,405	33,005	21,913	5,860
Totals	505,247	470,083	343,477	45,521

Note: There were 653,000 physicians in 1992. This table represents a selected group of this total. Excludes physicians in administration, medical teaching, and research. Figures in each row do not add up because of overlap.

Source: U.S. Department of Health and Human Services, Bureau of Health Professions.

INCREASED LIFE EXPECTANCY. Another demographic fact contributing to increased healthcare usage is a longer life. In fact, life expectancy in the United States has been on rise for a century. In just the last decade alone, the life expectancy for a male at birth has gone up more than 2 years, from 70 in 1980 to 72.1 in 1993. Similarly, a female's life expectancy at birth rose 1.5 years, from 77.4 to 78.9. These increases in longevity are due to advances in fighting the three leading causes of death

TABLE 1-3

Number of
Physician Contacts
per Year per
Person
(1990–1993)

	1990	1991	1992	1993
All persons	**5.5**	**5.6**	**5.9**	**6.0**
AGE				
Under 5 years	6.9	7.1	6.9	7.2
5—14 years	3.2	3.4	3.4	3.6
15—44 years	4.8	4.7	5	5
45—64	6.4	6.6	7.2	7.1
65—74 years	8.5	9.2	9.7	9.9
75 years +	10.1	12.3	12.1	12.3
SEX AND AGE				
Male				
Under 5	7.2	7.6	7.1	7.5
5—14	3.3	3.5	3.5	3.8
15—44	3.4	3.4	3.7	3.6
45—64	5.6	5.8	6.1	6.1
65—74	8	8.6	9.2	9.3
75 years +	10	11.6	12.2	11.7
Female				
Under 5	6.5	6.6	6.7	6.9
5—14	3.2	3.2	3.3	3.4
15—44	6	5.9	6.2	6.4
45—64	7.1	7.4	8.2	8.1
65—74	9	9.7	10.1	10.4
75 years +	10.2	12.7	12.1	12.8

ED: In all four faces
of Vendome the en
dash (—) and the em
dash (—) are very
close in size

We went over them
but we had en
dashes on this
galley page

Source: U.S. Department of Health and Human Services, 1994 National Health Interview Survey

in the United States—heart disease, cancer, and stroke—largely because
new technology and pharmaceuticals have helped many people survive
these formerly fatal diseases. Many more advances are likely to be discovered and implemented in the future as well, yet another sign that the
demand for health services can only grow further.

INCREASED USE OF HEALTH INSURANCE.   The increasing use of health insurance is another factor in explaining the boom in healthcare, as more and more people have come to rely on some form of insurance from a commercial insurance company, an employer-sponsored plan, or a government source such as Medicare or Medicaid. Whereas in 1985 only 204 million Americans had public or private health insurance, the Bureau of Census estimated that nearly 230 million Americans were covered by health insurance in 1995. Because of this explosion, a staggering amount of money annually floods the economy to pay for health services such as physician fees, hospitalizations, lab fees, and so on.

For example, according to the latest figures available from 1993, private insurance paid $84 billion in claims benefits for physician services alone, while Medicare and Medicaid payments added another $58 billion. As Table 1-1 showed, the per capita expenditure for healthcare will rise from nearly $4,000 per year in 1996 to more than $7,000 per year by the year 2005.

HEALTH-CONSCIOUSNESS FEVER.   Over the past two decades, the American population has been growing more conscious of the value of health and fitness. On one hand, as members of the baby boom genera-tion age, they have become more sensitive than any previous generation to growing "older"—and fighting it every step of the way. On the other hand, a continuous flood of new research clearly demonstrates the link between taking care of one's body and longevity. As a result of both trends, more and more people are recognizing that a long and healthful life depends on their own efforts to eat properly, exercise, sleep well, and reduce stress.

The ramifications of this increasing pursuit of good health are actual-ly contradictory. On one hand, people are staying in better shape and practicing proactive and preventative medicine. But on the other hand, many people are also getting more frequent checkups as they age or whenever a slight health or dental problem occurs. This trend has undoubtedly played a role in increasing healthcare expenditures, as more and more worried people have demanded—"just to be sure"—office visits, lab tests, blood tests, and many other routines that may not have been done in the past.

THE MEDICAL TESTING CRAZE.   The demand for more and more medical testing does not originate solely with patients. According to the *Complete Guide to Medical Tests* by H. Winter Griffith, M.D., medical tests have become extremely important—if not a requirement—in nearly every healthcare situation. One benefit of tests is that our increasingly sophisticated technology allows doctors to make a more accurate diagnosis of a patient's problem. Whereas many types of ailments or problems may have gone undetected in the past, they can be caught much earlier today through the use of sophisticated blood or urine tests, as well as high-tech imaging techniques such as MRIs.

Needless to say, the other benefit of tests (and the one that truly drives up their usage more than any other factor) is that tests provide protection for doctors against the risks of a lawsuit for medical malpractice. In the past, a doctor may have forgone a test to save money if the chances of a patient having a certain disease were remote; today such tests are automatically done so that doctors can protect themselves against mistakes and errors in judgment. Doctors with two years of experience and doctors with twenty years of experience both recognize that testing protects them against the vagaries of distrustful patients, nuisance suits, and perhaps an occasional wrong decision. Tests become part of a permanent record for each patient, thus proving that the doctor has made every attempt to ascertain the underlying problem and to treat it accordingly.

Testing has become so prolific that there are now thousands of types of tests—such as the more than 900 analyses on blood alone—and one hundred or more new tests are invented each year. Dr. Griffith estimates that nearly 10 billion tests are ordered by doctors each year for their patients, costing between $100 billion and $150 billion annually—that's nearly 1 out of every 3 of our healthcare dollars!

GOVERNMENT AND PRIVATE INSURANCE REGULATIONS. Another factor that points to continued growth in healthcare expenditures is the increase in medical regulations and rules from the federal and state governments, as well as from the thousands of commercial insurance companies. For example, Medicare and Medicaid laws now require many kinds of testing, second opinions, and record-keeping procedures—all aimed at limiting the skyrocketing costs of unnecessary medical care. Nevertheless, the overall effect of many regulations is that they end up adding to the costs they are trying to eliminate.

Many of these regulations are aimed at curbing abuse and fraud, both of which have unfortunately occurred in this otherwise respectable profession. Over the past decade, there have been many reports of doctors who falsely billed Medicare for services not rendered, as well as entire clinics such as one in a major metropolitan area that found people to file false worker's compensation claims supported by a doctor's fake diagnoses of injuries. Naturally, the doctors were keeping the insurance money for themselves until they were caught and prosecuted.

No matter how you look at these trends and figures, you will have a hard time not finding some niche to fill in the healthcare field if you so desire. Healthcare will most certainly continue to grow larger in the decades to come, with more and more services needed by a growing population of Americans, and supplied by an increasing number of health-care providers. The savvy entrepreneur knows that for each doctor in the profession and each consumer, a corresponding array of service personnel is needed, and therein lies your opportunity!

Overview of Three Healthcare Businesses

Although there are many careers you can enter in the allied medical fields, this book focuses on three that can be run as home-based or small businesses, either on a full-time or part-time basis. Each business offers a moderate to high income potential, and all indications are that each business will remain a solid opportunity over the next decade. Here is an overview of the three businesses to help you understand the essential differences between them before you jump into the specific chapters.

MEDICAL BILLING. Many people have heard about medical billing but are not quite sure what business it is. In a nutshell, medical billing is the business of getting healthcare providers paid. Most of this work involves filing insurance claims on behalf of doctors, chiropractors, thera-pists, dentists, and other healthcare providers to commercial insurance companies and government agencies such as Medicare and Medicaid. Over the past few years, the most successful medical billing businesses have expanded their services to include what is called "full practice man-agement," meaning that they handle all the bookkeeping and accounting functions for their doctor-clients, including patient statements, recording payments, preparing financial reports, and even advising the physicians on issues such as how to negotiate contracts with the growing number of managed care companies such as HMOs and PPOs that are trying to reign in doctors' fees.

Medical billing has become a "hot" business in the past few years, par-tially because of the advent and growth of electronic claims. Let's briefly explain this aspect of medical billing. Before computers, filing claims to insurance companies was a tedious and expensive process for doctors. A typical doctor who had several hundred patients, each with his or her own insurance company, was faced with a veritable quagmire in either let-ting patients file their own claims and waiting to get reimbursed before paying the doctor, or filling out the claims themselves to make sure they got done quickly and that the checks would be mailed directly to them. As a result, many doctors opted for the latter solution and filed the claims for their patients.

The problem was that each insurance company had its own rules and regulations, and, worse, the filing of claims had to be done using annoying paper forms with dozens of little boxes to fill in. Claims had to be either handwritten or typed, and many errors were made in filling out the claims. As a result, getting paid was a nightmare, and many healthcare providers who had agreed to handle claims for their patients simply gave up on collecting some of their money out of frustration or confusion. Some doctors literally lost thousands of dollars per month in unpaid claims.

The nightmare became even more critical for doctors in September 1990, when the federal government decided that Medicare recipients should not have to file their own claims. The government therefore legislated that it was the responsibility of *doctors* to file Medicare claims on behalf of their patients. Since the majority of people who see doctors are elderly, this meant that many doctors were literally swamped with Medicare claims to file, day in and day out.

Fortunately, over the course of the 1980s, more sophisticated software had brought about a new technology called "electronic claims processing" (often abbreviated ECP). With this technology, the doctor's office could use computers, special software, and a modem to handle the claims filing process. Electronic claims processing has many advantages, including simplifying the highly detailed record-keeping and accounting procedures used in medical offices. Most important, electronic claims substantially reduce the time it takes to prepare paper claims and the number of errors made—estimated to be as high as 30 percent—thereby speeding up the time it takes for doctors to receive reimbursements from the private insurance companies and government-run programs.

Unfortunately, many doctors' offices did not make the transition to electronic claims, usually because they did not have the computer equipment needed or the skilled personnel to use the software. In many cases, doctors simply did not understand the benefits of ECP. But in the late 1980s and early 1990s, as the cost of personal computers decreased and the benefits of ECP became more obvious, a new opportunity emerged for entrepreneurs to start independent medical billing businesses. The professional billing service takes over the filing of claims for doctors and moves them into the electronic twentieth century.

As mentioned earlier, handling electronic claims is just one side of running an independent medical billing service. Either right from the outset, or after getting a contract to handle just the claims, many billing services become involved with many other aspects of their clients' accounting needs.

The growth of managed care is the other key fueling independent billing agencies. Billers are literally becoming trusted financial advisors to their doctors, helping them decide the best ways to maintain their income in the face of severe reimbursement cutbacks from insurance companies and the dreaded monster of managed care plans.

Chapter 2 examines the details of starting your own independent medical billing service. You will find in this chapter a comprehensive explanation of how medical billing works, what knowledge and skills are required to run a billing service, and how to get started if you believe this business is for you. You will learn how health insurance works, how doctors' offices operate, and the steps to filing paper versus electronic claims and receiving payments. You will also get an introduction to the complex medical coding systems that you need to understand in processing claims for doctors.

The chapter especially emphasizes three issues that have been evolving since the early 1990s when the first edition of this book came out:

- The impact of managed care on both doctors and medical billing services. The chapter discusses the growth of HMOs, PPOs, IPAs, POSs, and MSOs and explains how such managed care arrangements are reducing physicians' incomes *and* thus how they are increasing the need for and potential success of independent billing services.

- The increasing level of sophistication and knowledge that it now takes to be successful in operating an independent medical billing service. Because of the growing complexity of running a doctor's office and the increased scrutiny of insurance companies to control costs, being successful in medical billing now requires a much higher level of insurance industry knowledge, computer skills, and marketing savvy to convince doctors to let you handle their financial affairs. The chapter therefore provides much advice about developing your industry knowledge as well as many inside tips on successful marketing strategies to get clients for your business.

- How to get into the medical billing business. Because of the popularity of medical billing, many people have invested money to buy software and training without being fully aware of what it takes to be successful in this business. Since I wrote the first edition of this book, literally dozens of people have personally called me to get advice about buying a medical billing "business opportunity" that would train them to get into the business within a few days. This chapter therefore explains how to evaluate the "biz opps" you will probably find out there. Unfortunately, some vendors take advantage of people interested in this profession, leading them to believe that medical billing is a get-rich-quick occupation. They use high-pressure tactics to get people to buy their software and training at extremely high prices. My goal here is to provide some general information on how to evaluate and purchase a good business opportunity that will truly help you succeed. I provide recommendations for vendors to work with and give you warnings about how to recognize unscrupulous business opportunity companies.

You will find in this chapter a large number of personal stories from people who got into medical billing and succeeded. As their stories show, you must work hard to learn this business and become a "medical reimbursement expert." But it doesn't stop there. Even if you begin to be successful, you will need to continue working hard to stay abreast of changes because there are constant new insurance rules and regulations, new technologies that will affect the profession, and new trends in managed care that doctors will want you to explain to them.

CLAIMS ASSISTANCE PROFESSIONAL.   The inverse, or flip side, of a medical billing service is a *claims assistance professional* (often abbreviated CAP, and pronounced "cap" just like the hat). A CAP works with consumers—not doctors. If you are unfamiliar with this profession, it is common to confuse medical billing and claims assistance. The two professions share a large body of knowledge, such as how health insurance works, but they are oriented to different audiences and require very different skills.

CAPs help two types of consumers:

1. Those who must submit their own health insurance claims to their insurance company. Because some doctors do not file insurance claims on behalf of their patients (except in the case of Medicare claims, which, as stated earlier, physicians are required to file), many people must submit their own claims each time they see their doctor, dentist, chiropractor, or psychologist. However, these people are often confused by the filing procedures or they simply want someone to handle the claims for them.

2. Those who have already filed a claim and had it denied or incorrectly paid by their insurance company. This audience is the majority of the CAP market because, knowingly or not, insurance companies

and Medicare make many mistakes when they evaluate claims for payment. Claims are often lost, delayed, underpaid, or completely denied, leaving consumers angry and upset, but not knowing what to do. A CAP therefore reviews all medical invoices and bills and makes sure that the client is not being cheated out of money he or she deserves. The CAP may appeal a denied claim or contest an erroneous bill from a doctor.

In essence, CAPs help the confused, the forlorn, and the just plain busy through the complex maze of the health insurance world. A good CAP is like a skilled tax preparer who assists his or her clients to file tax returns with the goal of maximizing their refunds. In the same sense, a skilled CAP reviews medical bills and payments and tries to maximize both the coverage and the reimbursements each client can obtain from his or her insurance carrier—be it Medicare or a private company.

Today's CAPs must understand doctor's office procedures, managed care, Medicare and Medicaid regulations, and the intricate details of increasingly complex insurance policies that often seem to contain double-talk when it comes to spelling out basic issues such as copayments, deductibles, coordination of benefits, stop-loss limits, and prior authorizations. To be a CAP, you must be exceptionally detail oriented, have good math skills, have excellent negotiation and communication skills, and be able to work well with many kinds of people, from naïve consumers to hard-core naysaying insurance bureaucrats. You must also have an action-oriented, fighting personality that believes in justice for the little guy, as well as perseverance, stick-to-itiveness, and a strong belief in the rights of patients. While running a CAP business does not necessarily require you to become heavily computer literate, you should be familiar with basic computer software so you can use your PC to maintain a database of your clients and word process all your correspondence.

Chapter 3 explains the career of a medical claims assistance professional, including the background and skills you need to get started, and how to market and price your service. You will meet several CAPs who have become successful running their own businesses. As you will see, this is one profession in which the practitioners have a true love for their work that far exceeds the usual and customary dedication found in other professions. Of the three careers in this book, being a CAP is by far the most people oriented.

MEDICAL TRANSCRIPTION SERVICE.   The third business covered in this book is medical transcription. In researching this field, hardly an interview went by in which I was not reminded that there is a serious shortage of transcriptionists in the United States. However, medical transcription is a rigorous and technical profession that requires extensive training and often a few years of experience before you can go off on your own. Medical transcriptionists are not just typists or secretaries; their skills are far more complex. They must have a good command of English grammar, *and* know thousands of words of highly technical medical vocabulary, *and* understand the garbled dictations of doctors who eat lunch while they dictate or doctors who have come from many parts of the world to practice in the United States, and for whom English is a second language, *and* be able to type 60 to 90 words per minute (or faster). As you can see, these are serious qualifications that are not easy to come by.

Because of these rigorous requirements though, medical transcription is an extremely valuable profession that is fast becoming a critical area of healthcare management. From routine patient visits and hospitalizations to complex surgeries and psychological exams, physicians are increasingly required by law and by ethics to prepare reports about their patients. In some cases also, such as accidents, lawsuits, and denied medical claims, doctors must prepare documents for insurance companies, police departments, employers, lawyers, and state-funded worker's compensation boards. Finally, in today's era of managed care, increasing numbers of doctors are also required to prepare authorization letters for patients who are referred to specialists outside of their network or HMO, as well as reports back to a primary care physician who is responsible for that patient within the network or HMO.

The transcriptionist's job is not easy. He or she must type up each report accurately from a dictated tape or digital recording, using proper English and the correct medical terminology, spelled correctly. In many cases, the transcriptionist must have reports back to the doctor or hospital within a quick turnaround time that may be as little as a few hours or perhaps one day.

Chapter 4 examines the world of medical transcription and shows you how to obtain training and preparation for this career. Note that, unlike the previous two businesses, which most people can start after just a few months of preparation, medical transcription requires more extensive preparation and education. Some people can enter the business with as little as six months of home study, but others may need one or more years of study if they do not have prior medical background.

Nevertheless, a career in medical transcription can be your ticket to independence, freedom, and financial self-sufficiency. You will meet several people in Chapter 4 who turned to a career in medical transcription with no previous medical background but who were able to achieve their goals within a reasonable time frame.

How to Use This Book

The next three chapters are the heart of this book and contain the essential information about the businesses profiled. Each chapter follows a roughly similar format and is divided into two major sections: **Background** and **Getting Started.**

In the Background section, you will find basic information about the business, including what the business does, how it works, the level of knowledge and skills you'll need, and information on the income and earnings potential. This section includes both the pros and cons of the business so you can truly understand what might await you if you decide to pursue this career. I have attempted to answer the question "Can I make a living doing this?" as well as "Will I enjoy this business?" The Background section ends with an informal 15-question checklist you can use to assess your feelings about the business and your chances of personal satisfaction and success.

In the second section of the chapter, Getting Started, you will find detailed information about how and where to find training, advice on hardware and software issues (as appropriate), tips for how to market your new business and determine your prices, and a final section on overcoming common start-up problems in that business. If after reading the first part of the chapter, you have decided that the business is not for you, you can probably skip or skim this second part of the chapter.

Scattered throughout each chapter are various "sidebar" features, based on interviews I conducted with people engaged in the business, or containing extra explanatory information. You will find many of these sidebars to contain the most valuable information in the chapter: personal stories of people who, just like you, decided to make that business their career. There is often no greater wisdom than that of someone who marched before you, although each person's experience will vary depending on his or her prior background, location, personal talent, and luck. Nevertheless, most of us can take inspiration from others who have made a success out of their own ventures.

The final chapter presents 10 steps to becoming an entrepreneur. To make remembering these steps easier, they are organized around a mnemonic device (a memory aid): DREAM BIG for $ & "smile face". Each letter or symbol in this acronym stands for one issue or activity you'll need to focus on as you get your business under way. This chapter is intended to serve as a reminder to seriously consider your decision, because many people think only about the income and earning potential without reflecting on whether they have the skills to be entrepreneurial or even whether they will truly enjoy the work they've chosen. I therefore urge you to read this last chapter where you'll find wisdom gleaned from many experts in the self-employment field.

A Note on the Choice of Businesses

I have chosen these three businesses for a variety of reasons. First, technically speaking, none requires a hard-core academic background prior to preparing for the business, such as a B.A. in biology, an R.N. degree, or an M.B.A. in health administration. Each business is more or less approachable by any hard-working, dedicated individual who has the entrepreneurial drive to operate his or her own business.

This is not to suggest that you can read this book today and be in business tomorrow. As in any profession or business, the more skills and background you have that relate to the business, the better off you are. If you have ever worked in a physician's office or an insurance company, or if you were a nurse or physician's assistant, or if you have had accounting or bookkeeping experience, or even computer consulting experience, you will have a leg up on those people who come into the healthcare field with absolutely no related background.

But I also want to convey that these skills are quite learnable. Most readers of this book should not have a problem learning about medical billing, claims assistance work, or medical transcription if they commit to studying the necessary subjects and make a sincere effort to run their business in a professional way.

Second, as mentioned earlier in this chapter, I also chose these three businesses because they appear to offer good potential for both personal satisfaction and a decent livelihood. While people are always reluctant to discuss their incomes, everyone interviewed for this book was optimistic and upbeat about what they were earning. Most answered affirmatively when asked if someone working full time at this profession could earn $30,000 to $60,000, or more.

None of these businesses is, however, a get-rich-quick operation (there are really none of those anyway). All require hard work, dedication, and even ambition, and there is still no guarantee. Running your own business is tough. You are the receptionist, marketing manager, sales agent, and professional running the shop. You *are* the business, and you will most likely need to work long hours to build up your company so that you are earning a decent income.

Last, I chose these businesses because I expect that they will be around for some time, and your initial investment of time and money to get into them will pay dividends for years. However, technology can change our world in the flash of an instant, and the medical field is particularly subject to technological advances. For example, voice recognition software is getting better and better and may change the medical transcription profession some day soon. Perhaps 5 or 10 years from now, doctors will be able to dictate their notes to a computer and specialized voice recognition software will automatically convert the speech into a perfect document. Politics too may change these professions. Perhaps our country will adopt a national healthcare plan that more or less abolishes health insurance claims, and both the medical billing and claims assistance businesses will fall by the wayside. Many changes are possible, but in reality, such changes are quite doubtful at this writing, so I feel confident in recommending these businesses to you.

Using Your PC

The title of this book suggests that these three businesses extensively utilize computers. However, the extent of computer usage varies greatly. In descending order of computerization, medical billing is very computer intensive and requires a fair knowledge of hardware and software. Medical transcription is less computer intensive and generally requires only a level of sophistication to operate basic word-processing software. Medical claims assistance turned out to be an industry that is only barely computerized, because, as you will see, insurance companies accept electronic claims only from doctors, not from individuals filing one claim at a time. A CAP must handle claims using the old tried-and-true paper forms.

In all, the computer skills necessary to be in these industries are not difficult to learn. Nevertheless, as you will see in each chapter, getting into one of these businesses means that you will likely need to do extensive marketing, so you can benefit from knowing how to use your PC to perform many general business functions. For example, if you can operate simple desktop publishing software, such as *Microsoft Publisher,* you can design your own brochures, newsletters, fliers, and other marketing documents. Developing such items yourself can often save you money because you can avoid hiring an outside designer or desktop publisher.

Similarly, knowing how to use contact management software, such as *Lotus Organizer* or *Symantec ACT!*, can help you keep better track of your appointments, schedules, meetings, and discussions with clients. If you bill by the hour, it helps to know how to use time management programs such as *Timeslips* to keep track of your productivity and to invoice your clients accurately.

Think of it this way: in today's market, if you are not using a computer to your best advantage, your competitor probably is, and that means you are likely losing opportunities or contracts that could be yours. So, regardless of which of the three businesses in this book you may start, you would be wise to use technology for all your important business functions. Throughout this book, I will refer you to a few such general business productivity programs that I believe to be the most useful.

Doing More Than One Businesses

Can you start more than one business? Most certainly. Several people I interviewed for this book practice two of these businesses at a time, particularly medical billing plus either CAP work or transcription.

For example, Linda Noel of Linda's Billing Service in Los Angeles does medical billing and medical transcription. As she explained, "I offer a personalized service which is the key to getting clients. It helps me be a full service agency, handling two areas of need for my clients." Linda's company is profiled in a sidebar in Chapter 2.

Lori A. Donnelly, founder of Donnelly Benefit Consultants in Bethlehem, Pennsylvania, likewise offers two businesses. Lori started out as a claims assistance professional and built that up as her primary business for six years. However, she eventually moved into medical billing when, quite by accident, an ambulance company saw one of Lori's advertisements in a newspaper and asked her to train someone to handle its claims processing. In thinking over the proposal, Lori realized that given how much she knew about insurance claims from her CAP business, she might as well do medical billing herself rather than train someone. So the ambulance company became her first client, and Lori continued from that point getting several more clients. She now has an ongoing medical billing practice that handles four doctors, and a CAP business that handles as many as 50 clients per month.

In general, it is wise to begin one business first and get it off the ground before expanding into another business. You don't want to confuse your clientele about which business you are really in. A doctor will be less likely to hire you if you walk into the office and say something like, "I am an expert in medical billing and would like to discuss how my company can improve your cash flow from insurance claims...but, oh, if you're not interested in that, I am also an expert transcriptionist." If you decide to offer more than one business, let it evolve over time.

As in any entrepreneurial venture, the sky is the limit for the ambitious, hardworking, and serious person. Whatever your goals, if you have an interest in the health professions, you will surely find something enticing for you in this book!

2

Medical Billing Services

Electronic medical billing services are riding a wave of change in U.S. healthcare. As the practice of medicine becomes more complex, and as insurance companies work overtime to figure out new ways to control costs, independent medical billing services are taking on even greater importance in the office operations of healthcare providers across the country.

In this chapter, we'll look at the basics of running a medical billing service, the pros and cons of getting into the business, and how to get started should you decide this field is for you. You'll learn about the complexities of the health insurance business, the increasing computerization of healthcare, and the advantages of electronic vs. paper claims. Most important, you'll get a sense of the emerging transition from traditional health insurance to managed care and how this revolution is affecting doctors professionally and financially. Through the sidebars in this chapter, you'll also meet many people who have started a home-based medical billing service. From their stories, you'll learn inside tips and advice on how to get your business off the ground and how to make it successful.

Medical billing is an excellent career or business opportunity for people with backgrounds in any of the following areas: accounting, law, computers (especially software), management, professional consulting, and general office administration. Of course, if you have experience working inside a doctor's office, you may already be quite familiar with this field, but it is not necessary to have this type of background to succeed. You'll learn why these backgrounds are so useful as you read the chapter.

Section I: Background

What Is a Medical Billing Service?

What exactly do medical billing services do? In simple terms, the main role of a medical billing service is to help healthcare providers of all kinds to get paid. Note that the term "healthcare provider" is the generic term commonly used to include medical doctors (M.Ds) of all types as well as chiropractors, physical therapists, dentists, psychologists, ambulance companies, suppliers of durable medical equipment (DME), and medical laboratories. (For simplicity in this chapter, the terms "doctor" and "physician" will sometimes be used interchangeably with "provider.")

A medical billing service essentially consists of two activities:

- Filing claims to the hundreds of private insurance companies and government-sponsored insurance programs (such as Medicare or Medicaid) in order to obtain reimbursement for medical services rendered to patients; and

- Sending statements to patients to obtain any necessary additional payments that their insurance has not covered.

In addition, a billing service that handles patient statements will often get involved in many other financial activities on behalf of its clients, such as managing the complete bookkeeping and accounting for the office, processing secondary insurance claims, following up on unpaid bills (soft collections), keeping track of accounts receivable owed to the doctor, producing reports to help a physician assess his or her financial status, and many other related tasks.

The distinction between these two types of activities is important to note. Some billing services just file claims and are often referred to as "just claims" businesses. In contrast, other billers handle the entire gamut of printing patient statements and maintaining all accounting and are therefore referred to as "full practice management" firms.

If you are interested in starting an independent medical billing service, you can choose to be either type of business; which one you choose depends on your background and skills, your goals, and your ability to get clients. This decision will be discussed in greater detail later in the chapter.

Why Is Medical Billing Attracting So Much Attention?

Medical billing services have actually been around for decades. As healthcare became more expensive in the United States between the 1940s and 1960s, and more people received health insurance plans from their employers, doctors had to resort to collecting from insurance companies and/or invoicing their patients. For this reason, there has long been a "cottage" industry of outside billing services that handled the bookkeeping for doctors and other types of healthcare providers. These billing services ranged from CPAs who specialized in medical practice management to women at home who did bookkeeping for a few doctors.

However, the medical billing profession has attracted a great deal of entrepreneurial attention in recent years for two reasons: (1) the growing feasibility and use of computers in "electronic data interchange" (EDI), which allows billing to be done from anywhere, and (2) the increasing complexity of healthcare that is driving doctors to seek help in managing their businesses. As part of the overview of this chapter, it is useful to look at each of these issues before going into the details about how to get started in your medical billing business. You cannot understand the medical billing industry without considering these two forces.

THE COMPUTERIZATION OF HEALTHCARE—THE EARLY YEARS Computers entered the health arena in the 1950s when more than 60 million Americans began receiving from their employers or buying their own health insurance to cover hospitalizations, surgical expenses, and physician care. To expedite the billing of health insurance claims, various data-processing companies with large mainframe computers made arrangements with hospitals and large medical practices to handle their claims. This was the beginning of computerized claims filing. Unfortunately, progress in expanding the number of claims filed by computer remained quite slow for the next 30 years, largely because of technological impediments in computer hardware and software, and a lack of vision of the role that computers could play in the process.

In the 1980s, several software companies began developing the capability to record claims using the new personal computers that were coming out at that time. This small step was largely focused on getting doctors to automate their offices. The manual typewriter could easily be replaced by a computer that could store patient records and invoices. Unfortunately, too many problems plagued the industry to allow it to take off: hardware limitations, bug-filled programs, slipshod software and hardware vendors, doctors who didn't understand the value of computerization, and dependence on floppy disks or magnetic tape that still had to be mailed to insurance companies.

In addition, one of the other major deterrents to computerization was that the format for computerizing claims was never standardized. This meant that doctors could not send a universal claim form to all insurance companies; each insurer had its own data format. A few software companies tried to resolve this problem by establishing themselves as "clearinghouses" or routing stations where claims of all kinds could be sent for "translation and editing," then forwarded to the appropriate insurer. Because of this problem, the conversion of the entire industry to a uniform "data interchange" standard remained a distant goal.

MEDICARE SPURS ON COMPUTERIZATION   The real impetus to continue computerizing the healthcare industry came from the skyrocketing costs of services from hospitals and doctors from the 1970s to the 1980s, especially in regard to medical care for the elderly. The major proponent of computerization turned out to be HCFA, the federal government agency responsible for administering Medicare, which is the program legislated under President Johnson to provide healthcare benefits for the elderly and certain others. The Medicare program took effect in 1966.

Between 1970 and 1980, HCFA realized that it would soon be faced with enormous growth in Medicare enrollment. By 1980, HCFA was already processing several hundred million claims on paper, and the task was clearly expensive and time consuming. In 1983, the agency began an aggressive campaign to shift hospitals and physicians to electronically transmitted claims to reduce costs and eliminate the backlog of paper claims. One of its smartest moves was to encourage the development of a standardized set of diagnosis codes and procedure codes so that doctors could easily list a patient's condition and what services they performed.

These codes replaced a hodge-podge system of coding that had previously blocked standardizing the electronic claims filing process.

As it turned out, HCFA's insight became the driving force for the industry. Its projections about future growth were right on target. By the end of the 1980s, Medicare was receiving nearly 500 million claims per year, 80 percent of which were from individual physicians, suppliers, and laboratories on behalf of their patients. Fortunately, Medicare's efforts to foster electronic claims processing began to pay off. By 1989, it was receiving 36 percent of its claims electronically; by 1991, this figure increased to 50 percent. In recent years, the percentage has been steadily rising, but it is still not 100 percent despite the easy availability of personal computers. At the time of this writing, HCFA was encouraging all insurance carriers (companies contracted by HCFA to process claims for Medicare Part B) to push for electronic filing from every doctor. Unfortunately, HCFA can only suggest this goal, because Congress has yet to pass a law requiring it. This means that hundreds of millions of Medicare claims still are done via paper claim forms mailed to the insurance intermediaries for processing.

COMMERCIAL INSURANCE COMPANIES SLOWLY JUMP ON BANDWAGON   Needless to say, millions of Americans are not part of Medicare and have their insurance through any of the hundreds of private insurance companies in the country or through a self-insured plan from their employer, often administered by a third party to whom the claims are sent. Although commercial and private insurance also generate hundreds of millions of claims per year, these insurance companies moved very slowly toward electronic claims. In fact, in the late 1970s and early 1980s, most private insurance companies resisted electronic claims, probably because of the expense to computerize their systems when the economic benefits were not clear.

The first significant support for electronic claims from commercial insurance companies came in 1981 when 11 of the biggest firms formed an association called the National Electronic Information Corp. (NEIC) to serve as a central clearinghouse for claims. By the late 1980s, NEIC began to play a stronger role and invited a larger segment of commercial insurers to join in taking claims electronically. Unfortunately, most commercial carriers still reacted cautiously. By 1990, although there were an estimated 3 billion claims filed annually to all insurers from hospitals, doctors, laboratories, and pharmacies, it was estimated that only 6 percent to 8 percent of commercial insurance claims from physicians were processed electronically, a mere drop in the bucket.

1990: WATERSHED YEAR FOR ELECTRONIC CLAIMS Electronic claims filing was given its most forceful push when Congress issued a directive that took effect in September 1990 requiring *all* physicians to file claims on behalf of their Medicare patients. Under the previous policy, doctors did not have to do so, and many left the paperwork to the patients to handle. Under the new policy, however, the burden for getting reimbursements from Medicare fell to the doctors.

Finding themselves suddenly deluged with claims that would not get reimbursed unless they did the filing themselves, many physicians were simply not prepared. In some cases, their offices were not computerized; and in other cases, they simply could not keep up with the volume of claims they had to file. Many physicians eagerly sought the services of outside billing experts.

This 1990 directive thus effectively started the revolution in medical billing, opening the door to many small and home-based businesses that foresaw an opportunity to provide a specialized service to doctors who could no longer manage their claims. Armed with more sophisticated hardware and software, some of these entrepreneurs began selling doctors the computers, software, and modems that would allow them to do claims filing on their own. More important, many other entrepreneurs saw an opportunity to sell claims filing, especially electronic claims filing, as a service they would perform for doctors. Thus originated the recent focus on independent medical billing services as a viable entrepreneurial endeavor.

ELECTRONIC VERSUS PAPER CLAIMS You are probably wondering at this point exactly what is involved in electronic claims filing. Let's describe how the process works and why it makes sense in today's health-care environment.

Before electronic claims, doctors and insurance companies used a slew of confusing paper forms to communicate with one other. Unfortunately, filing claims in this way was an enormously tedious process, usually performed by typing out and mailing paper forms to the various insurance companies covering the doctor's patients. The problem was, many insurance companies had their own paper forms, and filling them in often led to errors that would cause the claim to be rejected. This meant that doctors were not paid until the claim was corrected and sent back for processing. Even when a doctor's office purchased a computer and billing software, the office often simply recorded the patient information in the computer but printed the claims out on paper and mailed them to Medicare or the private insurance company. This process still did not ensure that the claims were error free, nor did it save much in the way of time and money.

With the advent of high-quality billing software and high-speed modems, the solution to this problem was clearly to make the process electronic. In simple terms, rather than fill out a paper form when a patient visits a doctor, electronic claims filing uses the computer throughout the entire process. All a biller needs to do is to type in the basic patient information, indicate date of service, place of service, diagnosis, and the procedures performed, then push a few buttons and send the claim via modem to the insurance company (sometimes via an intermediate routing station, which will be explained later) where it can be evaluated for payment.

The advantages of electronic claims over paper claims are significant. First, whereas a paper claim passes through many hands and is transferred from one location to the next via "snail mail," an electronic claim is keyboarded just once and can be sent from the doctor's or billing agency's office in seconds via modem to the insurance company. Paper claims also require a number of intermediary steps at the insurance company's office, because they need to be sorted, microfilmed, and keyboarded into the insurer's computer system. Electronic claims therefore save an enormous amount of time and labor.

Second, electronic claims save money in overhead costs in both preparation and processing time. Some estimates indicate that electronic filing saves from $3.00 to $12.00 per claim at the doctor's office, because of the speed at which they can be done and the reduction in errors. In essence, electronic claims save wasted salary that a billing clerk earns while filing claims by paper, claims that often contain errors and are rejected and returned. Meanwhile, at the other end, insurers are also recognizing that electronic claims save them money. HCFA estimates that it literally saves as much as $.50 per claim, amounting to hundreds of millions of dollars per year.

Third, electronic claims reduce the rejection rate because of fewer errors. Some estimates indicate that nearly one-third of paper claims contain errors and are rejected by insurers, because of either simple typing mistakes or coding errors made at the physician's office. Since a claim contains dozens of "fields" or units of information (name, address, policy number, diagnosis, procedures performed, etc.), it is easy to understand how such errors occur so frequently. Even worse, many rejected claims are never reprocessed at the doctor's office, because the billing clerk does not know what the mistake was or how to correct it. Some doctors have literally found entire desk drawers filled with rejected claims that were never resubmitted—amounting to tens of thousands of dollars in lost revenues.

In contrast, electronic claims cut down on rejected claims in a number of ways. Most billing software for electronic claims permanently stores a record for each patient a doctor has, so constant rekeying of this basic information is minimized, reducing the chances of mistakes and missing information. In addition, most high-quality medical billing software contains logical intelligence so that it can perform "error checking" on the claims. For example, the software can easily verify that all the blanks in the claim form are filled in, that the correct number of digits are used in each field (such as an ID #), and that a numeric code is not used where an alphabetic entry should be. Some software is also smart enough to catch illogical matches between diagnosis codes and procedure codes, such as a code indicating the doctor performed a hysterectomy on 10-year-old female. These kinds of mistakes really do happen!

Furthermore, as indicated earlier, many medical billers send their electronic claims first to a clearinghouse, whose software also checks them for errors and formats them according to the specifications of the insurance company to which they will be routed. Most clearinghouses provide an added service: If there is an error in the claim, the billing person can find out immediately—rather than weeks later by mail—because the clearinghouse electronically notifies him or her within hours or days that the claim contains a mistake. In this way, the claim can be corrected and resubmitted quickly.

All these advantages add up to a crucial benefit for healthcare providers: *electronic claims get processed more quickly at the insurance companies and are therefore paid much faster.* In other words, doctors can get paid sooner rather than later because the claims can be keyboarded more quickly, have fewer mistakes due to the editing and error checking they go through, and arrive earlier at the insurance companies. While paper claims often take 30 to 60 days to get paid, even if they are clean (i.e., without errors), electronic claims are usually paid within a few weeks, and sometimes in as little as 7 working days by commercial insurance companies. Medicare also gives priority status to electronic claims over paper claims. Since 1994, Medicare's policy has been that a clean claim that has been filed electronically may be paid in 14 days (but not before) and no later than 19 days, whereas paper claims must be held for a minimum of 27 days before they can be paid. (Note that, technically speaking, Medicare and insurance companies could pay electronic claims very fast, such as in just one or two days, but they intentionally sit on the claims for a minimum of 14 days to take advantage of the "float" on money. More will be said about this strategy later.)

The fast payment of electronic claims is critical to the financial survival of most doctors. Since a doctor usually gets as much as 80 percent of his or her gross earnings from Medicare or commercial insurance reimbursements, speeding up the payments can significantly improve cash flow. After all, wouldn't you rather wait just 20 to 25 days to get your insurance payments rather than 45 to 60 days?

Figures 2-1 and 2-2 contrast the process and timing for paper claims vs. electronic claims.

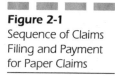

Figure 2-1

Sequence of Claims Filing and Payment for Paper Claims

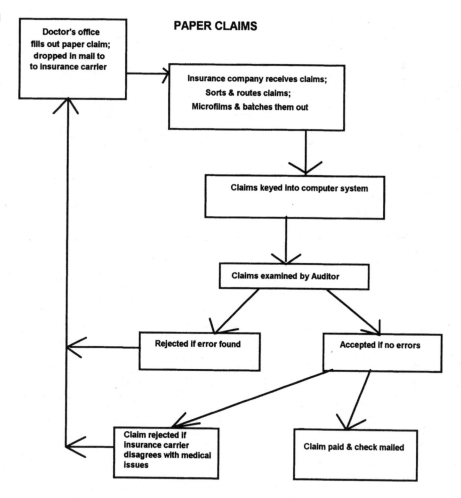

PAPER CLAIMS

Doctor's office fills out paper claim; dropped in mail to to insurance carrier

Insurance company receives claims; Sorts & routes claims; Microfilms & batches them out

Claims keyed into computer system

Claims examined by Auditor

Rejected if error found

Accepted if no errors

Claim rejected if insurance carrier disagrees with medical issues

Claim paid & check mailed

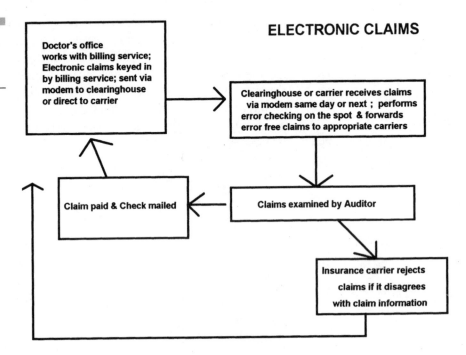

ELECTRONIC CLAIMS

Doctor's office works with billing service; Electronic claims keyed in by billing service; sent via modem to clearinghouse or direct to carrier

Clearinghouse or carrier receives claims via modem same day or next ; performs error checking on the spot & forwards error free claims to appropriate carriers

Claim paid & Check mailed

Claims examined by Auditor

Insurance carrier rejects claims if it disagrees with claim information

The Increasing Complexity of Healthcare

Electronic claims filing is only half the story behind the revolution in medical billing. The second factor driving the potential for independent medical billing services is the astonishing complexity of healthcare today, particularly in regard to the relationship between care and cost.

On one hand, the United States has long had the best medical care in the world and is capable of being the leader in taking care of its population. University and private research labs daily discover the secrets to conquering diseases of all kinds and invent new technologies to cure human ailments. Few doubt that U.S. doctors are the best trained and most sophisticated in the world. While some doctors go into business solely to make money, the vast majority love their work and eagerly want to take care of their patients to the best of their ability. For each patient seen with an illness or problem, they want to do whatever is necessary to cure the person and make sure he or she survives.

On the other hand, over the past 20 years, the cost of healthcare has skyrocketed far beyond belief, increasing at a rate ranging from 8 percent to 14 percent *per year* between 1980 and 1995. Worse, the projections for the

Business Profile: Jim Russell and Rich Russell

Jim Russell and Rich Russell are brothers who love music. Both have long been professional opera singers—but now they are also medical billers. They started their home-based billing business in 1995 after deciding that they needed to have a more consistent income to support their families, and more regular hours as well. They read the first edition of this book and decided to go into medical billing, purchasing a business opportunity from Medical Management Software, owned by Merry Schiff. Their firm, Hudson Valley Practice Management, is located in Rockland County, New York.

Getting their first client took some time (as it does for many people who enter the business). Jim explained to me:

It took nearly five months to get the first client; I believe our approach was too soft; we did a direct mail campaign but did not follow up with calls. Then we began cold calling with a goal of just getting an appointment to see the doctor and give ourselves a chance to do a presentation about the advantages of electronic claims. Most of the doctors had heard about ECP, but had not thought of converting.

Their first client was an audiologist, and since then some of the doctors who had received their direct mail pieces have also come on board. They now have more than half-a-dozen clients, including a social worker, a podiatrist, a chiropractor, and an ambulance service. Jim points out that their clients saw immediate results: "Before we took over, Medicare was taking five weeks to two months to pay, but with electronic claims, my clients get paid within three weeks." Jim also says that a friend of his who works at one of the largest insurance companies in the area, MetroHealth, tells him that the claims examiners get pulled off paper claims anytime the electronic claims department has a backlog. This shows the priority given to electronic claims in that company.

Jim and Rich charge from $3.00 to $3.50 per claim, except for the ambulance service, for which they charge $15.00 per claim. Jim explained that there is a good market among rural volunteer ambulance services that typically don't bill for insurance reimbursement because they are community funded. Jim seeks them out and shows them how his service can at least earn them money so that their public funding is replenished. It's a win/win situation for them both.

If you are doing just claims on a per claim fee basis, Jim recommends that you give much thought to the nature of your client's business. For example, a therapist who can bill for up to six patient visits on one claim form (with each visit averaging $90 to $100) is happy to pay you $3.00 or even $5.00 to do the work. In contrast, Jim points out that an optometrist who gets only $6.00 for eyeglasses isn't going to give you half his income for filing the claim. In short, it is useful to think about what type of doctor you are approaching and how his or her fees are structured.

After one year, Jim and Rich are discovering that doing just claims is not sufficient. Several of their clients are smaller practices, such as a social worker who does not own a computer nor does she have an interest in learning to use one. As a result, Jim and Rich are now moving toward full practice management for her. They send out patient invoices and they produce special financial reports to help her see her cash flow. Jim and Rich expect their medical billing business to go from just claims to full practice management for most of their clients in the near future.

future continue to show advancing costs. As noted in Chapter 1, the National Health Expenditure is expected to rise an average of 8 percent per year between 1996 and 2005.

This dichotomy between what doctors are capable of doing versus the need to control costs cannot be underestimated. The conflict is causing profound changes in our healthcare system, from the way consumers choose their healthcare to the way even the best doctors practice medicine. We are no longer living in the 1950s when the good family doctor made housecalls, nor are we living in the 1980s when doctors would not hesitate to perform test after test to find out what might be wrong with a patient. The 1990s has created the dawning of a new era in healthcare!

Needless to say, the most critical change is that insurance companies and Medicare are seeking to contain costs as much as possible. Doctors are being squeezed more and more to cut corners wherever and whenever they can. When they get a new patient, doctors must verify what insurance benefits that person has so they won't perform a service the person is not entitled to receive. When they decide on a treatment, they must make absolutely sure the patient needs it before doing it, often submitting their diagnosis and treatment strategy to a review panel within the patient's insurance company or health maintenance organization, which has the final word. In some instances, doctors are even told to avoid the use of expensive medical technology until the final moment.

When it comes to handling their billing, doctors are being asked to produce more paperwork justifying their fees, and to be more rigorous in specifying their diagnosis. For example, the 1996 numeric coding system used to indicate the doctor's diagnosis breaks down each illness into many detailed subcategories. It is no longer sufficient for a doctor to indicate on a claim form that the patient has diabetes; the claim form must use a specific code that tells the insurance company if the patient has diabetes with renal manifestations or diabetes with ophthalmic manifestations, and each one of these codes has "modifiers" to even more specifically identify the manifestation. A doctor practically needs a master's degree in medical coding today to please the insurance companies!

It is not an understatement to suggest that the practice of medicine has become a schizophrenic profession. On one hand, most doctors want and need to focus on the art of medicine, staying constantly abreast of new cures, new drugs, new medical technology, new treatments plans, and new research that can benefit their patients. This takes time; most doctors would truly prefer to see patients, read research and case studies, and perhaps take an occasional day off at home. Unfortunately, most doctors are being forced to spend inordinate amounts of their time paying attention to the *business* of medicine, lest they lose money. They must stay current with the rules and regulations of Medicare and commercial insurance reimbursement. They must understand how to code their invoices properly. And they must make sure they don't perform a service that their patient's insurance company won't allow. In short, these are not always good times to be a doctor!

To make matters worse, many doctors are losing income. In the boom years of the 1980s, when healthcare was rising at 10 percent or more per year, it was not unusual for a general practitioner to make between $200,000 and $250,000 per year, while many specialists made from $300,000 to $500,000. Today, most doctors can no longer maintain these incomes—or even a reasonable income—because of declining insurance reimbursements and increasing amounts of lost fees because of denied claims.

Under the rubric of containing costs, many doctors are literally being forced to become part of a Health Maintenance Organization (HMO), a Preferred Provider Organization (PPO), or another of the many forms of "managed care" networks. We examine these types of arrangements in greater detail later, but for now suffice it to say that managed care organizations are trimming doctors' incomes to the bone. Some managed care groups simply buy out a doctor's practice and pay him or her a modest salary to work onsite; others allow doctors to remain independent in their own offices but force them to accept fees that amount to as little as 15 cents on the dollar compared to what they formerly charged.

The significance of today's revolution in U.S. healthcare is enormous for anyone interested in medical billing. As doctors continue to fall under the cost gun and lose control of their practices and their incomes, they are increasingly turning to "professional practice managers," people who have the expertise to help them run the business side of their practice. This is where a skilled medical billing professional has an opportunity. A medical billing professional who has in-depth knowledge of the health insurance industry and reimbursement issues, a high level of familiarity with medical coding, reasonable computer skills, and the ability to handle money and to do accurate financial record keeping and projections can be a true savior to increasing numbers of today's busy healthcare providers.

You may be asking why the doctor's office staff can't handle all this for the doctor. Isn't that what he or she is paying them for? The truth is that the complexity and bureaucracy of running a medical practice go far beyond the capabilities of most office personnel. Obviously, some doctors' offices have a skilled billing person who has been on staff for 5, 10, or more years and so may understand Medicare and private insurance reimbursement issues. This kind of person may have even helped the office become computerized and he or she has learned the software, gone to coding classes, and attended Medicare seminars to stay abreast of reimbursement rules and regulations.

However, it is far more common that doctors' offices are staffed by people who do not have such skills or backgrounds. They are not experts in coding, filing claims, insurance regulations, or the ins and outs of managed care. Many such people don't know how to use a computer in a sophisticated way, such as required by medical billing and practice management software. Doctors' offices typically have a constant turnover of personnel, so there is little opportunity for a billing clerk to master the complexities of billing and insurance reimbursement if he or she stays for only eight months or a year. In some cases, a low-paid billing staff person has little motivation to file claims correctly or to follow up on unpaid claims and mistakes. As pointed out earlier, many doctors literally have $10,000 to $50,000 in outstanding claims in a drawer that were once rejected and never reprocessed correctly. Doctors have to write off this lost income. (The term "write off" means that the money is removed from their projected income on the balance sheet, by crediting what had been debited. It does not mean that doctors get a tax write-off for the lost income.)

Dr. Richard Wunneburger, founder and president of InfoHealth (a division of Synaps Corporation), a Texas software firm that produces and sells medical claims and practice management software and training, knows firsthand the problems that have eroded the joy of practicing medicine in the past decade. Richard was himself a physician in a small multidoctor practice in Colorado when he realized that he and his partners could not keep up with getting their claims filed and paid correctly. Being technically inclined, Dr. Wunneburger therefore learned computer programming, wrote his own software, and eventually went on to found InfoHealth to sell his software to doctors and independent medical billing services.

But as Dr. Wunneburger points out, even the best software is not enough, because most physicians and office staffs are not equipped to keep up with the business of healthcare and the complexities of health insurance. As he told me,

> The patient care side of medicine is changing dramatically and rapidly today; most doctors want to take care of their patients and learn new medical technology, but physicians today need to become very sophisticated about the business of healthcare. In fact, the need for business knowledge

is almost outdistancing the doctor's time and ability to practice medicine. Much of the business knowledge required has become so complicated and technical that a typical office staff cannot keep up with that knowledge and take care of their patients at the same time. Today's doctors have to depend more and more on business professionals. In my software company, we get a tremendous amount of support calls not about our software, but about the business issues. The truth is, doctors have chosen to be doctors but it's difficult to be a doctor and a businessman.

WHITE KNIGHTS: PROFESSIONAL BILLING SERVICES As you can see, there are two significant forces driving medical billing: the increasing benefits of filing electronically, which most doctors are still not doing, and the growing complexities of managing a practice in the face of tremendous pressures from insurance companies and the government to control costs. This is truly a time of opportunity for the savvy entrepreneur who is willing to work hard to become a true medical billing professional. Let's examine in greater detail now what you need to learn if you want to get into the business.

How Billing Services Work

To understand the details of medical billing and what you need to know to get into the business, I have divided the information into five sections:

- The traditional private health insurance industry (commercial insurance, self-insured plans, the Blues)
- The increasing role of managed care plans (HMOs, IPAs, PPOs, POSs, MSOs, etc.)
- The public health insurance programs (Medicare, Medicaid, Champus, Worker's Comp.)
- The operation of a typical medical office: paper claims versus electronic claims
- Advanced practice management functions done by billing agencies

Whatever your background or previous experience, I suggest you read each of these sections to be sure you have a complete understanding of the issues you will invariably deal with if you enter medical billing. This information is critical to your success, and it may take some time to fully understand if you do not have a medical or insurance background. You

Business Profile: Dave Shipton

Dave Shipton is the perfect example of a white knight medical biller. Dave started in medical billing in 1992, after Defense Department cutbacks eliminated his job and he found himself in his mid-50s seeking a new career. Dave originally formed his company, Business Medical Services, with a partner who had a medical background as a respiratory therapist, while Dave had extensive computer skills from nearly 35 years in the Air Force and as a special operations trainer in the aircraft industry. After one year though, his partner decided to leave to take a "real" job. Dave quickly realized that he had to master both sides of the job if he was to succeed. He applied himself and learned everything he could about health insurance reimbursement, coding, and the operation of a medical practice. He had originally purchased software from a business opportunity vendor but was disappointed with its clearinghouse and eventually switched to the software produced by Synaps, the company owned by Dr. Richard Wunneburger, mentioned earlier.

In the course of the next four years, Dave proceeded to build his company to the point of handling full practice management for eight medical practices, most of which included multiple doctors. Over this time, Dave became a trusted advisor to nearly every one of his clients because of his expertise in understanding billing and the effects of managed care on their practices. Because of his knowledge, he handles all insurance reimbursement issues for them, from filing claims and recording payments, to comparing fee schedules to be sure they are being paid accurately, to advising them how to maximize their earnings with special reports he prepares for them.

In particular, Dave closely follows the trends set by the HMOs and PPOs that have moved into his area, seeking out doctors to become part of their networks. He even guides his clients into knowing which managed care organizations to join, and which to avoid. When I spoke with Dave, he was even helping one of his clients, a pain management clinic with several doctors, to prepare a presentation to obtain the contract from a major insurance company to handle all of their subscribers who had chronic pain. Dave had played a leading role in finding the contact for the presentation and in preparing the bid to get the business for his client.

Dave agrees that the billing business is definitely changing. He says,

> I started out doing just claims for my first few clients, charging strictly on a per claim basis. In fact, I still have one doctor for whom I just do claims filing at $3.00 per claim, but now all my other doctors want me to handle as much as I can for them. I literally train some of my clients who are new doctors how to manage their practice. From me, they learn how to verify insurance coverages, how to get patients to sign payment coverage sheets, and even how to prepare their superbills.

Dave adds that the key to the business is building trust. Doctors have to believe that you can truly help them. "I consider this business a partnership," Dave says. "If you don't have that kind of relationship, you are just another biller."

Dave's advice is, "If you don't like hard work, don't get into this business." He adheres to a credo used by Calvin Coolidge: "Nothing in this world can take the place of persistence." It seems as if Dave's philosophy has paid off for him.

may also want to consult other sources of information, as this material can only skim the surface of many of these issues. A list of additional references and resources is presented in the section on training later in the chapter (page 120) and in Appendix A.

The Private Health Insurance Industry

Although you are probably somewhat familiar with the healthcare industry as a consumer, as a billing professional, you must have a sophisticated knowledge of it, especially the relationship between doctors and insurance companies. With literally thousands of different insurance programs in this country, and a constant stream of new ones, developing expertise in insurance reimbursement is a critical factor in your success.

Health insurance can be divided into two general categories: private and public. Private health insurance is offered by hundreds of large commercial companies. Private insurance also includes Blue Cross and Blue Shield plans that are typically run on a not-for-profit basis. Another major form of private insurance are self-insured plans, a type of group coverage usually sponsored by an employer. Rather than pay premiums to an insurer who bears the risk, the employer sets aside money on its own to pay the claims of its employees. Because of the sheer amount of paperwork, many employers hire what is called a "third party administrator" (TPA) to administer their self-insured plan. The administrator is sometimes an insurance company but could also be a professional management firm. Such contractual arrangements are also known as administrative services only (ASOs). A variation of ASOs are MPPs, "minimum premium plans." These are plans in which the employer self-insures up to a certain amount but then pays a commercial insurance company to assume the risk for all claims beyond that amount.

The fastest growing type of private insurance are "prepayment" plans that fall under the general term of "managed care." Managed care includes primarily Health Maintenance Organizations (HMOs) but also many other networks and arrangements. Many private health insurance companies, self-insured plans, and Blue Cross/Blue Shield plans have moved toward managed care plans.

Here are some important details about each of these insurance forms.

COMMERCIAL INSURANCE   Many people obtain their insurance from policies offered by private, profit-making insurance carriers. Such policies come in the form of either *individual* or *group* plans, with group policies being the larger category. The term "group policy" refers to the fact that the insurance is underwritten to cover a large group, such as all employees of a company, or all members of an association or fraternal organization. Each person insured may be covered as an individual or as a family. The term "individual policy" does not mean that the policy covers only one person; instead, it refers to the fact that only one individual purchased the insurance, as opposed to an entire group. The policy itself, of course, can cover either a single person or a family.

Group plans have three advantages over individual policies:

- The cost of group plans per person is usually lower, because the risk is spread out over many people.

- No individual member of a group plan may be canceled separately. The entire group must be canceled.

- When employees who are covered under a group plan retire or otherwise leave their company (assuming it has more than 25 employees), they may make use of a special clause that allows them to convert their group coverage to individual coverage. This was made possible through the Consolidated Omnibus Budget Reconciliation Act (COBRA) in 1986. (As you might recall, some of the rationale for COBRA was eliminated in 1996 when Congress passed new legislation that allowed for complete portability of health insurance when employees change jobs, regardless of preexisting conditions. This rectified the problem formerly created when a person left one company but was often not eligible for insurance until after three months on a new job.)

Note that many group policies are actually self-insured plans administered by a commercial carrier. In fact, a 1994 study by the Health Insurance Association of America estimated that 81 million Americans were covered under group policies and 7.1 million carried individual or family policies from commercial insurance companies. Of the 81 million people covered under a group policy, nearly 60 percent were covered under ASO or MPP arrangements, in which employers hired a commercial carrier to administer their insurance plan or assume the risk for higher-than-average claims.

Some commercial policies are "indemnity" plans, meaning that they reimburse (indemnify) the patient for covered services up to a certain limit specified in the policy, leaving it up to the doctor or hospital to collect from the patient. Other commercial policies reimburse physicians directly according to what the insurance company considers "usual and

customary" fees. However, these types of plans ar̃~~~~
into managed care arrangements, which will be dis̃~~~~

Commercial health insurance policies vary grea~~~~
not cover all illnesses or allow patients to see all ~~~~
providers, such as chiropractors. This is why doctors—~~~~
son—are increasingly double-checking each patient's i~~~~ ₚ~licy, a
process called *insurance verification and eligibility.*

In a typical commercial policy, the insurance holder, called the *sub-scriber,* pays an annual *premium.* The insurance does not pay for any healthcare until the subscriber's *deductible* is met. The deductible is the amount the person or family must pay entirely in each calendar or policy year before the insurance company will pay any claims. Deductibles usually range from $200 to $1,200 for an individual, and $600 to $3,600 for a family. (A deductible for a family is generally three times the amount of the deductible for an individual.)

Once the insurance company begins paying for claims, most policies pay or reimburse for only 70 percent or 80 percent of what the insurance company considers an appropriate fee. This is known as the *allowable* amount. (See the sidebar on page 41, "Understanding Reimbursement-Speak," for more details on this.) The other 20 percent or 30 percent paid by the patient is known as the *copayment.* Fortunately, many commercial policies cap the total copayment amounts that an individual or family must pay per year; these limits range from $1000 to $10,000 beyond the deductible. This is called a *stop-loss provision.* Once the subscriber reaches that limit, the insurer pays 100 percent of all covered charges. On the other hand, many commercial policies also have an annual and lifetime cap, limiting the charges that the insurer will pay. For instance, many dental policies limit the annual coverage to $1,000 and the lifetime coverage to $25,000.

In general, commercial health insurance policies are one of three types:

1. *Basic Plans* pay for limited services performed in a hospital, X-rays, lab tests, drugs and medications, and sometimes but not usually outpatient doctor's visits. Basic plans typically have low or no deductibles, but also low levels of benefits.

2. *Major Medical Plans* are designed to pay large amounts in the event of major illnesses or injuries. These plans sometimes do not cover minor health problems and office visits.

3. *Comprehensive Medical Plans* combine coverages for both Basic and Major Medical, plus outpatient services such as doctor's office visits for illnesses. However, policies differ greatly; one policy may cover

psychiatric benefits up to $1,000 per year for outpatient visits, but not reimburse for chiropractic treatment or eye examinations as another policy does.

Finally, note that there are two distinguishing characteristics of traditional commercial health insurance policies:

1. Most such individual and group commercial policies pay healthcare providers on a fee-for-service basis. This means that the insurance company pays for each procedure after it is performed. (However, as indicated earlier, the insurer may only pay an amount that it determines to be appropriate, regardless of how much the doctor wants to charge.) Subscribers are responsible for any copayment, or in some cases the physician will accept what the carrier reimburses as his or her full payment.

2. Under most traditional plans, patients can choose any doctor they want, anywhere they want. They do not need any authorization to see specialists or to go to emergency rooms.

Because of these characteristics, traditional commercial insurance has long been the preferred type of health insurance for many Americans.

BLUE CROSS AND BLUE SHIELD PLANS   Blue Cross originated in 1929 when a group of teachers contracted with Baylor Hospital in Texas to provide hospital care at a fixed monthly cost. This type of arrangement was different from the indemnity plans of commercial insurance based on fee for service. Over the next decade, such Blue Cross plans became successful in many other parts of the country. Similarly, Blue Shield was devised in 1938 by the American Medical Association as an insurance method to cover doctors' services for a fixed prepaid amount per month.

Since their origins, separate Blue Cross and Blue Shield organizations were established in nearly every state in the United States. Each organization had a national association that had to approve the plans established in each state. The names Blue Cross and Blue Shield were licensed from the national associations. In 1986, the two associations merged to form the Blue Cross and Blue Shield Association to manage the various state insurers.

Over the past decade, the two Blues in most states have also merged to form one organization to compete directly with commercial carriers. In the past few years, there have also been some mergers of BC/BS organizations across state lines.

Most Blue Cross/Blue Shield plans were set up to be not-for-profit. In exchange for this status, they were forbidden by state laws from canceling

Understanding Reimbursement-Speak

In general, there are four methods by which insurers determine how to pay physicians and other healthcare providers:

1. *UCR (Usual, Customary, and Reasonable)*. This method has long been used to monitor and control costs in fee-for-service healthcare. Under UCR, insurance carriers choose the *lowest* of three amounts from the following:

   - Usual fee—this is the "usual" amount a physician charges for a service. Insurance companies determine this amount by keeping records on doctors over each year and averaging out the median (50th percentile) charge.
   - Customary fee—this fee is determined from insurance company profiles, based on the 90th percentile of fees charged by all providers within the same specialty area in the same geographic location for a specific service.
   - Reasonable fee—this fee is the lesser of the billed fee (the amount the doctor would like to charge), the usual fee, the customary fee, or another fee that might be justified under special circumstances.

   For example, assume Doctor A submits a fee for $220, while the customary fee in that area is $225; this doctor will receive only the reasonable fee, based on 80 percent of $220 (assuming that the insurance is an 80/20 plan). Meanwhile, Doctor B submits a bill for $250 as her usual fee; this fee is higher than the customary fee of $225, so she will receive the customary amount, based on 80 percent of $225.

   From an insurer's perspective, the flaw with UCR is that it actually creates inflationary pressure on fees, because the system encourages doctors to charge higher fees on a regular basis to make sure that their *usual* fees are higher than the *customary* range. For this reason, of course, many doctors prefer to be paid according to UCR rates.

2. *Schedule of Benefits Method*. In this method, the insurance company maintains a table of fees for all procedures and pays only these allowable amounts, regardless of what the physician charges. If the doctor wants to charge more, the patient may need to make up the difference.

3. *Maximum Fee Schedule*. In this method, the insurance company maintains a table of maximum payment amounts for all procedures; the doctor must agree to accept that payment as his or her total reimbursement.

4. *Capitation*. Capitation is generally used in prepaid plans under managed care. The term originates from the Latin word meaning "head." Under capitation, a doctor receives a set fee per month per person enrolled in the healthcare plan, whether or not the person sees the doctor. Capitation takes advantage of statistical probabilities that the majority of a physician's patients won't all get sick at the same time or use more healthcare than mathematically predicted for people in that age group. The capitation amounts vary based on geography, age, sex, and experience rating per population group.

   In addition to these four methods, the Harvard School of Public Health developed another method at the request of the federal government, largely to curtail the high cost of Medicare. This method is known as RBRVS, which stands for Resource-Based Relative Value Scale. The RBRVS system takes three factors into account in determining a doctor's fee: (1) the physician's actual amount of work, (2) the provider's expenses (except malpractice), and (3) the cost of malpractice. The system is not simple, however, because each of these factors is multiplied by an index based on geographic location, and the total is then multiplied again by a "conversion" factor determined by Congress to account for inflation. RBRVS was introduced in 1992 and has been phased in for Medicare bills since then. It was expected that many commercial insurance companies would eventually adopt RBRVS, but in general, they have not done so.

coverage for an individual because of illness. They were usually required to obtain approval for rate increases as well.

Blue Cross and Blue Shield were pioneers in the concept of prepaid plans that have become the foundation for managed care today. In addition to their standard individual and group policies, many Blues negotiated contracts with providers in an area to become part of a network. The providers had to accept payment according to a fee schedule determined by the Blue, often 10 percent lower than what the company paid other providers who were not participating. In exchange, the providers were paid directly rather than having to seek payment from the patients. In some contracts, the doctors were penalized if they referred patients to specialists who were not part of the Blue network.

MANAGED CARE ORGANIZATIONS As you undoubtedly know, traditional commercial health insurance plans, including self-insured and Blue Cross/Blue Shield plans, are largely viewed by insurance companies as the cause for skyrocketing costs of healthcare in the past two decades. As a result, more and more commercial insurance companies, self-insured plans, and Blue Cross/Blue Shield insurers have moved toward offering some type of managed care arrangement in addition to their traditional indemnity plans.

The most common term you will hear in the context of managed care is HMO, or Health Maintenance Organization. HMOs originated in the 1930s and were fostered by the federal government in the early 1970s as a way to cut costs. However, HMOs did not truly take off until the mid-1980s through the early 1990s. There are now roughly between 600 and 700 HMOs in the country, although the exact figure is difficult to determine because of the variety of HMO operations.

In general, the distinguishing characteristics of HMOs include five basic precepts:

1. Providers are prepaid on a capitation basis; they receive fees each month per subscriber, regardless of whether the provider sees the patient.

2. Patients typically pay only a small copayment, such as $10 per visit, or none at all.

3. Care is highly controlled; patients usually see a primary physician first who must authorize visits to specialists.

4. Patients are either forbidden to see providers outside the HMO network unless absolutely medically necessary, or they are subject to higher copayments or no reimbursement at all when they do.

5. The HMO tries to cut costs through preventative care; patients may see doctors at no additional cost for regular checkups to catch any serious illnesses before they become aggravated.

Despite these five common precepts, the term HMO has been used to refer to many different types of healthcare arrangements. Some people call any managed care organization an HMO, although there are other types of arrangements—such as Preferred Provider Organizations (PPOs)—that are not the same.

In addition, HMOs can be operated in many different ways. In some cases, the HMO is owned by an insurance company, so belonging to this type of HMO is synonymous with being insured. In the other cases, the HMO is an independent business with which several private insurers have contracted to serve its subscribers.

In some arrangements, doctors are literally staff employees of the HMO, and they work solely at the HMO facility; they cannot see other patients. In other HMO models, the affiliated doctors maintain an independent practice but become part of a network of physicians who agree to take patients from that HMO; these doctors can also take patients from other HMOs or other traditional fee-for-service insurance plans.

As mentioned, PPOs are a related type of organization, but they differ in that they generally follow looser rules. A PPO usually consists of a network of physicians who agree to see patients who are insured under a certain plan. In general, the patients in a PPO have more flexibility in choosing their own doctors from among an extensive list of candidates. In some PPOs, the patients can see specialists without a referral from a primary care physician first, although some PPOs charge people a higher copayment for seeing a doctor who is not a member of the network. Unlike HMOs, which usually pay doctors on a prepaid capitated basis, doctors affiliated with a PPO are usually paid according to fee-for-service, but they must accept a discounted rate compared to their usual fees. They may charge the patient a copayment based on 20 percent of the allowable fee or sometimes a fixed amount such as $10 per visit.

In the past few years, there has been a flood of new types of HMOs and PPOs as the need to create profitable managed care programs has heated up. There are now so many different models and methods of managed care that the average consumer (and doctor) needs a scorecard to keep track of all the different types of arrangements and their affiliated terms. Here is a short glossary of managed care terms you may encounter:

HMO, staff model: Under this arrangement, doctors are employed by the HMO and are paid a salary.

HMO, group model: The HMO pays a large group of physicians representing all specialties, usually on a capitation rate, to handle all its subscribers. In some group models, physicians work at an HMO facility, but in others, they work at their own offices. Some group models allow physicians to see only HMO patients; others do not.

HMO, network model: The HMO contracts with two or more groups of independent physicians who handle patients at their own offices. Physicians may see only HMO patients.

IPA (Independent Practice Association): Under this arrangement, the HMO contracts with individual independent physicians or associations to care for its subscribers. Many IPAs are prepaid plans on a capitation basis. Under most IPAs, physicians may see non-HMO patients on a fee-for-service basis. In some IPAs, the physicians organize the association themselves and approach the HMO for a contract, rather than waiting to be approached by the HMO.

PPO (Preferred Provider Organization): This is a loose network of doctors who agree to participate in an insurance plan, usually at a predetermined fee-for-service rate established by the insurer, which pays the providers significantly less than the usual and customary fee. (However, some PPOs now pay on a capitated basis.) Doctors in PPOs can usually see other nonmember patients in their own practices.

EPO (Exclusive Provider Organization): This is an extreme version of a PPO, almost like an HMO. Patients cannot see doctors who are outside the network selected by the insurer, or they must pay 100 percent of costs. Providers are reimbursed according to fee-for-service at a predetermined rate.

POS (Point of Service Plan): Also a hybrid between a PPO and an HMO, this type of plan requires patients to have a primary doctor who oversees their care and determines which specialists are necessary. If a patient seeks care from a participating provider, he or she pays little or nothing and may not file any claims. Care provided by out-of-network providers is reimbursed at a much lower rate (i.e., with higher copayments). The reimbursement to providers may be fee-for-service or capitation.

MSO (Managed Service Organization): The newest arrangement at this time, MSOs are managed care arrangements started by hospitals that form their own group of doctors. They want doctors to see patients in their own offices, but to use the hospital for lab work, X-rays, and so on.

All in all, understanding managed care can be very difficult for the neophyte, as the definitions of each type of arrangement change all the time. In fact, some medical professionals say that the powerful insurance companies proliferate many different types of plans to intentionally confuse consumers and take advantage of their inability to compare among health plans and be smart consumers. (Despite my own extensive experience as a researcher in healthcare and medical billing, I too find the diversity of managed care plans and the lack of standards so confusing that I agree with this conjecture.)

There is no doubt that managed care will continue to evolve over the next decade. According to recent surveys, in 1994, more than 50 million Americans—about 20 percent of the population—already belonged to some type of HMO and that number has risen by 1996 to almost 30 percent. California was the leader in HMOs, with 40 percent of its population enrolled in one, followed by Oregon (38%), Maryland (36%), and Arizona (35%). Meanwhile, surveys indicate that more than 45 million Americans belonged to PPOs in 1994.

See Table 2-1 for some interesting statistics on HMO and PPO enrollments in each state. See Table 2-2 for a list indicating HMO ownership in early 1995. See Figure 2-3 for a graph showing the breakdown of HMO models as of January 1995.

SUMMARY: PRIVATE INSURANCE VERSUS DOCTORS   From its modern beginnings in the early twentieth century, private insurance has been a boon for doctors. Because of the tremendous explosion in the American population, and the growth of corporations throughout the 1950s, 1960s, 1970s, and 1980s, group insurance became a standard benefit offered by most employers and demanded by employees. At the same time, most insurers created affordable individual policies for those people who did not have access to group coverage. As a result, doctors experienced several decades of consistent, patient growth, during most of which they were paid handsomely on a fee-for-service basis.

Table 2-3 shows the extent of this growth by indicating the increases in insurance payments among all types of private insurance between 1950 and 1993. Notice the sharp rise in payments between 1960 and 1980, and the steady rise each year from 1981 to 1989, after which the annual increases began to shrink substantially. This decrease marks the beginning of the effects of managed care.

As Table 2-3 makes clear, insurance companies have been trying to hold down costs, particularly physicians' fees, since 1990. Three factors had driven the cost of private insurance sky high in the 1980s: (1) consumers had

TABLE 2-1

Number of HMOs, PPOs, and POSs Per State—1994

	Number of HMOs*	Market Share*	Number of PPOs**	Market Share**	Number of POSs***
Alabama	8	10%	29	34.5%	2
Alaska	0	0	3	3.1	0
Arizona	20	35.8	30	16.5	1
Arkansas	6	3.8	9	2.5	2
California	36	38.3	84	23.4	5
Colorado	12	24.4	33	50.9	1
Connecticut	14	27.4	16	4.6	1
Delaware	6	20.5	6	1.2	1
District of Columbia	2	25.6	7	12.6	0
Florida	36	20.1	78	22.2	11
Georgia	11	8.8	39	13.3	4
Hawaii	7	23.2	6	40.7	0
Idaho	2	1.2	2	0.2	0
Illinois	27	16.9	50	24.4	2
Indiana	12	7.4	37	15.9	2
Iowa	3	4.1	13	8.9	0
Kansas	10	10.9	21	15.1	2
Kentucky	7	12.1	16	11.6	2
Louisiana	11	7.0	30	15.5	2
Maine	3	6.2	6	0.8	0
Maryland	16	36.2	21	21.1	3
Massachusetts	16	35.2	23	7.6	7
Michigan	17	20.2	28	7.7	5
Minnesota	9	26.6	14	32.9	1
Mississippi	1	0.3	10	22.8	1
Missouri	18	14.7	31	22.5	4
Montana	1	1.5	1	0.2	0
Nebraska	5	9.5	11	33.2	0

TABLE 2-1

Number of HMOs, PPOs, and POSs Per State—1994   (Continued)

	Number of HMOs[*]	Market Share[*]	Number of PPOs[**]	Market Share[**]	Number of POSs[***]
Nevada	7	14.7	20	18.5	1
New Hampshire	3	17.0	5	3.3	1
New Jersey	14	16.9	23	13.1	3
New Mexico	6	17.4	7	2.4	0
New York	33	24.3	23	3.8	4
North Carolina	12	8.3	24	11.2	3
North Dakota	2	1.1	0	0	0
Ohio	31	19.2	47	19.7	9
Oklahoma	6	7.3	20	12.9	4
Oregon	7	37.5	13	15.6	1
Pennsylvania	19	21.5	56	13.8	8
Rhode Island	3	28.8	3	9.6	0
South Carolina	4	4.2	18	11.6	2
South Dakota	1	2.9	3	1.6	0
Tennessee	17	16.2	37	31.8	4
Texas	31	9.7	67	28.7	9
Utah	8	19.2	11	8.6	1
Vermont	1	12.6	1	0.3	0
Virginia	13	8.4	19	7.9	4
Washington	11	16.4	21	24.1	2
West Virginia	0	0	7	4.2	1
Wisconsin	27	24.2	26	11.2	2
Wyoming	0	0	0	0	0
TOTAL	572		1105		118

[*] *Source:* Group Health Association of America, National Directory of HMOs

[**] *Source:* American Managed Care and Review Association (AMCRA) Foundation

[***] *Source:* American Managed Care and Review Association (AMCRA) Foundation

TABLE 2-2

HMO Ownership as of January 1, 1995

Total Plans	625
Insurance companies	154
National managed care chain	124
Blue Cross/Blue Shield	88
Independently owned	67
Hospital or hospital alliance	43
Corporation	26
Physician/hospital joint venture	19
Physician/medical group	18
Cooperative	10
University	10
County/state government	8
Private non-profit	8
Managed care company	7
Local non-profit	5
Health system joint venture	2
Hospital/university	2
Multiple owner types	2
National chain and physician group	2
Insurance company/hospital	1
National managed care chain/hospital	1
State medical association	1
Other	9
Unknown	18

Source: American Managed Care and Review Association (AMCRA) Foundation

Figure 2-3
Breakdown of HMO
Model Types—
January 1995

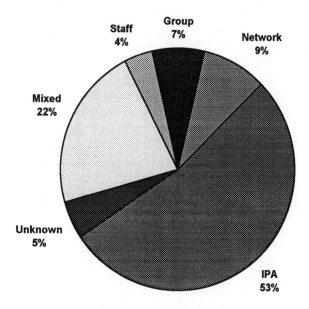

great expectations of healthcare and demanded more services; (2) new technology created improvements in healthcare, but at increased costs; and (3) providers and consumers were not given incentives to contain costs. These factors have slowly prompted private insurers to rethink their policies and to devise new ways to constrain fees. In a sense, one might say that private insurers today are seeking retribution for the extravagances doctors enjoyed in past decades.

The significance of this transition for anyone wanting to get into medical billing can be seen in the confused eyes and smaller pocketbooks of most physicians today. Many of them can no longer afford to practice independently and "according to their own wits," the way they probably imagined it when they went to medical school. Instead, they are being forced to reduce their costs, kowtow to insurance companies, and join dozens of PPOs and HMOs in order to keep their patients (who themselves have been "encouraged" to switch to these types of plans by their employers to save money).

Mary Vandegrift, owner of a successful billing service called AccuMed Solutions, Inc., in Columbia, Maryland, notes that some of her doctors have signed up with as many as a dozen HMOs, and one of her doctors was a member of 17 managed care organizations. In terms of income, Mary also related to me that one of her clients, a specialist, used to make over $300,000 per year but has barely made more than $150,000 in the past few years and is now nearly broke because of her huge expenses.

TABLE 2-3

Private Health Insurance Claims Payments by Type of Insurer 1950–1993 (numbers are in billions)

Year	Total	Percentage Change from Previous Year(s)	Breakdown of Total*		
			Insurance Companies	Self-Insured and HMOs	Blue Cross/ Blue Shield
1950	$1.3		$0.8	NA	$0.6
1955	3.1	138	1.8	NA	1.4
1960	5.7	84	3.0	NA	2.6
1965	9.6	68	5.2	NA	4.5
1970	17.2	79	9.1	NA	8.1
1975	32.1	87	16.5	NA	16.9
1980	76.3	138	37.0	16.2	25.5
1981	85.9	13	41.6	18.9	29.2
1982	97.1	13	49.2	21.6	32.2
1983	104.1	7	51.7	24.1	34.4
1984	107.5	3	56.0	26.1	35.7
1985	117.6	9	60.0	32.5	37.5
1986	128.5	9	64.3	36.8	40.6
1987	151.7	18	72.5	56.5	44.5
1988	171.1	13	83.0	62.8	48.2
1989	194.5	14	89.4	79.8	50.7
1990	208.9	7	92.5	93.4	55.9
1991	223.0	7	97.6	112.0	60.0
1992	245.5	10	104.8	131.1	63.1
1993	253.5	3	103.6	144.7	62.0

*Numbers may not add up because of rounding.

Source: Health Insurance Association of America, Annual Survey of Health Insurance Companies; Blue Cross/Blue Shield Association, Group Health Association of America, Inc.

This is not to suggest that all HMOs or PPOs hurt doctors or restrict their income to the point of poverty. In many cases, doctors can continue to charge on a fee-for-service basis and earn decent incomes. For example, many specialists who are part of an HMO are allowed to charge fee-for-service; it is only the primary care physician who must accept capitation.

But, as Mary says, "There are some good HMOs out there...and some very bad ones!" She points to the financial risks many doctors unknowingly take when they agree to become part of a capitated prepayment HMO plan. For example, Mary told me about one of her doctors who is affiliated with an HMO plan and paid on a capitation basis. The rules of the HMO are quite complex, but the doctor effectively receives only a $5.00 capitation payment per month. This amount can end up being even less, due to what is called a "withhold." If the patient uses the services of the doctor more than statistically expected for that year, the insurer keeps some of the capitation payments as compensation. In Mary's analysis of this situation, some of her clients are "losing their shirts!"

Perhaps it is now becoming even clearer to you the many ways that a professional medical billing service can help its clients when it comes to private healthcare insurance reimbursement. First, the professional biller can attend to business while the doctor attends to medicine. This makes sense, because doctors typically don't learn business skills such as marketing, accounting, and financial analysis. Second, the billing service can make sure that reimbursements are expedited by using electronic claims filing, which usually obtains payments for the physician within a few weeks rather than months. Third, the professional biller can pay attention to the many different fee structures that a typical doctor today must track when he or she belongs to many different kinds of managed care plans. As indicated earlier, if a doctor belongs to a dozen or more HMOs and PPOs and each has its own fee structure, each claim must bill for the correct amount.

Fourth, the professional biller can keep track of the write-offs, the amounts above allowable fees that PPOs and HMOs do not let doctors charge their members. These amounts must be credited from the doctor's accounts receivable. Most doctors want to keep track of how much they have to write off each month, and the professional biller can provide this information. Finally, in cases of HMOs that pay by capitation, the professional biller can compare how much the doctor earns in monthly capitated fees versus how much he or she might have been able to bill if the claims had been charged on a fee-for-service basis. In this way, the professional biller can advise the client if it is worthwhile to continue to be a member of the HMO.

Some healthcare industry watchers predict that HMOs have had their heyday and will soon fall by the wayside. In 1995 and 1996, many HMOs reported unprofitable years, and several of the country's largest ones merged with others. More important though, many consumers have become leery of HMOs because of the reported poor quality of health-care they provide. Many industry experts say there is an inherent conflict of interest that exists among doctors affiliated with HMOs: doctors are supposed to do what's best for their patients, but HMOs restrict their ability to do so because of their cost-saving rules and regulations. Ultimately, many people are predicting that, given the American love for independence and freedom of choice, PPO-type plans will eventually win out

Business Profile: Mary Vandegrift and Candis Ruiz

Mary Vandegrift started a medical billing business in 1993 after a long career with IBM. In the beginning, she tapped into her computer background to sell computer systems to medical offices, but she did not enjoy the sales aspect of her job. Mary eventually met a neighbor, Candis Ruiz, whose background in insurance sales seemed to be the perfect match. Together they formed a partnership that has taken off beyond their dreams. They eventually purchased software and additional training from Santiago SDS, Inc.

Mary and Candis now serve more than a dozen practices, for whom they mostly do full practice management. They are very involved with their clients, handling their billing and advising them on many financial issues arising out of the inherent problems of managed care. As discussed in the previous section, Mary has had several of her clients experience a notable shrinkage in income over the past two years, and so she has learned to make sophisticated financial projections to analyze the value of joining certain HMOs. As Mary says,

Our job is almost like auditing; we have to keep track of the fees they are paid compared to how much they might have gotten. We try to stay on top of what HMOs are doing business-wise, and to become knowledgeable if not experts on every aspect of healthcare that we can. If it's a problem for the doctor, we consider it to be our problem. We take that headache off them so they can be doctors.

One of the most interesting strategies Mary has pursued is to recruit other professionals to be part of her team. She has introduced her clients to insurance people, accountants, lawyers, and others who can help the doctors improve their business. Mary realized this was a useful idea because, as she puts it, "Doctors don't have a sphere of influence outside of other doctors for business information. We go in and help them increase their patient load, improve their records management, verify that they are coding properly, and even take care of their office supply problems." At the moment, Mary and Candis use the experts to increase the professionalism of their service, but at some point in the future, they may organize this idea into a consortium of professionals that would work with all their clients as a group, while they share in their fees.

because they allow patients to choose their own physicians and make decisions based on their personal preferences, even if it costs them more to go outside the PPO network.

Public Health Insurance Programs

The two largest public health insurance programs are the federally run Medicare and the combined federal/state-run Medicaid programs. Public health insurance also includes CHAMPUS (the Civilian Health and Medical Program of the Uniformed Services), Veterans Medical Care, FEHBP (Federal Employees Health Benefits Program), and various other local government-run plans. Here are details about the major public health programs.

MEDICARE   The federal government began Medicare in 1966 to assist elderly and disabled citizens (typically on a fixed income) who faced rapidly rising costs in medical and hospital care. Medicare falls under the aegis of the Social Security Administration but is run by the Health Care Financing Administration (HCFA), an agency of the Department of Health and Human Services. Today roughly 37 million Americans are covered by Medicare. Table 2-4 shows the growth of Medicare in terms of enrollees and claims paid between 1983 and 1995 (the latest detailed information available).

Medicare coverage is divided into two parts, as follows:

1. **Part A** covers hospitalization, skilled nursing facilities, home health-care, and hospice care. Part A of Medicare is automatic and free of charge for almost every American over the age of 65 and the permanently disabled. It is financed through payroll taxes for Social Security. Each eligible subscriber pays a deductible ($760 in 1997, but it increases slightly every year) for each hospitalization, and then Medicare picks up the tab for 60 days of inpatient hospital care during the benefit period. In general, billing services are not involved with filing claims for Part A services, because hospitals process these claims through Medicare "intermediaries" in each state, which are sometimes insurance carriers or sometimes data-processing centers.

2. **Part B** of Medicare pays for inpatient or outpatient doctor's services performed in a hospital, clinic, doctor's office, or home. It also covers surgical services and supplies, diagnostic tests, laboratory tests, X-rays, ambulance transportation, physical and occupational therapy, blood (after 3 pints), outpatient mental health services, artificial limbs, and

durable medical equipment (DME). Part B of Medicare is voluntary, but most Americans sign up for it, paying a monthly premium ($43.80 in 1997, with increases each year) that is deducted from their Social Security checks. In general, Part B insurance covers the subscriber for 80 percent of what Medicare determines to be "allowable" charges in a given geographic area and specialty, according to its own fee schedule. The beneficiary is then responsible for an annual deductible ($100 in 1996), and for a copayment.

TABLE 2-4

Medical Enrollment and Benefit Payments (Parts A and B) (fiscal years 1967–1995)

	Hospital and/or Medical Insurance Part A + B		Hospital Insurance Part A		Supplementary Medical Insurance Part B	
	Number of enrolled persons (millions)	Benefit payments ($billions)	Number of enrolled persons (millions)	Benefit payments ($billions)	Number of enrolled persons (millions)	Benefit payments ($billions)
1967	19.5	$ 3.1	19.5	$ 2.5	17.9	$ 0.7
1970	20.5	6.8	20.4	4.8	19.6	1.9
1975	25.0	14.1	24.6	10.4	23.9	3.8
1980	28.5	33.9	28.1	23.8	27.4	10.1
1985	31.1	69.5	30.6	47.7	29.9	21.8
1986	31.8	74.1	31.2	48.9	30.6	25.2
1987	32.4	79.8	31.9	49.8	31.2	29.9
1988	32.9	85.5	32.4	51.9	31.6	33.7
1989	33.6	94.3	33.1	57.4	32.1	36.9
1990	34.2	108.7	33.7	66.2	32.6	42.5
1991	34.9	113.9	34.4	68.5	33.2	45.5
1992	35.6	129.2	36.2	80.6	35.4	48.6
1993	36.3	142.9	N/A	N/A	N/A	N/A
1994	36.9	159.3	N/A	N/A	N/A	N/A
1995	37.6	190.0	N/A	N/A	N/A	N/A

Source: U.S. Department of Health and Human Services, Health Care Financing Administration, Bureau of Data Management and Strategy.

One of the primary markets for professional independent billing services are physicians and other healthcare providers who have many Medicare patients, because, as indicated earlier, these doctors must file Part B claims for their patients. Part B claims are processed through insurance companies in each state that have been contracted to handle Medicare claims. In many states, these carriers are the Blue Cross/Blue Shield insurer, but this aspect of their business is separate from their commercial insurance. These contracted intermediary companies change from time to time, so I have not listed them in this book; you can find a current list of them in the official Medicare handbook published each year, available from the Social Security Administration or on the Internet at www.hcfa.gov. If you are just learning about medical billing, you need to know about the specific Medicare carriers in your state.

In addition to Medicare Parts A and B, many Medicare enrollees supplement their health insurance with an additional policy called Medicare Supplement Insurance, but usually referred to as *Medigap* because it fills in the gaps between Part A and B deductibles, copayments, and uncovered services. Medigap policies are purchased from commercial insurers, associations, and organizations such as the American Association of Retired Persons (AARP). When Medigap policies first appeared, insurance companies offered dozens of types of plans, causing a tremendous amount of confusion among Medicare enrollees. As a result, the federal government stepped in to regulate Medigap, standardizing the policies to just 10 choices, called Plans A to J. Every insurer that sells Medigap policies must sell the basic Plan A, plus a number of other plans. These plans differ in terms of what they cover and how much they pay for as a supplement to Medicare Parts A and B. For example, most of the plans will pay the Part A deductible and the copayments that Medicare normally requires for hospitalizations, skilled nursing facilities, and so on. Table 2-5 summarizes the 10 plans.

Understanding Medicare and Medigap is critical to a billing service. Doctors (and hence their billing service) must know a person's Medicare/Medigap coverage, and if any exceptions apply. For example, for most people over 65, Medicare is likely their primary coverage, with a Medigap policy providing "secondary" coverage. In many states, the claims for such individuals can be filed electronically: the Medicare carrier will pay its share and then automatically forward the claim electronically to the Medigap secondary insurer for payment. This means that the patient never has to hand over cash to the doctor, and the billing service needs to file the claim only once.

However, Medicare coverage can also be confusing. You must make sure that the person has only one Medigap plan, to avoid duplication of

TABLE 2-5

Standard Medigap Policies

Basic Benefits are included in all plans:

- Hospitalization—Part A coinsurance plus coverage for 365 additional days after Medicare benefits end
- Medical expenses—Part B coinsurance (generally 20% of Medicare-approved expenses)
- Blood: First three pints of blood each year.

Plan A	Plan B	Plan C	Plan D	Plan E	Plan F	Plan G	Plan H	Plan I	Plan J
Basic Benefits	Basic Benefits	Basic Benefits	Basic Benefits	Basic Benefits	Basic Benefits	Basic Benefits	Basic Benefits	Basic Benefits	Basic Benefits
		Skilled Nursing Coinsurance	Skilled Nursing Coinsurance	Skilled Nursing Coinsurance	Skilled Nursing Coinsurance	Skilled Nursing Coinsurance	Skilled Nursing Coinsurance	Skilled Nursing Coinsurance	Skilled Nursing Coinsurance
	Part A Deductible	Part A Deductible	Part A Deductible	Part A Deductible	Part A Deductible	Part A Deductible	Part A Deductible	Part A Deductible	Part A Deductible
		Part B Deductible			Part B Deductible				Part B Deductible
					Part B Excess (100%)	Part B Excess (100%)		Part B Excess (100%)	Part B Excess (100%)
		Foreign Emergency Travel	Foreign Emergency Travel	Foreign Emergency Travel	Foreign Emergency Travel	Foreign Emergency Travel	Foreign Emergency Travel	Foreign Emergency Travel	Foreign Emergency Travel
			At-Home Recovery			At-Home Recovery		At-Home Recovery	At-Home Recovery
							Basic Drugs ($1,250)	Basic Drugs ($1,250)	Basic Drugs ($1,250)
				Preventive Care					Preventive Care

Note: All plans may not be available in every state.

benefits. (Before the new law restricting Mediga~~p~~ icy, some people actually made money on their several policies that would pay their deducti~~ble~~ would thus pocket the excess as profit.)

Another glitch can be finding out that ~~for~~ ~~some~~ Medicare is not their primary insurer. This can happen when ~~the~~ ~~patient~~ is still employed and has health coverage from his or her company. In this case, the employer policy is primary to Medicare. Similarly, Medicare is a second payer whenever the claim involves a work-related injury, an automobile or other accident, and in a few other circumstances.

Another vital aspect of Medicare reimbursement that a professional biller must understand is the distinction between *participating* and *non-participating* providers. Similar to the way that many old Blue Shield plans worked, doctors may or may not accept Medicare's fee schedule. There are pros and cons to each side.

Once per year, doctors must decide either to participate in Medicare, thus becoming a PAR (participating) physician by "taking assignment," or to not participate, called a NON-PAR.

- ■ PAR—Taking assignment means that the doctor accepts the allowable fee determined by Medicare as his or her full payment for services rendered to the Medicare patient. This means that he or she cannot charge the patient the difference between the standard fee and the allowable amount. In return for this cooperation, Medicare will mail its check directly to the doctor, saving the physician the risk of collecting from the patient. Note: remember that Medicare will then pay the physician only 80 percent of the allowable amount, and the patient *must* be billed for the remaining 20 percent copayment.

- ■ NON-PAR—In contrast, doctors can choose not to participate in Medicare. They must file claims for patients, but they can charge patients up to 115 percent more than Medicare allows (this is called the *limiting charge*). However, there is a major penalty for not participating: Medicare will mail the check to the patient, so the physician must collect his or her fees directly from the patient—a potentially risky venture.

Table 2-6 compares one patient who sees Dr. Smith, a participating provider, with a patient who sees Dr. Jones, a non-participating provider. Assume that both patients are treated for the exact same problem and both doctors practice in the same geographic area.

2-6

ple of Difference in Charges Between a Participating Provider and a Non-Participating
vider Under Medicare

	Customary Charge	Limiting Charge	Medicare Allowable Amount	Paid by Medicare	Balance Due from Patient	Write-off
Dr. Smith (PAR)	$300.00 (disallowed)	N/A	$159.52	$127.62 directly to doctor	$31.90	$140.48
Dr. Jones (NON-PAR)	$300.00	$183.44	$159.52	$127.62 directly to patient	$55.82	$116.56

Explanation

Dr. Smith has agreed to be a PAR provider and so is willing to accept the Medicare allowable amount as total payment. His patient owes only $31.90 because Dr. Smith accepts $159.52 as the full fee rather than his usual fee of $300. Dr. Smith receives 80% of $159.52, hence $127.62, and so must collect $31.90 from the patient either at the time of visit or after Medicare pays him. He receives the check directly from Medicare. He must also write off the $140.48 difference between his usual fee and the Medicare approved amount.

Dr. Jones is a NON-PAR provider. She is able to collect $183.44 because she is allowed to charge 15% more than the Medicare allowable amount. Medicare pays 80% of the allowable amount, hence $127.62 to the patient, so the patient must pay the $55.82 difference to Dr. Jones. Note that Dr. Jones can ask the patient to pay the entire $183.44 up front since Medicare will reimburse the patient later.

As mentioned in the sidebar on page 41, "Understanding Reimbursement-Speak," Medicare has been phasing in a new fee schedule called RBRVS to replace the UCR method. A billing service that offers full practice management will need to understand this new fee schedule, the distinction between PARs and NON-PARs, and the differences between billed amounts, allowable amounts, limiting charges, Medicare-paid amounts (80 percent), copayment amounts (20 percent), and write-off amounts. Got it?

A NOTE ON MEDICARE HMOS In recent years, Medicare has endorsed the HMO concept as a way to cut its own costs and has therefore contracted with a variety of HMO facilities to take over the care of Medicare members. Under these Medicare-HMO models, the subscriber must continue to pay the Medicare Part B premium to HCFA, but the person will generally not pay any deductibles for Part A services or any 20 percent copayments for Part B services, thus potentially saving a lot of money, especially if the person does not have Medigap coverage or is very ill.

Some Medicare HMOs are of the pure type, in which the person cannot see doctors outside the network. These plans, called "lock-ins," require patients to obtain all covered care through a primary care physician and referrals to specialists. Other Medicare HMO plans operate with more flexibility. If the patient goes outside the network, the HMO will not pay, but Medicare will (in which case the patient will usually need to pay any deductibles plus the 20 percent copayments). These types of plans are good for seniors who live in different states at different times of the year or who want to continue using a particular physician.

Certain extra benefits make Medicare HMOs more attractive than "regular" Medicare. Many HMOs provide routine preventative checkups, eye examinations and glasses, hearing aids, and discounted prescription drugs. Because of the lower costs to patients and the extra benefits, it is now estimated that millions of Medicare enrollees have opted to join a Medicare approved HMO rather than continuing to see independent physicians on a fee-for-service basis.

However, as I write this book, there have been many reports from dissatisfied consumers in Medicare HMOs. Many people have complained that their HMOs do not give them quality care, that their primary physician refuses to let them see a specialist, and so on. In each state, there is a "peer review organization" (PRO), a panel of doctors who are paid by the federal government to monitor problems in Medicare. However, filing complaints to PROs is slow and time consuming.

Again, you will need to be familiar with these issues should you get into the medical billing business.

MEDICAID Medicaid is administered jointly by HCFA and each state government, according to general guidelines established by federal law. Medicaid assists those whose incomes are below certain levels. In 1995, an estimated 36.2 million people utilized Medicaid, of which more than 17 million were dependent children. Note also that many Medicare members who cannot afford Medigap secondary insurance can be covered by Medicaid, which pays deductibles and copayments for them. These people are often called *Medi-Medi* crossovers. (Note if you are doing electronic claims filing: just as Medicare can send secondary claims electronically to many Medigap insurers, it can also forward the claims electronically to the appropriate Medicaid carrier. This relatively new process has facilitated the electronic filing of millions of Medicare claims that also require secondary payers.)

Many physicians do not accept Medicaid patients because the allowable amounts for billed charges are typically as low as 30 percent to 35 percent of the usual and customary fees the physician charges. For many physicians, this makes treating Medicaid patients almost a losing proposition.

Medicaid claims are processed differently in each state, either through an insurance carrier such as a Blue or a computer service company that handles the claims for HCFA. Medicaid regulations are very strict regarding what kinds of medical services are covered, and what the allowable fees are.

CHAMPUS   CHAMPUS is the Civilian Health and Medical Program of the Uniformed Services, a healthcare program for dependents of active military personnel, as well as retired military personnel and their families. Under CHAMPUS, covered persons can use civilian doctors for medical care and have a portion of the care paid for by the federal government. At age 65, CHAMPUS beneficiaries are transferred to the Medicare program.

WORKER'S COMPENSATION   Worker's compensation covers medical expenses and disability benefits when an illness or injury results directly from work. Employers with more than a certain number of employees are required to carry this insurance from a carrier of their choice.

Worker's comp. claims are more complex than standard claims, as they require second opinion reviews and many kinds of reports filed by doctors to verify the injuries. If you do billing for worker's comp. claims, it is recommended that you charge more because they take longer.

How a Doctor's Office Works

How a billing service works is directly tied into how a doctor's office works. If you have no background working in a doctor's office, you will be surprised by how many elements are involved. For this reason, this section reviews the operation of a typical physician's office.

To begin, most healthcare practitioners have one or more office personnel who handle the reception work; provide some patient support; and perhaps work on the claims filing, billing, and accounting functions. The person may be called "office manager," "receptionist," "business assistant," or there may be one of each. These office personnel may be a major impediment to your signing on a doctor—or they may be your allies. We discuss this issue in the "Marketing Guidelines" section later in the chapter.

Business Profile: Heidi Kollmorgen and Susan Kruger

Heidi Kollmorgen and Susan Kruger are partners in H/D Medical Receivables, Inc., in Cleveland, Ohio. Heidi started the business after doing billing for a doctor's office in-house for eight years; little by little, she realized that she preferred to be her own boss. Like many parents today, she also wanted to be available at home for her two children, Haley and Dylan. Through careful planning, she left her job and opened up her own company to handle "just claims," purchasing software from Medical Management Software and Merry Schiff. Her first client turned out to be her former employer, who had not found someone to replace her. While getting that contract was a cinch, Heidi told me that getting additional contracts with doctors has not been easy, as few physicians in her city have been willing to outsource billing.

Heidi therefore jumped at the chance to work with Susan when they met at their community club. Susan had worked as a hospital administrator and at a bank in marketing, so she had excellent skills in making appointments to see doctors and presenting their sales pitch. Her primary strategy is to become friendly with the office staff, as they are the gatekeepers to the doctor. Even when the office tells Susan it is not interested in hiring out its billing, Susan continues to drop in and make small talk about the newest medical coding procedures and what might be happening in healthcare at the time. As Susan says, "It's all in your manner; if you don't present yourself as a know it all, you can truly build a rapport with the office staff, and when the time is ripe, they even get behind you because you make their life easier."

Heidi and Susan say that after a few years, they were fortunate in finding several doctors who were in desperate need of their services for full practice management. They cite a major reason for this: the fact that as HMOs have become more and more common in the Cleveland area, doctors have to spend much of their time arranging referrals for their patients to specialists. Referrals require dictating medical reports and making many phone calls, functions for which the doctor relies on the office staff for support. This is why outsourcing the billing ultimately improves the conditions in a doctor's office for the office staff. Their time becomes free to help the doctor, instead of doing the billing and handling calls from patients asking about their invoices. Only in one case when Susan and Heidi took over the billing did an office staff person lose her job; in all the other cases, the office staff have been reassigned to patient relations and other office work.

Heidi and Susan now focus on full practice management. They file claims electronically and track each client's receivables, including comparing what the doctor receives from capitated payments versus fee-for-service payments. Heidi was also working with a group of doctors to help them organize and negotiate proactively with an HMO before being swallowed up by one. In building her business, Heidi believes that experience makes a difference: "The more you learn about practice management and gain experience, the better living you will earn."

THE BACKGROUND WORK   Assuming the doctor's office is independently run (not a staff HMO model), the following background events typically occur just to log the patient in.

1. When a patient first sees the physician (or dentist), he or she is asked to complete a *patient registration form*. This form includes the patient's vital statistics: name, address, sex, phone number, employer, primary insurer, member number, secondary insurer if any, and so on. The patient also usually signs a *release and assignment of benefits form* that allows the doctor to release information about the diagnosis and treatment to the insurance company so that he or she may bill the insurer directly and receive the payment. This form may be part of the registration form or it might be a separate form. Figure 2-4 shows a typical patient registration form.

2. If necessary, the patient fills out a *pre-authorization form* (also called a *pre-certification form*), which is used to specify information about a planned procedure or service that requires approval in advance by the insurance carrier, Medicare, or Medicaid. If the physician fails to obtain this approval, he or she may be denied payment by the insurance carrier or Medicare. Many insurance companies now have 800 phone numbers for physicians to use in emergencies when immediate authorization is necessary.

In the coming years, the process of checking eligibility and pre-authorizing treatments may be done via computer. Several software companies are developing systems that would allow the doctor's office or the outside billing service to use a modem to check the patient's insurance coverage and/or obtain approval for a service. Such new technology is an important step toward computerizing the medical industry and speeding up the doctor's ability to treat patients. It may also be likely that an independent billing service can either sell this software as part of its service, or do the work for doctors by phone whenever the physician gets a new patient.

3. The next form, usually called the *superbill* (also referred to as the fee ticket, visit slip, or encounter form) is used to record the purpose of the patient visit and billing information. The form contains blanks for the patient's name and other information and then lists the most common diagnostic and procedure codes used by that doctor. These codes are now required by all insurance carriers to demarcate why the patient saw the doctor and what services the doctor performed (more details about these coding systems appear later in the chapter). Since there are thousands of possible diagnosis codes and procedure codes, each office usually designs and prints its own superbills listing only the codes the doctor most commonly uses in his or her specialty. The superbill also serves as a payment receipt if the patient has to file his or her own claims.

Figures 2-5A and 2-5B show typical superbills.

Figure 2-4

Patient Registration
Form (Courtesy of
Dave Shipton)

**Corrected
art to come**

NAME:_____, SOCIAL SECURITY: _____

ADDRESS:_____
          (Street)   **(City)**   **(State)**   **(Zip Code)**

PHONE:(___) ___-_____, BIRTHDATE:___/___/___(Month, Day, Year), AGE:_____, SEX _____

STATUS: Married___, Single___, Other___, EMPLOYED: Yes___, No___, Full Time___, Part Time___,

EMPLOYER:_____ PHONE:(___) ___-_____

ADDRESS:_____
          (Street)   **(City)**   **(State)**   **(Zip Code)**

PRIMARY INSURANCE INFORMATION

NAME:_____, SOCIALSECURITY#:_____
(Policy Holder) (the primary person the insurance policy is assigned to) (If same as line 1, PRINT "SAME")

ADDRESS:_____
          (Street)   **(City)**   **(State)**   **(Zip Code)**

PHONE:(___) ___-_____, BIRTHDATE:___/___/___(Month, Day, Year), AGE:_____, SEX _____

PATIENT'S RELATIONSHIP TO INSURED: Self___, Spouse___, Child___, Other___,

INSURANCE COMPANY:_____, POLICY NUMBER_____

GROUP NUMBER:_____, PLAN:_____, CERTIFICATE NUMBER:_____

ADDRESS_____
          (Street)   **(City)**   **(State)**   **(Zip Code)**

SECONDARY INSURANCE INFORMATION

NAME:_____, SOCIAL SECURITY #:_____
(Secondary Policy, another person who may be responsible for payment) (If same as line 1, PRINT "SAME)

ADDRESS:_____
          (Street)   **(City)**   **(State)**   **(Zip Code)**

PHONE:(___) ___-_____, BIRTHDATE:___/___/___(Month, Day, Year), AGE:_____, SEX _____

INSUREDS RELATIONSHIP TO PATIENT: Self___, Spouse___, Child___, Other___,

INSURANCE COMPANY:_____, POLICY NUMBER_____

GROUP NUMBER:_____, PLAN:_____, CERTIFICATE NUMBER:_____

ADDRESS_____
          (Street)   **(City)**   **(State)**   **(Zip Code)**

PLEASE READ AND SIGN THE FOLLOWING STATEMENT

I authorize the release of any medical or other information necessary to process insurance claims. I authorize payment of medical benefits to the physician or supplier for services described in the insurance claim. I understand that some Commercial Insurance plans (Metropolitian, Prudential, Aetna, PPO, HMO, etc.) may not cover the total cost of treatment (due to the nature of the insurance plan or that some treatment(s) may be considered medically unnecessary by the insurance company) and that <u>I am responsible</u> for any <u>copayment</u>, <u>deductable</u> and <u>other charges</u> not covered by my primary or secondary insurance plan(s). Medicare Patients, I understand that <u>I am responsible</u> for the <u>deductable</u> and <u>copayment</u> applied to my Medicare Insurance coverage.

SIGNATURE_____ DATE_____

ALL INFORMATION IS KEPT STRICTLY CONFIDENTIAL

Anytown Cardiology

Pt. Name (LAST)	(FIRST)	Date of Birth	Insurance Type	Date of Service	Doctor's Name

DIAGNOSIS CODES

		#
Angina Pectoris (NOS)	413.9	
Aortic Stenosis	747.22	
Aortic Valve Prolapse	424.1	
Atrial Fibrillation	427.31	
Atrial Flutter	427.32	
Cardiac Dysrhythmia (NOS)	427.9	
Cardiomyopathy, Idiopathic	425.4	
CV Insufficiency (Carotid, WO CVA)	433.10	
CV Insufficiency (NOS)	437.1	
Cong. Heart Disease (NOS)	746.9	
Congestive Heart Failure	428.0	
COPD (NOS)	496	
Coronary Atherosclerosis, unsp.	414.00	
Diabetes W/ Insulin Depend.	250.01	
Diabetes Wo/ Insulin Depend.	250.00	
Emphysema	492.8	
Fistula, Arteriovenous	414.19	
Heart/Renal Failure (NOS)	404.90	
Hyperlipidemia (NOS)	272.4	
Hypertension, Uncontr (NOS)	401.9	
Hypertensive Cardiomyopathy	402.91	
Ischemic Heart Disease	414.8	
Mitral Insufficiency /Prolapse	424.0	
Mitral Valve Stenosis	394.0	
Mitral/Aortic Valve Insuff.	396.3	
Myocardial Infarction	411.89	
Myocarditis, Viral	422.91	
Post CV Disease	438	
Pulmonary Artery Stenosis	747.3	
Rheumatic Heart Disease	391.9	
Supraventricular Tach.	427.0	
Tricuspid Insufficiency	397.0	

Consultations

Office Cons. prob. focused 15 min	99241	
Office Cons. expanded 30 min	99242	
Office Cons. detailed 40 min	99243	
Office Cons. compreh, mod. 60 min	99244	
Office Cons. compreh, high 80 min	99245	

Follow-up Office Visits

Minimal 5 min	99211	
Focused 10 min	99212	
Expanded, low complex, 15 min	99213	
Detailed, mod. complex, 25 min	99214	
Comprehen, high complex, 40 min	99215	

Referring Physician

September 27, 1996 © Priority Medical Management

PROCEDURES
Electrocardiography

EKG	93000	
CV stress, test & report	93015	
CV stress, report only	93018	
Holter	93224	
Holter removal	93225	
Holter (with printout)	93230	
Holter (with printout) removal	93231	

Ultrasound

Abdominal aorta	76700	
Duplex scan of aorta	93978	

Echocardiography

2D complete	93307	
Doppler complete	93320	
Echo stress	93350	

Abdominal aorta	76705	
Duplex scan, carotid bilateral	93880	
Carotid flow scan	93875	

PVP

Duplex scan of lower aorta	93925	
Duplex scan of extremity veins	93970	

Pulmonary Function Tests

Spirometry	94060	
Membrane diffusion capacity	94725	
Residual capacity	94240	
Breathing response to CO2	94400	
Maldistribution of inspired gas	94350	
Airway closing volume	94370	
CO diffusing capacity	94720	
Thoracic gas volume	94260	
All of the above	PFT	

Vascular Studies

CV arterial, bilateral	93875	
Venous study, bilateral	93965	
Extremity arteries, single level	93922	
Extremity arteries, multi-level	93923	
Extremity arteries, lower, with stress	93924	

Other

Routine venipuncture	36415	
Handling fee	99000	

Notes

Figure 2-5A   Superbill for a typical cardiology practice (Courtesy of Neal A. Kling, Priority Medical Management, Poway, CA)

Peachblossom Family Practice

Name: Last	First		Date of Birth		Account Type	Date of Service		Dr's Name	

NEW		X-RAY		PROCEDURES		SUTURES/CASTING	
Focused	99201	Abdomen	74020	Audiometry	92552	*Requires Accident Report!*	
Expanded	99202	Abdomen (KUB)	74000	Colonoscopy	45378	Simple? Intermediate?	S I
Detailed	99203	Ankle	73610	CV stress test	93015	Enter *length* and *location*	
Comp. (45 Mins)	99204	Cervical spine	72040	EKG	93000		
Initial OB	Z1032	Chest (2 views)	71020	Endoscopy, upper	43235		
		Elbow	73080	Holter monitor	93230		
ESTABLISHED		Face	70150	Holter removal	93231		
Minimal	99211	Femur	73550	IV therapy	90780	Casting supplies	A4580
Focused	99212	Finger	73140	Nerve study	95904		
Expanded	99213	Foot	73630	Pulmo aide	94640		
Detailed	99214	Forearm	73090	Spirometry P&P	SPIRO		
Comp. (45 Mins)	99215	Hand	73130	**LAB (IN OFFICE)**			
OB Prenatal	Z1034	Hips, bilateral	73520	Glucose	82947		
OB Postpartum	Z1038	Hip	73510	Hemoglobin	85018		
		Knee	73562	Hemoccult stool	82270		
INJECTIONS		Lumbosacral	72110	Pregnancy, urine	81025		
Ancef	J0690	Neck, soft tissue	70360	Urine dipstick	81002		
B12 Complex	J3500	Pelvis	72190	Venipuncture	36415		
Demerol	J2175	Ribs, bilateral	71111				
Depoprovera	J1055	Ribs, unilateral	71101				
Dexamethasone	J1100	Sacro-iliac	72202			**SUPPLIES**	
Diphenhydramine 50mg	J1200	Sacrum & Coccyx	72220	**LAB (OUTSIDE)**		Ace bandage	A4460
Droperidol	J1790	Shoulder	73030	Afetoprotein	82105	Gauze pads	A4200
Epinephrine	J0170	Sinus series	70220	Arthritis panel	ARTH	4" roller bandage	A4202
Estradiol Valerate 40mg	J0970	Skull series	70260	Blood lipoprotein assay	83718	Electrodes	A4556
Furosemide 20mg	J1940	Thoracic Spine	72070	CBC	85025	Irrigation tray	A4320
Gentamicin 80mg	J1580	Tibia/fibula	73590	Culture, throat	87060	Surgical tray	A4550
Glycophyprolate 0.2	X6258	Toes	73660	Culture, urine	87086		
Keflin 1gr	J1890	Wrist	73110	Culture, vaginal	87070	**SURGICAL**	
Lidocaine 1%	J2000	**ULTRASOUND**		Estrogens, total	82672	Biopsy, skin	11100
Lincocin 300mg	J2010	Abdominal	76700	GC & Chlamydia	87110	Cryotherapy	17340
Marcaine HCL 0.25%	J0670	Breast(s)	76645	Hepatitis panel	80059	Debridement, burn	16020
Methylprednisolone 40	J1030	OB	76805	HTLV or HIV test	86689	Debridement, skin	11041
Methylprednisolone 80	J1040	Pelvic (Non-OB)	76856	Lipids profile	80061	Destr. les., face	17000
Penicillin 600,000	J0560	Prostate	76856	Liver function screen	LIVER	Destr. les. - nonfacial	17100
Penicillin 1.2 Mil	J0570	Renal	76770	Mono test	86317	Excision of nail	11750
Penicillin 2.4 Mil	J0580	Scrotum	76870	O&P, stool	87177	I&D, seb. cyst	10060
Phenergan	J2550	Thyroid	76536	Older adult profile	OLD	I&D, hematoma	10140
Progesterone 50mg	J2675	**PVP**		Pap smear	88150	Inj. trigger pts.	20550
Rocephin	J0696	Dup. scan lower aorta	93925	Pap smear, abnormal	88151	Removal, cerumen	69210
Triamcinolone	J3301	Sup. scan extrem. veins	93970	PAP test (prostate)	84066	Rem. for. obj., eye	65205
Toradol	J1885	**VASCULAR STUDIES**		Pregnancy, serum	84703	Rem. FO eye embedded	65210
Valium	J3360	Abdominal aorta	76705	Prenatal panel	80055	Removal FO, nose	30300
Versed	90782	Carotid, duplex	93880	Prolactin assay	84146	Removal, skin tags	11200
Vistaril	J3410	Extr. arter. upper	93922	Protein electroph.	84165	Removal, warts	17110
		Extr. arter. lower	93923	PSA	84153	**NORPLANT**	
IMMUNIZATIONS		Extr. art. low w/stress	93924	RPR	86592	Insertion	11975
DTP	90701	Cerebrovascular	93875	Rubella	86762	Norplant kit	X1520
DT	90702	Venous, lower	93965	Sedimentation rate	85651	Surgical tray	A4550
Gamma Globulin	J1470	**OTHER DRUGS**		SMAC	80018	Anesthesia	J2000
Hepatitis B	9074?	Acet. w/Cod 300mg	99070	T4 test	84436	Removal	11976
HIB	90737	Chlorzoxazone 500mg		T7 (Thyroid panel)	80091	**PHYSICAL THERAPY**	
Influenza	90724	Diphenhydramine		Toxoplasma	80090	Hot/Cold packs	97010
Mantoux Test	86580	Elavil Amitriptyline 10mg		Urinalysis, micro	81000	TENS unit	64550
MMR	90707	Ibuprophen 200mg #30				TENS unit leads	E0730
Polio	90712	Naprosyn 500mg #20		**ECHOCARDIO**		Ultrasound	UL95
Tetanus Toxoid	90703	Pediazol 600mg		2D, comp	93307		
STEROID INJECTIONS		Podophilin		Doppler, comp	93320		
Small joint	20600	Robaxin 750mg #20		Echo stress	93350		
Medium joint	20605	Seldane 60mg					
Large joint	20610	Tylenol 500mg #30					
		Valium 5mg #30					

	ICD9 Code		ICD9 Code		ICD9 Code	Ded.Remain	Payments
1		3		5			
2		4		6			

September 27, 1996 © Priority Medical Management, Poway, CA

Figure 2-5B Superbill for a typical family practice physician (Courtesy of Neal A. Kling, Priority Medical Management, Poway, CA)

It may be that in several years, the paper superbill will be replaced by some form of computerized record that the doctor or office staff keys in, perhaps on a portable or laptop computer device specially made for this purpose. If you become a billing service, you should pay attention to such technological developments, as they may bring in further opportunities for services you can offer your clients in helping them computerize many current paper-based operations.

After the patient visit, the doctor passes the superbill to the front office staff, and the insurance process and patient billing get under way. In some cases, the billing person will ask the patient to pay the fee at the time the service is rendered, and it is then up to the patient to obtain reimbursement from his or her insurance. In the case of Medicare, the doctor's office must file the claim on behalf of the patient. If the physician is a PAR provider, the patient usually makes no payment at this time or only the 20 percent copayment (unless he or she has Medicaid or Medigap insurance as the secondary payer).

Next, processing the superbill depends on whether the office still uses a paper-based method of accounting and claim filing, or is computerized and does its own claim filing, or uses an outside billing service. Here's a comparison of paper accounting systems versus electronic accounting systems including electronic claims, regardless of whether the electronic accounting is done at the doctor's office or by an independent billing service.

PAPER CLAIMS AND ACCOUNTING

Step 1—Paper. If the office is paper based, the billing clerk refers to the superbill and types out a preprinted paper claim form, called the HCFA 1500 (pronounced Hick-fah fifteen hundred). This is now the universal claim form required and accepted by every insurance company and Medicare for filing medical claims other than hospitalizations. (Hospitals, emergency care clinics, and certain other types of healthcare providers use a different form, called the UB92.) Dentists use another form, called the ADA form that, like the HCFA 1500, indicates the diagnosis and procedures the dentist performed.

   The HCFA 1500 and ADA form are shown in Figures 2-6 and 2-7. The accompanying sidebar explains how the HCFA 1500 form came about.

Step 2—Paper. Depending on the doctor's office, the claim form may get typed out the same day as the patient's visit or the clerk may wait several days before completing many forms all at once. As noted earlier in the chapter, paper claim forms are then mailed to the insurance carriers

The HCFA 1500

The story behind the HCFA 1500 is important to know. It familiarizes you with some terminology and sheds light on why the healthcare industry has been slow to implement efficient procedures in the health insurance arena.

In the past, claims filing was a nightmare. Nearly every commercial insurance company, as well as Medicare, Medicaid, and Blue Cross/Blue Shield, had its own unique paper claim form. Keeping track of which form was to be used for which carrier was a major job. Every form had its particular requirements for reporting the doctor's diagnosis, the procedures performed, and the fee.

In the early 1980s, the American Medical Association established a task force to develop a standardized form that would be acceptable to the various government agencies and to the commercial carriers. The result of its work was the Uniform Health Insurance Claim Form, called the HCFA 1500, issued originally in 1984. In 1990, the form was revised to eliminate the spaces in which doctors would write an explanation of unusual services or circumstances to justify their fee. The new version, called the Red Form (since it is printed in red ink), allows spaces only for standard codes representing the diagnosis and the procedure performed. The Red Form also requires patients to provide information about any secondary insurance carrier so that the primary carrier will not duplicate any benefits paid.

Most medical billing software programs print HCFA 1500 claim forms. Of course, the goal is to file electronically and completely abandon the paper form.

via U.S. mail. Meanwhile, to track the patient's account, the billing clerk also writes the charges for the visit in a daily log (often called a "pegboard system") or on a patient ledger card that serves as a record of that person's accounts. Figure 2-8 shows an example of a patient ledger card.

Step 3—Paper. The mailed claim form eventually arrives at the insurer's office, where it is opened, screened, assigned a control number, microfilmed for record keeping, and then manually entered into a computer by a claims examiner. If it contains no errors, the physician receives payment for the claim in 30 to 90 days. However, if the claim contains errors, such as missing information or an incorrect or unacceptable diagnosis or procedure code, it is denied and returned to the doctor's office for correction. It may take several months before the claim can be corrected and resubmitted.

Many people with inside knowledge of how insurance companies work point out that many insurers "lose" claims and take months to "find" them (or never do). In fact, it is common knowledge in the business that commercial insurers took advantage of the perception of many errors in paper claim forms so as to delay paying claims as long as possible. Each day a provider was not paid was money in the bank for the insurers, on which they earned interest. It was also com-

PLEASE
DO NOT
STAPLE
IN THIS
AREA

TOPFORM DATA, INC. (800) 834-7470

| | PICA | | | | | | HEALTH INSURANCE CLAIM FORM | PICA | |

| 1. MEDICARE | MEDICAID | CHAMPUS | CHAMPVA | GROUP HEALTH PLAN | FECA BLK LUNG | OTHER | 1a. INSURED'S I.D. NUMBER | (FOR PROGRAM IN ITEM 1) |

(Medicare #) (Medicaid #) (Sponsor's SSN) (VA File #) (SSN or ID) (SSN) (ID)

2. PATIENT'S NAME (Last Name, First Name, Middle Initial)

3. PATIENT'S BIRTH DATE MM DD YY   SEX M   F

4. INSURED'S NAME (Last Name, First Name, Middle Initial)

5. PATIENT'S ADDRESS (No., Street)

6. PATIENT RELATIONSHIP TO INSURED
Self □ Spouse □ Child □ Other □

7. INSURED'S ADDRESS (No., Street)

CITY   STATE

8. PATIENT STATUS
Single □ Married □ Other □

CITY   STATE

ZIP CODE   TELEPHONE (Include Area Code)

Employed □ Full-Time Student □ Part-Time Student □

ZIP CODE   TELEPHONE (Include Area Code)

9. OTHER INSURED'S NAME (Last Name, First Name, Middle Initial)

10. IS PATIENT'S CONDITION RELATED TO:

11. INSURED'S POLICY GROUP OR FECA NUMBER

a. OTHER INSURED'S POLICY OR GROUP NUMBER

a. EMPLOYMENT? (CURRENT OR PREVIOUS)
□ YES □ NO

a. INSURED'S DATE OF BIRTH MM DD YY   SEX M   F

b. OTHER INSURED'S DATE OF BIRTH MM DD YY   SEX M   F

b. AUTO ACCIDENT?
□ YES □ NO   PLACE (State)

b. EMPLOYER'S NAME OR SCHOOL NAME

c. EMPLOYER'S NAME OR SCHOOL NAME

c. OTHER ACCIDENT?
□ YES □ NO

c. INSURANCE PLAN NAME OR PROGRAM NAME

d. INSURANCE PLAN NAME OR PROGRAM NAME

10d. RESERVED FOR LOCAL USE

d. IS THERE ANOTHER HEALTH BENEFIT PLAN?
□ YES □ NO   If yes, return to and complete item 9 a-d.

READ BACK OF FORM BEFORE COMPLETING & SIGNING THIS FORM.
12. PATIENT'S OR AUTHORIZED PERSON'S SIGNATURE I authorize the release of any medical or other information necessary to process this claim. I also request payment of government benefits either to myself or to the party who accepts assignment below.

SIGNED _____ DATE _____

13. INSURED'S OR AUTHORIZED PERSON'S SIGNATURE I authorize payment of medical benefits to the undersigned physician or supplier for services described below.

SIGNED _____

14. DATE OF CURRENT: MM DD YY   ILLNESS (First symptom) OR INJURY (Accident) OR PREGNANCY (LMP)

15. IF PATIENT HAS HAD SAME OR SIMILAR ILLNESS. GIVE FIRST DATE MM DD YY

16. DATES PATIENT UNABLE TO WORK IN CURRENT OCCUPATION
FROM MM DD YY   TO MM DD YY

17. NAME OF REFERRING PHYSICIAN OR OTHER SOURCE

17a. I.D. NUMBER OF REFERRING PHYSICIAN

18. HOSPITALIZATION DATES RELATED TO CURRENT SERVICES
FROM MM DD YY   TO MM DD YY

19. RESERVED FOR LOCAL USE

20. OUTSIDE LAB? □ YES □ NO $ CHARGES

21. DIAGNOSIS OR NATURE OF ILLNESS OR INJURY. (RELATE ITEMS 1,2,3, OR 4 TO ITEM 24E BY LINE)
1. L___ . ___   3. L___ . ___
2. L___ . ___   4. L___ . ___

22. MEDICAID RESUBMISSION CODE   ORIGINAL REF. NO.

23. PRIOR AUTHORIZATION NUMBER

24.	A				B	C	D	E	F	G	H	I	J	K
	DATE(S) OF SERVICE From MM DD YY		To MM DD YY		Place of Service	Type of Service	PROCEDURES, SERVICES, OR SUPPLIES (Explain Unusual Circumstances) CPT/HCPCS MODIFIER	DIAGNOSIS CODE	$ CHARGES	DAYS OR UNITS	EPSDT Family Plan	EMG	COB	RESERVED FOR LOCAL USE
1														
2														
3														
4														
5														
6														

25. FEDERAL TAX I.D. NUMBER   SSN □ EIN □

26. PATIENT'S ACCOUNT NO.

27. ACCEPT ASSIGNMENT? (For govt. claims, see back) □ YES □ NO

28. TOTAL CHARGE $

29. AMOUNT PAID $

30. BALANCE DUE $

31. SIGNATURE OF PHYSICIAN OR SUPPLIER INCLUDING DEGREES OR CREDENTIALS (I certify that the statements on the reverse apply to this bill and are made a part thereof.)

SIGNED _____ DATE _____

32. NAME AND ADDRESS OF FACILITY WHERE SERVICES WERE RENDERED (If other than home or office)

33. PHYSICIAN'S, SUPPLIER'S BILLING NAME, ADDRESS, ZIP CODE & PHONE #

PIN#   GRP#

REORDER ITEM #1117

(APPROVED BY AMA COUNCIL ON MEDICAL SERVICE 8/88)
APPROVED OMB-0938-0008

PLEASE PRINT OR TYPE

FORM HCFA-1500 (12-90)
FORM OWCP-1500   FORM RRB-1500

Figure 2-6   HCFA 1500 Claim Form

ATTENDING DENTIST'S STATEMENT

CARRIER NAME AND ADDRESS

CHECK ONE:

_____ DENTIST'S PRE-TREATMENT ESTIMATE

_____ DENTIST'S STATEMENT OF ACTUAL SERVICES

PATIENT COVERAGE INFORMATION

| 1. PATIENT NAME — FIRST / M.I. / LAST | 2. RELATIONSHIP TO INSURED — SELF / SPOUSE / CHILD / OTHER | 3. SEX — M / F | 4. PATIENT BIRTHDATE — MO. / DAY / YEAR | 5. IF FULL TIME STUDENT — SCHOOL / CITY |

6. EMPLOYEE/SUBSCRIBER NAME AND MAILING ADDRESS | 7. EMPLOYEE/SUBSCRIBER SOC. SEC. OR I.D. NUMBER | 8. EMPLOYEE/SUBSCRIBER BIRTHDATE — MO. / DAY / YEAR | 9. EMPLOYER (COMPANY) NAME AND ADDRESS | 10. GROUP NUMBER

11. IS PATIENT COVERED BY ANOTHER PLAN OF BENEFITS? — DENTAL _____ MEDICAL _____ | 12-A. NAME AND ADDRESS OF CARRIER(S) | 12-B. GROUP NO.(S) | 13. NAME AND ADDRESS OF EMPLOYER

14-A. EMPLOYEE/SUBSCRIBER NAME (IF DIFFERENT THAN PATIENT'S) | 14-B. EMPLOYEE/SUBSCRIBER SOC. SEC. OR I.D. NUMBER | 14-C. EMPLOYEE/SUBSCRIBER BIRTHDATE — MO. / DAY / YEAR | 15. RELATIONSHIP TO INSURED — SELF / SPOUSE / PARENT / OTHER _____

I HAVE REVIEWED THE FOLLOWING TREATMENT PLAN. I AUTHORIZE RELEASE OF ANY INFORMATION RELATING TO THIS CLAIM. I UNDERSTAND THAT I AM RESPONSIBLE FOR ALL COSTS OF DENTAL TREATMENT.

▶ SIGNED (PATIENT, OR PARENT IF MINOR) _____ DATE _____

I HEREBY AUTHORIZE PAYMENT OF THE DENTAL BENEFITS OTHERWISE PAYABLE TO ME DIRECTLY TO THE BELOW NAMED DENTAL ENTITY.

▶ SIGNED (INSURED PERSON) _____ DATE _____

BILLING DENTIST

16. NAME OF BILLING DENTIST OR DENTAL ENTITY

17. ADDRESS WHERE PAYMENT SHOULD BE REMITTED

CITY, STATE, ZIP

18. DENTIST SOC. SEC. OR T.I.N. | 19. DENTIST LICENSE NO. | 20. DENTIST PHONE NO.

21. FIRST VISIT DATE CURRENT SERIES | 22. PLACE OF TREATMENT — OFFICE / HOSP. / ECF / OTHER | 23. RADIOGRAPHS OR MODELS ENCLOSED? NO YES HOW MANY?

24. IS TREATMENT RESULT OF OCCUPATIONAL ILLNESS OR INJURY? NO YES | IF YES, ENTER BRIEF DESCRIPTION AND DATES.

25. IS TREATMENT RESULT OF AUTO ACCIDENT?

26. OTHER ACCIDENT?

27. ARE ANY SERVICES COVERED BY ANOTHER PLAN?

28. IF PROSTHESIS, IS THIS INITIAL PLACEMENT? | (IF NO, REASON FOR REPLACEMENT) | 29. DATE OF PRIOR PLACEMENT

30. IS TREATMENT FOR ORTHODONTICS? | IF SERVICES ALREADY COMMENCED, ENTER: | DATE APPLIANCES PLACED | MOS. TREATMENT REMAINING

IDENTIFY MISSING TEETH WITH "X"

FACIAL / LINGUAL / FACIAL — UPPER / LOWER / RIGHT / LEFT / PERMANENT / PRIMARY

TOOTH # OR LETTER	SURFACE	31. EXAMINATION AND TREATMENT PLAN - LIST IN ORDER FROM TOOTH NO. 1 THROUGH TOOTH NO. 32 - USE CHARTING SYSTEM SHOWN. DESCRIPTION OF SERVICE (INCLUDING X-RAYS, PROPHYLAXIS, MATERIALS USED, ETC.)	DATE SERVICES PERFORMED MO. DAY YEAR	PROCEDURE NUMBER	FEE	FOR ADMINISTRATIVE USE ONLY

32. REMARKS FOR UNUSUAL SERVICES

I HEREBY CERTIFY THAT THE PROCEDURES AS INDICATED BY DATE HAVE BEEN COMPLETED AND THAT THE FEES SUBMITTED ARE THE ACTUAL FEES I HAVE CHARGED AND INTEND TO COLLECT FOR THOSE PROCEDURES.

SIGNED (TREATING DENTIST) _____ LICENSE NUMBER _____ DATE _____

TOTAL FEE CHARGED	
MAX ALLOWABLE	
DEDUCTIBLE	
CARRIER %	
CARRIER PAYS	
PATIENT PAYS	

Form Approved by the
AMERICAN DENTAL ASSOCIATION
1990

TOPFORM DATA, INC. • (800) 854-7470   Reorder Item #1116

Figure 2-7   ADA Dental Claim Forms

Figure 2-8
Patient Ledger Card

					Credits	
Date	**Code**	**Description**	**Charge**	**Payments**	**Adjustments**	**Current Balance**

Statement

John Doe Patient
1234 Main Street
Springfield, IL

OV - Office Visit
OS - Office Surgery
TC - Telephone Consultation
FA - Failed Appointment
RP - Report

HOSP - Hospital Visit
HS – Hospital Surgery
SA - Surgical Assistant
ER - Emergency Room

ROA - Received on Account
NC - No Charge
INS - Insurance payment

mon knowledge that claims examiners at insurance companies would never check claims and correct minor errors if they found some. Claims with even the slightest error, such as no check mark in the male/female box for a patient named Edward, would be rejected. (I guess there are female Edwards; one never knows!) The result was a very high rate of rejection.

Step 4—Paper. When a claim has no errors and is approved, the insurer sends out a document called an Explanation of Benefits (EOB) to the patient and a copy of it to the physician. For Medicare, the patient is mailed an Explanation of Medicare Benefits (EOMB), while the physician receives a computerized report.

The EOB or EOMB shows the amount charged, the amount allowed, and the amount paid for each procedure. Remember that Medicare and most commercial insurance policies pay only 80 percent of the allowable fee for physician services, leaving the patient responsible for the 20 percent coinsurance. If the physician has accepted assignment, he or she receives the check directly. If not, the patient receives the check.

Next, in a traditional paper accounting system, the billing clerk must log payments onto each patient's ledger, and to a daily accounts receivable journal that keeps track of the day's cash flow. To remind patients about their due balances and copayments, the clerk also sends out a monthly statement to each patient, often by simply photocopying the ledger cards showing the balance due—a time-consuming task that can take a billing clerk hours.

Step 5—Paper. If the patient has secondary insurance, another paper HCFA 1500 form must now be filed. This form must be accompanied by a copy of the EOB from the primary insurer showing how much it paid, so the secondary insurer does not duplicate any payments. It might take another 30 days to receive the remainder due from a secondary insurer.

These steps describe the billing and accounting operation of many medical offices that continue to operate manually or are only partially computerized. As mentioned earlier, some offices use computers to do their accounting but print out the HCFA 1500 forms and mail them on paper for insurance reimbursement rather than doing electronic claims processing using communications software and a modem.

However, filing paper claims is a risky business. Between the expense and effort required to fill them out, and the lengthy time delay to get them reimbursed, combined with the anxiety of dealing with our unpredictable postal service and insurance companies that love to deny claims, continuing to use paper claims is like throwing money away. Few people doubt that the days of paper claims are numbered.

ELECTRONIC CLAIMS AND ACCOUNTING In an office that utilizes computerized accounting systems and electronic claims processing, patients still fill out a registration form and doctors still use paper superbills (although, as pointed out, these paper forms may also become computerized very shortly). The procedure differs in the steps that occur after the superbill is prepared. A clerk in the office or the independent medical billing service does the following:

Step 1—Electronic. The first step in an electronic office is to set up the software. The setup work is perhaps the most time-consuming phase for a medical billing service, but once it is done, electronic claims processing and accounting take considerably less time than handling paper forms and are virtually error free.

Most medical billing software programs today are easy to use. They may be DOS-based or Windows-based. In either type, there is usually a "main menu" of basic functions from which you select your commands. Each main menu command then leads to "submenus" with more detailed commands, just like programs such as *Microsoft Word for Windows* with the commands across the top that you access by pointing at and clicking your mouse, or in the popular DOS-based *WordPerfect 5.1* with its many function key commands.

To help visualize these programs, look at Figures 2-9 and 2-10. Included with this book is a CD-ROM that contains demonstration software from a selection of vendors.

- Figure 2-9 shows a few screen shots from the program *Claims Manager* produced by InfoHealth. This program is a full practice management software package that handles all basic accounting functions as well as electronic claims filing.

- Figure 2-10 shows a few screen shots from the program *Lytec Medical for Windows*, produced by Lytec Systems (and resold by several business opportunity vendors). This software is also a full practice management program that handles accounting functions and electronic filing.

Whichever software you use, the setup procedures are quite similar because you need to store the same type of information. All software involves creating database "records" for each patient, doctor in the practice, and insurance company to be billed by the practice. You usually can also create a database of the commonly used diagnostic and procedure codes (or the software may already have the procedure codes stored in it from the AMA, which owns the copyright on these codes). If the software you are using performs accounting and practice management functions, the setup also includes entering the existing account balances for each established patient.

For example, when you first get a client, you will need to enter all current patients, including their name, address, Social Security number, the primary and secondary insurance company, the plan ID number and the group number, the employer, and a variety of other data. Table 2-7 shows a list of the patient fields that are typically required in a software package for patient data.

Similarly, you need to create a database record for every provider in the practice, including his or her address, tax ID number, and other special ID numbers sometimes assigned by Medicare and Medicaid.

Figure 2-9
Sample Screens from
InfoHealth Claims
Manager Software

```
                    SYSTEM MENU
       _____

       D - Daily Functions
       E - End of Day Reports
       R - Reports & Forms
       C - Claims Processing
       M - Month End Processing
       P - Practice Analysis
       L - Login Options
       S - System Services


[Esc] - Exit                    [F1] - Help
```

```
Account Frederick Morgan          Patient Number 00002-00000   05/31/96
Patient Frederick Morgan          Doctor 02     Billcode 21     08/19/96
                                  InsCo  0003   Codeset  A04I   14:25:20
— Code —— Diagnosis ————————————
1. *  246.8  Thyroid Disease                  Insurance amount:    30.00
2.                                                                  0.00
3.              _____            30.00
4.             |          Reimbursement Calculator     |          30.00
               |                                        |
— Code —       | Insurance charges #       ====>  30.00 | Pos  Tos  DxRf
1. *99213.00.  | Insurance allowed ============>   22.80 | OF   1I   1
               | Primary pmt (02P) #         18.24      |
2.             | Other pmts   (02P) #                   |
               | Deductible remaining                   |
3.             | Insurance write off (02C) =======>  7.20 |
               |                                        |
4.             | Amount insurance remaining (07C) ===>  4.56 |
               | Amount patient responsible (01D) ===>      |
5.             |                                        |
               | [F2]=Store              [Esc]=Exit     |
6.              _____

7.

[Esc]=Exit   [F1]=Help   [F2]=Store
```

As mentioned earlier, one advantage of today's sophisticated medical billing software is that keying information involves error checking. For example, the software will block you from keying in an alphabetic character if the field accepts only numeric characters, or it may beep if you have keyed in only nine digits where ten are expected.

Assuming that the setup has been done correctly at this point, you are ready to begin taking superbills from your clients and turning them into electronic claims.

Step 2—Electronic. This step involves getting the superbill document from the physician. Some billing services pick up the documents from their clients on a daily or weekly basis; others have the doctor fax them.

Note: several vendors sell programs that allow you to "download" superbill information from the computer in the doctor's office, assuming the staff has keyboarded it. For example, the best program of this kind is called *Data-Link,* available from ClaimTek Systems, a

Patients

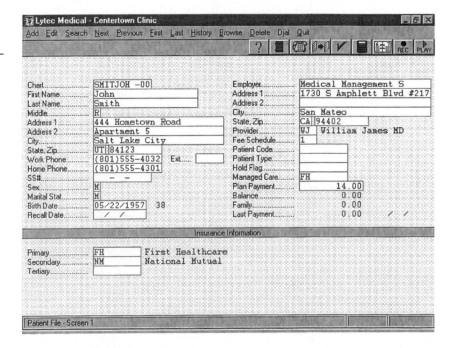

Figure 2-10
Sample Screens
from Lytec Medical
for Windows

Patients - (Insurance Information) - Zoom

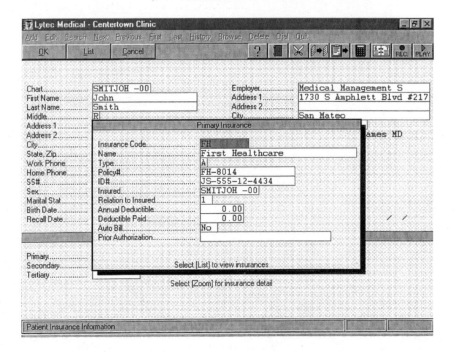

74

Figure 2-10
Sample Screens
from Lytec Medical
for Windows
(Continued)

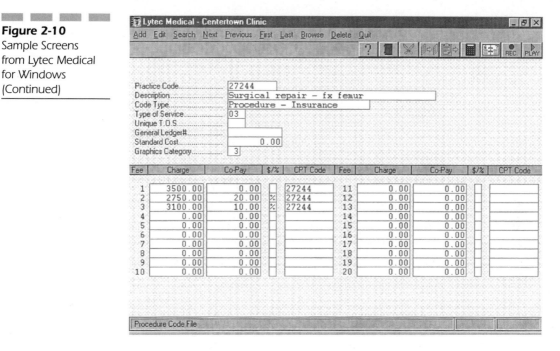

Figure 2-10
Sample Screens
from Lytec Medical
for Windows
(Continued)

business opportunity vendor in Portland, Oregon. *Data-Link* allows the doctor's office to key in some of the data; the outside billing service then uses *PCAnywhere!* software to tap into the doctor's computer and retrieve the data; the service can then process all the claims and do the accounting at night, delivering updated data back to the doctor's computer in the morning. While some people question the logic of these types of arrangements (why would the doctor pay you when his or her staff is still doing some of the work?), you should consider such linking software in the context of how it might serve your business. In other words, some billing service owners believe it will help them get clients; others think that it will not.

Step 3—Electronic. The next step for a billing service is to key in the data for all the superbills collected. Every billing service I have interviewed estimates that data entry takes less than one minute per patient, because today's software is so easy to use and prompts for the fields of information needed to complete the claim. (The exception is new patients, when you need to go through the setup routine, which takes longer.) For the standard claim, you simply need to key in the patient code or name, the diagnosis codes, procedure codes, fees, date

TABLE 2-7

Fields to Keyboard for a Typical Patient Record

Last name

First name

Middle initial

Address 1

Address 2

City

State

Zip code

Home phone

Work phone

Date of birth

Sex

Patient category (private, insurance, Medicare, Medicaid, worker's comp.)

Primary physician's code

Location of service (office = 1, hospital = 2, branch office = 3, home = 4, etc.)

Referring physician

Facility of services

Is the condition related to employment? (Y/N)

Is the condition related to an accident? (Y/N)

Date of accident

State in which accident occurred

Date of illness/injury/or pregnancy

Date first consulted doctor

Date of similar previous injury

Date of admission to hospital

Date of discharge from hospital

Disability from date

TABLE 2-7

Fields to Keyboard for a Typical Patient Record (Continued)

Disability to date

First insurance carrier

Insured person's ID #

Is the insured person related to the patient? (Y/N)

Accepts assignment (Y/N)

Bill the carrier (Y/N)

Patient's signature on file (Y/N)

Pay benefits to patient (Y/N)

Insured person's name (if different from patient)

Medicare coverage

Secondary insurance company

Second insurance related to insured

Accept assignment from second insured (Y/N)

Bill other carrier (Y/N)

Medicare other policy prefix

Marital status

Employment status (full-time, part-time, retired, no)

Student status (full, part, no)

Prior authorization #

Recall date/time

First diagnosis

Second diagnosis

Third diagnosis

Fourth diagnosis

Primary responsible party (name)

Secondary responsible party

of service, location of service, and a few additional fields. Many software programs store the data, so all you need to do is press a Function key or click on the mouse and a list pops up, from which you can highlight the entry rather than typing it.

Step 4—Electronic. After you have keyboarded the day's claims, you usually go back to your main menu and select the function for "batch" electronic claims filing. This allows you to send an entire group of claims all at one time. The software may first prepare a summary printout of the claims to transmit so that you can verify the report before going online; this also serves as a record for you. Some software also compresses the data file to increase transmission speed.

Step 5—Electronic. The next step is the actual transmission of the claims to the insurance companies over the phone lines using a communications component of your billing software and a modem. Note that most billing services do not transmit directly to each and every insurance company, but rather to a central clearinghouse that acts as a routing station between the billing service and the insurers. One reason for this is that the data format standards among insurance companies still differ, just as they do with paper claims. Where one company wants a ten-digit number with trailing zeros, another wants leading zeros. (Medicare has recently implemented a standard electronic data format policy that will apply to all Medicare intermediaries throughout the country.)

Clearinghouses rectify the discrepancies among insurance company data preferences by translating from the language of your software to the language required by each insurer in a matter of seconds. Claims for your local Medicare are translated one way, while claims for Aetna or another commercial carrier are translated into its respective data format.

Do you need a clearinghouse? In some cases, no. A billing service can transmit directly to a local carrier such as Blue Cross or a regional Medicare carrier. In fact, many Medicare intermediaries give away free software to facilitate filing electronic claims directly to them. However, in the long run, most billing services that handle many claims from a variety of doctors choose to use a clearinghouse because it saves them time and confusion. By going through a single clearinghouse, you do not need to work with more than one medical billing software package, and all your data are stored in one program.

Furthermore, clearinghouses serve another vital purpose as well: *online* error checking. As pointed out earlier, the quality and comprehensiveness of error checking at the clearinghouse significantly reduces the error rate on incomplete or inaccurate claims to practically zero.

However, clearinghouses are not free. Most charge between $0.35 and $0.50 per claim, and some also have an annual registration fee plus a per doctor fee. Also, to make sure you know how to use the software and dial them up, they usually require that you take a simple test by sending in 20 or so claims to prove that you can code and transmit correctly. See the sidebar "Clearing the Air About Clearinghouses" on page 80 for more information.

Step 6—Electronic. After receiving the claims, the clearinghouse notifies you (usually within minutes while online) about the claims received and processed to each insurance carrier, and those rejected because of errors. You can then make a paper copy of this report, called an Audit/Edit Report or Sender Log, for your records. In many cases, you can make an immediate correction on certain rejected claims and resubmit them the same day. However, if an error is due to coding, you are best advised to confer with your doctor's office before resubmitting the claim.

Insurers process clean electronic claims within 7 to 15 days, and clean Medicare claims are reimbursed in 14 to 19 days for PAR providers. Because of the error checking that occurs in both the keying-in phase and when you are online with the clearinghouse, filing claims electronically is significantly faster and less prone to mistakes than filing paper claims.

Practice Management Functions

If you perform practice management for your clients, your software will invariably make all the other functions you need to do more efficient. Let's examine the additional functions you might perform in the way of full practice management.

Whenever a claim is paid and the physician receives the EOB and a check, you will continue to track each patient's account. Many billing services do this by arranging for the office staff to forward them copies of all EOBs that come in each day, so they can key in the payments and adjust the accounts. This may be done through the mail or by fax. To simplify the process, some doctors even agree to have the insurance companies send the EOBs and checks directly to their billing service. Of course, you must establish a significant amount of trust for this to occur.

Clearing the Air About Clearinghouses

Clearinghouses are confusing to most people new to medical billing. One way to understand them is to realize that although the HCFA 1500 standardized the paper claim, electronic claims are still not universally formatted. Clearinghouses are the solution to the chaos that would occur if doctors had to send electronic claims to each different insurance company their patients had. Another way to think about clearinghouses is the purpose they serve for the insurance companies themselves. Given that there are hundreds of insurers in the country, and each one has its own proprietary computer system and data demands, a clearinghouse is the only way that doctors and billing services can communicate with them.

When electronic claims are sent, the data are "formatted" a certain way according to the insurance company's needs. Here's an example from Frank Haraksin, president and founder of Electronic Translations and Transmittals Corporation (commonly known as ET&T). As Frank told me, "Some insurers take a data field and do what they need with it. In one case, a Blue I worked with wanted a plan code to occupy a certain field in its system. That was fine, but another insurer wanted a blank space there."

In order to be useful, a clearinghouse needs to make contracts with as many insurance companies as it can if it wants to accept claims from billers and doctors throughout the country. This means that a lot of programming goes into making a clearinghouse successful. In return, clearinghouses make money from both sides of the fence. Insurance companies pay them a per claim fee for transmitting the claims electronically to them, saving the insurers money on processing paper claims. Doctors and independent billing agencies usually pay a per claim fee as well to compensate the clearinghouse for taking their claims and transmitting them to the insurance companies.

The competition among clearinghouses for customers (like you) has heated up in recent years. Frank Haraksin estimates that there are now about 30 clearinghouses battling for your business, and the industry may be due for a shakedown. In fact, in the most recent years, several clearinghouses have been purchased by other companies. The company formerly called ETS in Atlanta was purchased by Equifax, Inc., which, in turn, was purchased by National Data Corporation, a large conglomerate of information service companies. As Chris Heller, Account Manager for National Data Corporation's Health EDI Services reminds readers, "The advantage of a clearinghouse is the edits that it can perform to increase the chances of being paid to nearly 100 percent. When you send a claim to a clearinghouse, you get immediate online information about the claim; you know if it was accepted or rejected."

When you buy your medical billing software, you may be told to work with a certain clearinghouse that has contracted with your software company to handle its claims. Note that you may not need to work with that particular clearinghouse. In most cases, you can shop around to find a clearinghouse that might offer a better deal. For example, Frank Haraksin points out that his company ET&T is very competitive with other clearinghouses. Frank indicates that ET&T has no annual sign up fee and no per doctor fees; its only charges are per claim (and there is no fee if your claim is rejected at the clearinghouse for incompleteness). Frank also indicates that because his company is small, it can get you online more quickly than some other clearinghouses. His company accepts any billing software format, such as *Medisoft* or *Lytec.* See Appendix A for information about clearinghouses.

BLUE SHIELD OF CALIFORNIA

PROVIDER #: 0000000
PAGE #: 1 OF 1

PERF PROV	SERV DATE	POS	MOS	PROC	BILLED	ALLOWED	DEDUCT	COINS	PROV. PD.	RC-AMT
NAME		31	HIC 123-432-000A						ASG	Y
0PL1234B0			1 908456z9							
	052496		1	96115	300.00	159.52	0.00	31.90	127.62	CO-42 140.48
PT RESP	31.90		CLAIM TOTALS		300.00	159.52	0.00	31.90	127.62	127.62 NET

CLAIM INFORMATION FORWARDED TO: MEDI-CAL

NAME		31	HIC 123-432-000A						ASG	Y
0PL1234B0			1 908456z9							
	052696		1	90820	150.00	98.14	0.00	19.63	78.51	CO-42 51.86
PT RESP	19.63		CLAIM TOTALS		150.00	98.14	0.00	19.63	78.51	78.51 NET

CLAIM INFORMATION FORWARDED TO: MEDI-CAL

NAME		31	HIC 123-432-000A						ASG	Y
0PL1234B0			1 908456z9							
	052796		1	96115	300.00	159.52	0.00	31.90	127.62	CO-42 140.48
PT RESP	31.90		CLAIM TOTALS		300.00	159.52	0.00	31.90	127.62	127.62 NET

CLAIM INFORMATION FORWARDED TO: BLUE CROSS OF CALIFORNIA

TOTALS	TOTAL CLAIMS				TOTAL BILLED	TOTAL ALLOWED	TOTAL DEDUCT	TOTAL COINS	TOTAL PROV. PD.	AMOUNT OF CHECK
	3				750.00	417.18	0.00	83.43	333.75	333.75

Figure 2-11   Example of Medicare Remittance Notice

In the case of Medicare, the local carrier for Medicare sends doctors a long list showing all claims processed in the most recent batch. The list summarizes each claim, including the original fee billed, the allowable amount, the amount paid, the coinsurance, and the required write-off. This is called a remittance notice. Figure 2-11 shows what this report looks like.

Your first step is therefore to key in all the data from the EOBs and any Medicare remittance lists. This is done in the accounts receivable module that full practice management software contains. You begin by looking up each patient's record and keying in the amount paid based on the EOB or the Medicare remittance notice. Most medical billing software automates a portion of this record-keeping function, such as calculating the 20 percent coinsurance payment and the write-off once you enter the amount paid.

If the patient is a managed care patient on a capitated payment, the EOB will so indicate and show that the original fee is denied. You therefore need to go into the accounts receivable module and record a write-off for the fee-for-service charge that was originally posted. These postings eventually allow you to compare how much the doctor would have earned if the patients had been fee-for-service versus the amount of capitated payments you received from that HMO. Obviously, the doctor may come out ahead with some patients and behind on others, so you must calculate profitability by taking into account many patients over months of time. Some software, such as *Lytec Medical for Windows,* has a specific module for managed care patients. As Lytec points out in its manual:

> Please be aware that insurance companies making capitated payments as part of a managed care plan need to be billed just like any other insurance company. These insurance companies still need to know how often and why a patient is getting healthcare treatment. Before entering transactions into the Changes and Payment screen, you will need to add a managed care adjustment code in the procedure code file and also modify the existing procedure codes.

Many industry experts expect that electronic funds transfer from insurance companies right into providers' bank accounts will become more common. If so, this improvement may substantially automate the posting of payments and write-offs. You may not even need to key in the amounts; updating the accounts receivable records will be done automatically when you log on to capture the notification of payments to your doctor's bank.

As discussed throughout this chapter, a billing service offering complete practice management will likely become involved in many additional functions related to the doctor's business. These can include

- Printing out monthly statements for patients showing their past payments and balances due. Most medical billing programs make this process fast and easy. You can often add a customized comment, such as "Balance due over 60 days; please remit today." (My dentist adds a "quote of the day" from a famous philosopher.)

- Preparing financial reports for doctors showing the status of their cash flow and analyzing the major factors of their business, including aged balances (showing which patients are delinquent in their payments for 30, 60, and 90 days or more), and insurance aged balances (showing which insurance companies are delinquent for 30, 60, and 90 days or more). Many doctors also like to get reports showing which procedures generate the most income, which clients see them most frequently, what percentage of their fees is generated from referrals, and so on. Most current state-of-the art billing software allows you to provide a variety of sophisticated financial summaries, as well as visual data in the form of pie graphs, bar graphs, and so on. Figures 2-12 through 2-14 show samples of two reports and a graph that many practice management software packages can produce.

- Advising the doctor about the correct use of diagnostic and procedure codes that determine how much reimbursement the physician receives. Many doctors code incorrectly or unintentionally "down-code," meaning that they use a code that pays less than they could receive for a service. In addition, doctors do not have the time to keep up with the changes in coding that Medicare and other insurance firms regularly implement; and in many cases, the doctor's staff also does not stay abreast of new coding requirements. The professional billing service that is current with coding procedures can therefore play an important role in ensuring that doctors are properly reimbursed for services rendered.

- As stated throughout this chapter, another important practice management function for a billing service is analyzing the doctor's practice and making recommendations about managed care options, such as whether to join certain HMOs and PPOs. As you have seen in several of the business profiles in this chapter, some billing services even become involved in preparing proposals on behalf of their clients to handle the patients of a certain HMO. Most qualified billing services will prepare financial analysis reports showing their client patient usage under capitated fees as well as comparisons of capitated fees received versus fee-for-service fees written off.

As you can readily see, a professional billing service offering electronic claims filing and full practice management can alleviate many problems for a medical practice. Working hand in hand with the doctor's office staff, a good billing service can serve the interests of the doctor and the patients. This explains why billing services are increasingly able to sign on a growing number of healthcare providers who are no longer able to pay attention to their business.

Page 1   DIAGNOSIS STATISTICS for Month 7 Ending July 31, 1996
          Order:NAME Range:ALL RECORDS

CODE	DESCRIPTION	DEPT	********* MONTH TOTALS *********		********** YTD TOTALS **********		NUM
			FREQ / RATIO	CHARGE / RATIO	FREQ / RATIO	CHARGE / RATIO	

Physician 01 - Anderson, Robert H., M.D.

CODE	DESCRIPTION	DEPT	FREQ / RATIO	CHARGE / RATIO	FREQ / RATIO	CHARGE / RATIO	NUM
491.0	BRONCHITIS	2	3 / 37.50%	147.00 / 42.73%	5 / 8.06%	192.00 / 9.55%	44
382.9	OTITIS MEDIA	2	1 / 12.50%	0.00 / 0.00%	3 / 4.84%	0.00 / 0.00%	4
844.9	SPRAIN, KNEE	2	2 / 25.00%	130.00 / 37.79%	2 / 3.23%	130.00 / 6.47%	13
463	TONSILLITIS	2	1 / 12.50%	32.00 / 9.30%	5 / 8.06%	132.00 / 6.57%	1
***** TOTAL CHARGES			8 /100.00%	344.00 /100.00%	62 /100.00%	2010.35 /100.00%	

Physician 02 - Barr, John S., M.D.

CODE	DESCRIPTION	DEPT	FREQ / RATIO	CHARGE / RATIO	FREQ / RATIO	CHARGE / RATIO	NUM
493.9	ASTHMA, ALLERGIC NOS	2	1 / 11.11%	127.00 / 28.05%	1 / 3.03%	127.00 / 12.60%	45
276.5	DEHYDRATION	2	2 / 22.22%	0.00 / 0.00%	2 / 6.06%	0.00 / 0.00%	34
276.9	ELECTROLYTE IMBAL.	2	1 / 11.11%	0.00 / 0.00%	1 / 3.03%	0.00 / 0.00%	28
401.9	HYPERTENSION	2	2 / 22.22%	136.80 / 30.21%	2 / 6.06%	136.80 / 13.57%	15
844.9	SPRAIN, KNEE	2	1 / 11.11%	45.00 / 9.94%	4 / 12.12%	121.40 / 12.05%	13
435.9	TIA	2	2 / 22.22%	144.00 / 31.80%	2 / 6.06%	144.00 / 14.29%	12
***** TOTAL CHARGES			9 /100.00%	452.80 /100.00%	33 /100.00%	1007.80 /100.00%	

Physician 03 - Martin, J. F., M.D.

CODE	DESCRIPTION	DEPT	FREQ / RATIO	CHARGE / RATIO	FREQ / RATIO	CHARGE / RATIO	NUM
311	DEPRESSION	2	2 / 66.67%	125.00 / 69.25%	2 / 8.33%	125.00 / 10.11%	27
044.9	SPRAIN, KNEE	2	1 / 33.33%	55.50 / 30.75%	1 / 4.17%	55.50 / 4.49%	52
***** TOTAL CHARGES			3 /100.00%	180.50 /100.00%	24 /100.00%	1236.45 /100.00%	

Practice totals

CODE	DESCRIPTION	DEPT	FREQ / RATIO	CHARGE / RATIO	FREQ / RATIO	CHARGE / RATIO	NUM
493.9	ASTHMA, ALLERGIC NOS	2	1 / 5.00%	127.00 / 12.99%	1 / 0.73%	127.00 / 2.30%	45
491.0	BRONCHITIS	2	3 / 15.00%	147.00 / 15.04%	5 / 3.65%	192.00 / 3.47%	44
276.5	DEHYDRATION	2	2 / 10.00%	0.00 / 0.00%	3 / 2.19%	0.00 / 0.00%	34
311	DEPRESSION	2	2 / 10.00%	125.00 / 12.79%	3 / 2.19%	175.00 / 3.16%	27
276.9	ELECTROLYTE IMBAL.	2	1 / 5.00%	0.00 / 0.00%	2 / 1.46%	0.00 / 0.00%	28
401.9	HYPERTENSION	2	2 / 10.00%	136.80 / 14.00%	9 / 6.57%	439.30 / 7.94%	15
382.9	OTITIS MEDIA	2	1 / 5.00%	0.00 / 0.00%	3 / 2.19%	0.00 / 0.00%	4
844.9	SPRAIN, KNEE	2	3 / 15.00%	175.00 / 17.91%	6 / 4.38%	251.40 / 4.54%	13
044.9	SPRAIN, KNEE	2	1 / 5.00%	55.50 / 5.68%	2 / 1.46%	78.30 / 1.41%	52
435.9	TIA	2	2 / 10.00%	144.00 / 14.73%	4 / 2.92%	209.00 / 3.78%	12
463	TONSILLITIS	2	1 / 5.00%	32.00 / 3.27%	15 / 10.95%	704.45 / 12.73%	1
***** TOTAL CHARGES			20 /100.00%	977.30 /100.00%	137 /100.00%	5533.60 /100.00%	

Figure 2-12   Example of a Tabular Report—Practice Analysis by Diagnosis Frequency

Aging Report Summary

Type	Past due -> 0 - 30	-> -> -> 31-60	-> -> -> 61-90	-> -> 91+
Patient Accnt's	2524.00	652.00	829.00	332.00
%	58%	15%	19%	08%
Insurance	7924.00	879.00	321.00	212.00
%	85%	09%	03%	02%
Totals	10,448.00	1,531.00	1,150.00	544.00

```
Total patient receivables:   $ 4337.00
Total insurance receivables: $ 9336.00
Total receivables:           $13,673.00
```

Corrected art tk

Figure 2-13 Example of a Tabular Report—Aging Report Summary

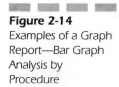

Figure 2-14
Examples of a Graph
Report—Bar Graph
Analysis by
Procedure

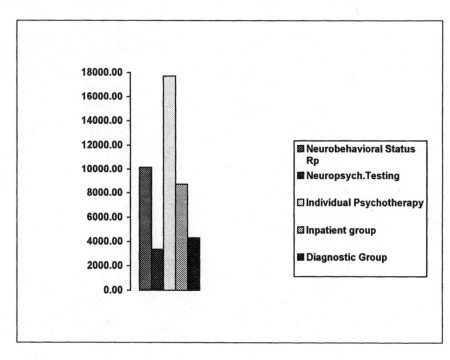

Business Profile: Sheryl Telles and Kathy Allocco

Sheryl Telles and Kathy Allocco worked for a local physician for many years; between them, they had more than 35 years of experience in medical management. The day came, however, when they saw opportunity knocking at their door. Prompted by the increasing use of managed care arrangements in Arizona, the two set up their company, Arizona MedLink Provider Resources, in Scottsdale to help doctors preserve their independence. Fortunately, they were able to tap into their combined skills: Sheryl has a medical coding background while Kathy knows billing and insurance. Sheryl also does medical transcription as part of her business, subcontracting out the work. The software they use is from Medisoft.

At first, they had no clients and a lot of apprehension about the future; but keeping focused on their skills, their friendship, their dream, the firm got its first client in seven weeks, after doing a brochure and targeted marketing letter. They also arranged for an interview in a local business journal that helped them get free publicity. Within one year, it seemed that they were well on the way to success. Kathy and Sheryl now handle full practice management functions for 13 practices (many of which involve multiple doctors), and their goal is to pick up an additional practice per month. They service a variety of clients, including podiatrists, family practitioners, psychiatrists, orthopedic surgeons, and chiropractors. For their work, Kathy and Sheryl charge a percentage of everything they collect, which is common for full practice management billing services. They also have two employees and moved from Sheryl's home office to a 3000-square-foot office.

Kathy and Sheryl speak about medical billing from the heart. As they related to me, "In Arizona, the choice for doctors about how to practice is being taken out of their hands. Doctors are being told what to do and how to do it. They are being forced to join dozens of different HMOs and MSOs. There are even some sneaky insurance companies that establish lucrative fee-for-service PPO plans that doctors want to join, but the insurer then makes the doctor join their HMO too, in which the doctor is paid at a *very low* capitated rate, as little as $3 per patient. This is also bad for consumers, because the patients who are on that $3 capitated plan often get treated by phone. The doctor literally can't afford to see them."

Kathy and Sheryl point out that doctors need to keep careful track of whatever they do today, because insurers will question everything and frequently deny payments. Because of the proliferation of insurance plans, doctors can get confused; they can do X in the office and get paid, but they can't do Y.

Kathy and Sheryl have a formal partnership agreement, created for them by a lawyer. When asked why each didn't go into business for herself instead of working together, Kathy told me, "You can always hire employees who have the skills you lack, but for us, the question was, did we want to do it alone? We decided that we would rather work together and reap the rewards."

One key to their success is that they function exceptionally well together. They admit to having experienced an occasional disagreement over business strategy, but they are able to resolve their differences through discussion and negotiation. They also highly value their long-standing friendship, which prevents them from ruining their relationship over a business squabble.

When I interviewed them, Kathy and Sheryl were in the midst of developing a new clearinghouse that would handle eligibility requests on a nationwide basis. Whenever a doctor needs to verify a patient's insurance and its coverages (deductibles, copayments, procedures covered, etc.), the information can be requested via modem through Sheryl and Kathy's clearinghouse to insurance companies nationwide. Their new company is called EDI Pathway, and their partner in that business is Noreen Sachs. Information about reaching them is found under "Clearinghouses" in Appendix A.

Knowledge and Skills Needed to Run a Medical Billing Business

Some home businesses are easy to start, while others require an extensive range of skills and knowledge. On a scale of 1 to 10, with 10 being the measure of highest difficulty, medical billing is now probably between 7 and 10, depending on your background and personal style. In researching this book, I met billing service owners who were able to jump right in, although they had no medical experience or knowledge. The most successful people I interviewed usually had a professional background involving one of the following: healthcare, nursing, banking, insurance, finance, administrative work, computer consulting, or marketing.

Regardless of your background, to be successful in medical billing, you will need to learn three areas to develop your knowledge and skills. You need

- A moderate knowledge of medical coding procedures
- A moderate to high level of knowledge and skills with computers and software
- A high level of knowledge and skills in marketing and sales to get clients

Each of these areas can be mastered in a few months, but the greater the slope of your learning curve, the longer it will take you to get your business off and running.

Of course, dedication, persistence, and personal outlook have much to do with your ability to traverse the hurdles. If you enter your new business venture thinking you cannot learn what it takes to succeed, or that you can handle only half the task, you will almost certainly fulfill only that limited vision of yourself. You may find that you have to s-t-r-e-t-c-h your thinking and your commitment if you are to succeed.

After reading the following sections, which cover the various areas of knowledge and skills needed for medical billing (except for the insurance business and the business of medicine, which this chapter has already covered), try the following informal method of charting your challenge. First, choose a unit of time with which you feel comfortable learning something new; perhaps it's one month, three months, or six months. Then, for each skill/knowledge area, plot your starting point on a scale of 1 to 10.

For example, if you have a medical background and some computer skills, but no marketing or selling experience, you might give yourself an 8 for Medical Knowledge, a 4 for Computer Knowledge, and a 2 for Business Knowledge. Then, using those numbers as your starting points, plot your learning curve for each area over the course of time you have allocated. Figure 2-15 shows how the learning curves might differ for a person with a nursing or medical front office background versus a person with sales experience but no medical background.

The purpose of this informal exercise is to help you become conscious of your strengths as well as those areas in which you will need to concentrate some effort. If you find that you have a low learning curve in only one area, you may be more inclined to move your business plans along quickly. On the other hand, if you find that you have two or three very steep curves, it may be better for you to improve your knowledge and skills in those areas before moving ahead in your business or investing in software or a business opportunity. Remember, do this exercise after you have read the following sections that present a brief preview of each knowledge or skill base you need.

Figure 2-15
Plotting Your
Learning Curve

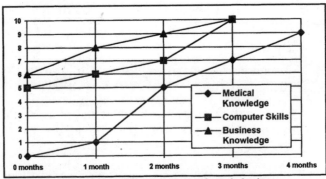

Graph for   entrepreneur with previous experience in business

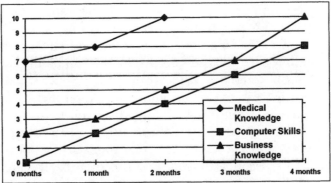

Graph for a person with medical background such as a nurse

Area 1: Knowledge of Medical Coding

Earlier in this chapter, I referred to two sets of codes used by insurance carriers and the medical community. These codes are a kind of shorthand for the doctor's diagnosis of the patient's problems and for the services he or she performs. These coding systems have come to the foreground of the health insurance industry in recent years because of increased computerization. Being familiar with them—and even becoming an expert in coding—is critical to your ability to get clients. Rising healthcare costs and a growing reluctance on the part of insurance companies to overpay for services or to pay for needless procedures have created a greater emphasis on identifying the precise diagnosis and procedures.

Here is a brief review of the two coding systems.

ICD-9-CM DIAGNOSIS CODES   Prior to 1988, healthcare professionals described the reason for their encounter with a patient by writing out longhand the patient's complaints, condition, injury, symptoms, and diagnosis. However, the 1988 Medicare Catastrophic Coverage Act instituted the ICD-9-CM coding system, which had to that point been in only limited usage. The ICD-9-CM stands for International Classification of Diseases, 9th Revision, Clinical Modification. ICD-9-CM is now mandated for all Medicare and Medicaid claims and nearly all commercial insurance claims.

Originally devised to improve statistical recordkeeping on the spread of diseases by the World Health Organization (WHO), the ICD-9-CM codes have been tailored for clinical use in the United States. (WHO updates the codes every 10 years, but HCFA and the U.S. Public Health Service issue annual changes and addenda.) The codes are usually printed in two volumes. The first volume is a "tabular" list; it contains the numerical listings of disease codes from 001.0 through 999.9 (plus some additional "V" codes for vaccinations, some types of exams, treatments and other issues, as well as a section of "E" codes for causes of external injuries such as traffic and boating accidents). The second volume is an alphabetic listing of diseases. Physicians and billers often need to use one or the other volume to look up a code.

Figures 2-16 and 2-17 show a page from each of these volumes.

The ICD-9 codes are used to facilitate automation of the claims process and payments. Doctors must follow strict requirements in utilizing the ICD-9-CM codes to supply proof that the services performed (which are the basis for the insurance paid) are backed up by an appropriate and cor-

◆ ● **800.3 Closed with other and unspecified intracranial hemorrhage**

◆ ● **800.4 Closed with intracranial injury of other and unspecified nature**

● **800.5 Open without mention of intracranial injury**

● **800.6 Open with cerebral laceration and contusion**

● **800.7 Open with subarachnoid, subdural, and extradural hemorrhage**

◆ ● **800.8 Open with other and unspecified intracranial hemorrhage**

◆ ● **800.9 Open with intracranial injury of other and unspecified nature**

● **801 Fracture of base of skull**

Requires fifth-digit. See beginning of section 800-804 for codes and definitions. 🏛

INCLUDES	fossa:	sinus:
	anterior	ethmoid
	middle	frontal
	posterior	sphenoid bone
	occiput bone	temporal bone
	orbital roof	

● **801.0 Closed without mention of intracranial injury**

● **801.1 Closed with cerebral laceration and contusion** ·

● **801.2 Closed with subarachnoid, subdural, and extradural hemorrhage**

◆ ● **801.3 Closed with other and unspecified intracranial hemorrhage**

◆ ● **801.4 Closed with intracranial injury of other and unspecified nature**

● **801.5 Open without mention of intracranial injury**

● **801.6 Open with cerebral laceration and contusion**

● **801.7 Open with subarachnoid, subdural, and extradural hemorrhage**

◆ ● **801.8 Open with other and unspecified intracranial hemorrhage**

◆ ● **801.9 Open with intracranial injury of other and unspecified nature**

● **802 Fracture of face bones**

Requires fifth-digit. See beginning of section 800-804 for codes and definitions. 🏛

802.0 Nasal bones, closed

802.1 Nasal bones, open

● **802.2 Mandible, closed**

Inferior maxilla　　　Lower jaw (bone)

◆ **802.20 Unspecified site**

802.21 Condylar process

802.22 Subcondylar

802.23 Coronoid process

◆ **802.24 Ramus, unspecified**

802.25 Angle of jaw

802.26 Symphysis of body

802.27 Alveolar border of body

◆ **802.28 Body, other and unspecified**

◆ **802.29 Multiple sites**

● **802.3 Mandible, open**

◆ **802.30 Unspecified site**

802.31 Condylar process

802.32 Subcondylar

802.33 Coronoid process

◆ **802.34 Ramus, unspecified**

802.35 Angle of jaw

802.36 Symphysis of body

802.37 Alveolar border of body

◆ **802.38 Body, other and unspecified**

◆ **802.39 Multiple sites**

802.4 Malar and maxillary bones, closed

Superior maxilla	Zygoma
Upper jaw (bone)	Zygomatic arch

802.5 Malar and maxillary bones, open

802.6 Orbital floor (blow-out), closed

802.7 Orbital floor (blow-out), open

◆ **802.8 Other facial bones, closed**

Alveolus	Palate
Orbit:	
NOS	
part other than roof or floor	

EXCLUDES	orbital:
	floor (802.6)
	roof (801.0-801.9)

◆ **802.9 Other facial bones, open**

● **803 Other and unqualified skull fractures**

Requires fifth-digit. See beginning of section 800-804 for codes and definitions. 🏛

INCLUDES	skull NOS	skull multiple NOS

● **803.0 Closed without mention of intracranial injury**

● **803.1 Closed with cerebral laceration and contusion**

● **803.2 Closed with subarachnoid, subdural, and extradural hemorrhage**

◆ ● **803.3 Closed with other and unspecified intracranial hemorrhage**

◆ ● **803.4 Closed with intracranial injury of other and unspecified nature**

● **803.5 Open without mention of intracranial injury**

● **803.6 Open with cerebral laceration and contusion**

● **803.7 Open with subarachnoid, subdural, and extradural hemorrhage**

◆ ● **803.8 Open with other and unspecified intracranial hemorrhage**

◆ ● **803.9 Open with intracranial injury of other and unspecified nature**

● **804 Multiple fractures involving skull or face with other bones**

Requires fifth-digit. See beginning of section 800-804 for codes and definitions. 🏛

● **804.0 Closed without mention of intracranial injury**

● **804.1 Closed with cerebral laceration and contusion**

● **804.2 Closed with subarachnoid, subdural, and extradural hemorrhage**

◆ ● **804.3 Closed with other and unspecified intracranial hemorrhage**

◆ ● **804.4 Closed with intracranial injury of other and unspecified nature**

● **804.5 Open without mention of intracranial injury**

● **804.6 Open with cerebral laceration and contusion**

● **804.7 Open with subarachnoid, subdural, and extradural hemorrage**

◆ ● **804.8 Open with other and unspecified intracranial hemorrhage**

◆ ● **804.9 Open with intracranial injury of other and unspecified nature**

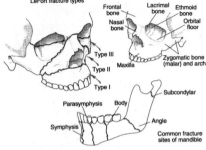

LeFort fracture types

Frontal bone / Lacrimal bone / Ethmoid bone / Nasal bone / Orbital floor / Type III / Zygomatic bone (malar) and arch / Type II / Maxilla / Type I / Subcondylar / Parasymphysis / Body / Symphysis / Angle / Common fracture sites of mandible

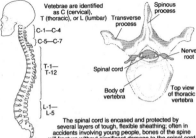

Vetebrae are identified as C (cervical), T (thoracic), or L (lumbar) / Transverse process / Spinous process / C-1—C-4 / C-5—C-7 / T-1—T-12 / Spinal cord / Nerve root / Body of vertebra / Top view of thoracic vertebra / L-1—L-5 / The spinal cord is encased and protected by several layers of tough, flexible sheathing; often in accidents involving young people, bones of the spine will fracture without significant damage to the spinal cord

🏛 Unpublicized government change　　● Additional digit(s) required　　◆ Nonspecific code　　❚ Not a primary diagnosis

Figure 2-16　　ICD-9-CM Tabular Listing

History — *continued*
  irradiation V15.3
  leukemia V10.60
    lymphoid V10.61
    monocytic V10.63
    myeloid V10.62
    specified type NEC V10.69
  little or no prenatal care V23.7
  lymphosarcoma V10.71
  malaria V12.03
  malignant neoplasm (of) V10.9
    accessory sinus V10.22
    adrenal V10.88
    anus V10.06
    bile duct V10.09
    bladder V10.51
    bone V10.81
    brain V10.85
    breast V10.3
    bronchus V10.11
    cervix uteri V10.41
    colon V10.05
    connective tissue NEC V10.89
    corpus uteri V10.42
    digestive system V10.00
      specified part NEC V10.09
    duodenum V10.09
    endocrine gland NEC V10.88
    esophagus V10.03
    eye V10.84
    fallopian tube V10.44
    female genital organ V10.40
      specified site NEC V10.44
    gallbladder V10.09
    gastrointestinal tract V10.00
    gum V10.02
    hematopoietic NEC V10.79
    hypopharynx V10.02
    ileum V10.09
    intrathoracic organs NEC V10.20
    jejunum V10.09
    kidney V10.52
    large intestine V10.05
    larynx V10.21
    lip V10.02
    liver V10.07
    lung V10.11
    lymphatic NEC V10.79
    lymph glands or nodes NEC V10.79
    male genital organ V10.45
      specified site NEC V10.49
    mediastinum V10.29
    melanoma (of skin) V10.82
    middle ear V10.22
    mouth V10.02
      specified part NEC V10.02
    nasal cavities V10.22
    nasopharynx V10.02
    nervous system NEC V10.86
    nose V10.22
    oropharynx V10.02
    ovary V10.43
    pancreas V10.09
    parathyroid V10.88
    penis V10.49
    pharynx V10.02
    pineal V10.88
    pituitary V10.88
    placenta V10.44
    pleura V10.29
    prostate V10.46
    rectosigmoid junction V10.06
    rectum V10.06
    respiratory organs NEC V10.20
    salivary gland V10.02
    skin V10.83
      melanoma V10.82
    small intestine NEC V10.09
    soft tissue NEC V10.89
    specified site NEC V10.89
    stomach V10.04
    testis V10.47
    thymus V10.29
    thyroid V10.87
    tongue V10.01
    trachea V10.12
    ureter V10.59

History — *continued*
  malignant neoplasm — *continued*
    urethra V10.59
    urinary organ V10.50
    uterine adnexa V10.44
    uterus V10.42
    vagina V10.44
    vulva V10.44
  manic-depressive psychosis V11.1
  mental disorder V11.9
    affective type V11.1
    manic-depressive V11.1
    neurosis V11.2
    schizophrenia V11.0
    specified type NEC V11.8
  metabolic disorder V12.2
  musculoskeletal disorder NEC V13.5
  myocardial infarction 412
  neglect (emotional) V15.42   ◆
  nervous system disorder V12.4
  neurosis V11.2
  noncompliance with medical treatment V15.81
  nutritional deficiency V12.1
  obstetric disorder V13.2
    affecting management of current pregnancy
      V23.4
  parasitic disease V12.00
    specified NEC V12.09
  perinatal problems V13.7
  physical abuse V15.41   ◆
  poisoning V15.6
  poliomyelitis V12.02
  polyps, colonic V12.72
  poor obstetric V23.4
  psychiatric disorder V11.9
    affective type V11.1
    manic-depressive V11.1
    neurosis V11.2
    schizophrenia V11.0
    specified type NEC V11.8
  psychological trauma V15.49   ◇
    emotional abuse V15.42   ▼
    neglect V15.42
    physical abuse V15.41
    rape V15.41   ▲
  psychoneurosis V11.2
  radiation therapy V15.3
  rape V15.41   ◆
  respiratory system disease V12.6
  reticulosarcoma V10.71
  schizophrenia V11.0
  skin disease V13.3
  smoking (tobacco) V15.82
  subcutaneous tissue disease V13.3
  surgery (major) to
    great vessels V15.1
    heart V15.1
    major organs NEC V15.2
  thrombophlebitis V12.52
  thrombosis V12.51
  tobacco use V15.82
  trophoblastic disease V13.1
    affecting management of pregnancy V23.1
  tuberculosis V12.01
  ulcer, peptic V12.71
  urinary system disorder V13.00
    calculi V13.01
    specified NEC V13.09
HIV infection (disease) (illness) — *see* Human
  immunodeficiency virus (disease) (illness)
  (infection)
Hives (bold) (*see also* Urticaria) 708.9
Hoarseness 784.49
Hobnail liver — *see* Cirrhosis, portal
Hobo, hoboism V60.0
Hodgkins
  disease (M9650/3) 201.9
    lymphocytic
      depletion (M9653/3) 201.7
        diffuse fibrosis (M9654/3) 201.7
        reticular type (M9655/3) 201.7
      predominance (M9651/3) 201.4
    lymphocytic-histiocytic predominance
      (M9651/3) 201.4
    mixed cellularity (M9652/3) 201.6
    nodular sclerosis (M9656/3) 201.5
      cellular phase (M9657/3) 201.5

Hodgkins — *continued*
  granuloma (M9661/3) 201.1
  lymphogranulomatosis (M9650/3) 201.9
  lymphoma (M9650/3) 201.9
  lymphosarcoma (M9650/3) 201.9
  paragranuloma (M9660/3) 201.0
  sarcoma (M9662/3) 201.2
Hodgson's disease (aneurysmal dilatation of
  aorta) 441.9
  ruptured 441.5
Hodi-potsy 111.0
Hoffa (-Kastert) disease or syndrome
  (liposynovitis prepatellaris) 272.8
Hoffman's syndrome 244.9 *[359.5]*
Hoffmann-Bouveret syndrome (paroxysmal
  tachycardia) 427.2
Hole
  macula 362.54
  optic disc, crater-like 377.22
  retina (macula) 362.54
    round 361.31
      with detachment 361.01
Holla disease (*see also* Spherocytosis) 282.0
Holländer-Simons syndrome (progressive
  lipodystrophy) 272.6
Hollow foot (congenital) 754.71
  acquired 736.73
Holmes' syndrome (visual disorientation) 368.16
Holoprosencephaly 742.2
  due to
    trisomy 13 758.1
    trisomy 18 758.2
Holthouse's hernia — *see* Hernia, inguinal
Homesickness 309.89
Homocystinemia 270.4
Homocystinuria 270.4
Homologous serum jaundice (prophylactic)
  (therapeutic) — *see* Hepatitis, viral
Homosexuality — *omit code*
  ego-dystonic 302.0
  pedophilic 302.2
  problems with 302.0
Homozygous Hb-S disease 282.61
Honeycomb lung 518.89
  congenital 748.4
Hong Kong ear 117.3
HOOD (hereditary osteo-onychodyplasia) 756.89
Hooded
  clitoris 752.49
  penis 752.69   ◇
Hookworm (anemia) (disease) (infestation) —
  see Ancylostomiasis
Hoppe-Goldflam syndrome 358.0
Hordeolum (external) (eyelid) 373.11
  internal 373.12
Horn
  cutaneous 702.8
    cheek 702.8
    eyelid 702.8
    penis 702.8
  iliac 756.89
  nail 703.8
    congenital 757.5
  papillary 700
Horner's
  syndrome (*see also* Neuropathy, peripheral,
    autonomic) 337.9
    traumatic 954.0
  teeth 520.4
Horseshoe kidney (congenital) 753.3
Horton's
  disease (temporal arteritis) 446.5
  headache or neuralgia 346.2
Hospice care V66.7   ◆
Hospitalism (in children) NEC 309.83
Hourglass contraction, contracture
  bladder 596.8
  gallbladder 575.2
    congenital 751.69
  stomach 536.8
    congenital 750.7
    psychogenic 306.4

Figure 2-17   *ICD-9-CM Alphabetic Listing*

91

responding diagnosis. Physicians must use the most specific level of coding possible. This generally means using a four- or five-digit code rather than a three-digit code. As the ICD-9-CM warns, "Claims submitted with three- or four-digit codes where four- and five-digit codes are available may be returned to you by the Medicare carrier for proper coding It is recognized that a very specific diagnosis may not be known at the time of the initial encounter. However, that is not an acceptable reason to submit a three-digit code when four or five digits are available.."

Physicians are also not supposed to choose codes based on "probable," "suspected," or "questionable" hypotheses. When a physician does not know the diagnosis, codes that represent a description of the symptoms or a "family history of" classification must be used. There are also rules about which codes must come first (e.g., the primary diagnosis), how many codes are allowed (e.g., up to four), how to code late effects (effects that appear before a no-longer acute cause), as well codes that apply to where the service was performed, the frequency of the service, and level of service provided.

As you can imagine, understanding and working with the ICD-9 diagnosis codes require some knowledge of medical terminology. Although billing services are not responsible for the original coding itself (the doctor is), your professionalism is enhanced when you know the codes of the specialties you hope to service. (In other words, don't walk into a specialist's office without first learning which codes are commonly used in that specialty.)

Remember: knowing the coding can also pay off by giving you an additional service to offer. Many billing services that know coding well can offer to review a doctor's superbill to make sure it is up to date and that the doctor is getting reimbursed at the highest level. This increases your value to physicians. Caution: don't attempt to formally advise physicians about coding or to change codes yourself; it could open you up to malpractice suits. However, if you discuss the coding with your client and tell him or her what you believe to be a better code to use, the physician can consider your opinion and make the decision.

PROCEDURES CODES Procedure codes are similar to diagnosis codes, in that they are a shorthand for the services performed by the doctor. Prior to 1983, there were more than 120 different procedure coding systems in the United States. For each of the insurance companies they dealt with, doctors had to be familiar with the codes currently in use. This is one reason that doctors began giving their patients the responsibility for filing claims themselves.

Medicare and HCFA established the current coding system in 1983, largely based on codes recommended by the American Medical Association. Most commercial insurance companies now use this same coding system. The codes are complex and are updated each year. For example, in 1992, there was a major change in the way physicians were instructed to code the nature of the patient/doctor contact when reporting to Medicare; many insurance companies have also adopted this same system.

The coding system is divided into three levels, with the top level being the most utilized. This level is called the CPT-4, which stands for Current Procedural Terminology, Fourth Edition. The CPT is a listing of more than 7,000 codes representing services performed by medical personnel of all kinds. Updated and published each year by the American Medical Association, the CPT keeps track of all currently accepted medical procedures.

The main body of the CPT codes is divided into six sections; each section represents a broad field of medicine, such as shown in the following list. Each of these sections contains hundreds of specific procedures, each with a unique five-digit *numeric* code:

Evaluation and Management	99200 to 99499
Anesthesiology	00100 to 01999
Surgery	10000 to 69999
Radiology, Nuclear Medicine, and Diagnostic Ultrasound	70000 to 79999
Pathology and Laboratory	80000 to 89999
Medicine	90000 to 99199

Remember that most healthcare providers do not use all these codes, because they typically specialize. Most physicians commonly work with about 100 codes on a daily basis; these are the codes that they preprint on their superbill.

Although using the procedural codes is straightforward, several areas often cause confusion for doctors and billing specialists. One area in particular is the Evaluation and Management Codes (E/M). These codes were completely revised in 1992 for Medicare, but now commercial carriers have adopted them as well. The E/M codes are complex, with dozens of different codes that apply either to new or established patients. ("New" patients are those whom the doctor has not seen in at least three years.) The codes also take into account the location of the visit (e.g., office, home, hospital, clinic) and many other specific issues. There are also a variety of two-digit supplemental codes, called modifiers, that the physician must append to a

Evaluation and Management Codes

The Evaluation and Management Codes (E/M) define the physician/patient contact in terms of the time, depth of diagnosis, and level of decision making and thinking required for that meeting. Naturally, a 5-minute visit to diagnose a sore throat and take a throat culture does not cost as much as a 45-minute visit to suture a wound. The technical and intellectual requirements are substantially different.

The E/M codes were devised and went into effect in 1992 to classify the work of doctors for Medicare billing. Commercial carriers require these codes now as well. The new codes replace the old six-level "Visit" codes for reporting service using the nomenclature of *brief, limited, intermediate,* and *comprehensive* with a more complex hierarchical system divided into many categories and subcategories. For example, there are categories, such as office visits, hospital inpatient visits, consultations, emergency department services, critical care services, nursing facility services, rest home services, home services, case management services, preventive care services, and newborn care. These categories are further divided into two or more subcategories, such as office visit—New Patient vs. Established Patient, or Hospital Inpatient Visits—Initial Visit versus Subsequent Visit.

These subcategories are then further divided into levels of services, selected according to seven components, as follows:

Key Components (these carry the most weight)
- History (4 types: problem focused, expanded problem focused, detailed, comprehensive)
- Examination (4 types: problem focused, expanded problem focused, detailed, comprehensive)
- Medical Decision Making (4 subcategories: straightforward, low complexity, moderate complexity, and high complexity)

Contributory Factors
- Counseling (discussions with family/patient over diagnosis, prognosis, risks of treatment, importance of compliance with treatment, risk factor reduction, and patient/family education)
- Coordination of Care (a patient encounter with other providers or agencies)
- Nature of Presenting Problem (5 levels: minimal, self-limited or minor, low severity, moderate severity, and high severity)

Additional Factor
- Time (face-to-face time versus unit/floor time)

As you can imagine, for a doctor to arrive at a decision combining all these factors to convey which type of service he or she provided is not a simple issue. The Medical Decision Making subcategory alone requires an entire table to determine which level of decision making was used, as shown in Table 2-8.

Despite the effort that doctors must exert to properly select an E/M code, insurance carriers have also developed their own standards, so in some cases, the coding is an exercise in futility.

primary code to indicate extra services, such as special prolonged time, concurrent care (more than one doctor attending), repetitive service for chronic care, and so on. The sidebar on "Evaluation and Management Codes" will give you some idea of CPT coding.

These coding complexities can make the work of a neophyte billing service quite confusing, yet they are extremely important. Just as with diagnosis codes, if a doctor has chosen the wrong code or reports a procedure that does not correspond to a diagnosis, the claim will be rejected, delayed, or downcoded.

LEVEL II AND III CODES. As stated earlier, the CPT codes are just the top level of the procedural codes. Below CPT are two additional sets. The entire system is referred to as HCPCS (pronounced HicPics), which stands for HCFA Common Procedure Coding System. The Level II codes, called the National Codes, are used to bill Medicare for many items not listed in the CPT codes, such as medical supplies. CPT has only a few dozen codes to bill for supplies while there are several thousand codes in the Level II book for items such as gauze pads and syringes, as well as drugs, injections, and durable medical equipment (DME) that may be sold or rented to patients. All these items must be coded as part of a physician's services.

The Level II codes are five-digit alphanumerics, ranging from A0000 to V5999. These codes are revised each year, and there are usually hundreds of additions, deletions, and changes that billers must learn by purchasing

TABLE 2-8

Decision-Making Factors Influencing E/M Codes

Number of Diagnoses or Management Options	Amount and/or Complexity of Data to be Reviewed	Risk of Complications and/or Morbidity or Mortality	Type of Decision Making
Minimal	Minimal or none	Minimal	Straightforward
Limited	Limited	Low	Low complexity
Multiple	Moderate	Moderate	Moderate complexity
Extensive	Extensive	High	High complexity

a new edition of the HCPCS book and by reading Medicare bulletins and books on coding. A list of Level II codes follows:

Transportation Services	A0000—A0999
Chiropractic Services	A2000
Medical and Surgical Supplies	A4000—A5500
Miscellaneous and Experimental	A9000—A9300
Enteral and Parenteral Therapy	B4000—B9999
Dental Procedures	D0000—D9999
Durable Medical Equipment (DME)	E0000—E1830
G Codes for Procedures	G0001—G0062
Drugs Administered Other Than Oral Method	J0000—J8999
Chemotherapy	J9000—J9999
Orthotic Procedures	L0000—L4999
Prosthetic Procedures	L5000—L9999
Medical Services	M0000—M9999
Pathology and Laboratory	P0000—P9999
Temporary Codes	Q0000—Q9999
Diagnostic Radiology	R0000—R5999
Vision Services	V0000—V2799
Hearing Services	V5000—V5900

The lowest level of procedure coding is called the HCPCS Local Level 3. These codes are alphanumeric, ranging from W0000 to Z0000. They are established by the local Medicare office in each state and vary greatly. Local codes are used to describe new procedures that one Medicare office may recognize. Local codes will likely be used less and less, because Medicare is trying to standardize its benefits for all citizens.

While this three-tier program of coding makes it easy to identify exactly what transpired between doctor and patient, it takes time to master and may be confusing to all but the most experienced coders. With hundreds of coding changes each year, it goes without saying that the entire CPT/HCPCS system is hard to keep up with. As a result, there are many professional books intended for teaching doctors how to use the codes.

A billing service that knows coding has a significant advantage in the market. This is not to suggest that you need to memorize codes; becom-

Business Profile: Nancie Lee Cummins; Medical Management Billing

Nancie Lee Cummins got into medical billing from a background selling group health and life insurance to employers. With her knowledge of the healthcare industry, she felt that medical billing was the right business for her. To purchase her software and learn the details of the business, she went to a trade show for business opportunities and evaluated several offers, finally selecting Medical Management Software from Merry Schiff.

After her training, she immediately began marketing—and it paid off. She sent out 25 letters, from which one doctor responded and hired her. That client eventually referred another doctor to Nancie, and now all her clients have come from referrals.

Nancie now has six practices and is expecting to sign a 10-provider IPA outpatient mental healthcare facility. She attributes her success to the excellent training and support she received from Merry Schiff and to the referrals she has gotten. She also believes that specializing in billing for mental health practitioners, such as clinical psychologists and social workers, has been effective for her business.

In Nancie's view, medical billing is a professional business that must be treated with integrity. She says,

> If you get into this business, you have to work hard at it. You have to constantly read and educate yourself. Your knowledge is what makes the difference for your clients. For example, let's say you are coding a depression, and the doctor gives you a code for "general" depression, you need to know that this code will kick out (get denied) because it is not specific enough. The insurance company wants to know if it's single incident or multiple, what type, and so on. It may be that the doctor coded it incorrectly. While a worker's comp insurance might have taken the code, if it's a Medicare patient, the code should have one or two more digits to make it work. Many doctors simply don't know this; they give wrong codes, or they use old coding books.

To keep up on her training, Nancie goes to Medicare workshops whenever they are available. She also doesn't hesitate to call Medicare and ask questions when necessary. She finds the Medicare staff quite willing to help her, and in fact, she gets even better service when she says that she's a biller.

For most of her clients, Nancie performs full practice management. She files claims electronically, prints out and mails patient invoices, and prepares many financial reports. Because of managed care, she finds her responsibilities growing. For example, she has helped her doctors prepare proposals for HMOs and PPOs, and when we spoke, she was working with another potential client as he set up an MSO.

Nancie's expertise once prevented one of her doctors from making a costly error. The doctor was part of several clinics and believed that he was losing money in one of them. Nancie produced a report for him that proved that he was actually making more money in that clinic in less time than he was making at the clinic he had thought was his best choice. He decided to continue seeing patients in the first clinic, thanks to Nancie.

ing familiar with them is sufficient. Your goal is to appear professional when you speak with any potential client. Be sure to review the codes in that doctor's specialty before trying to sell your billing expertise. Be sure you stay up to date with Medicare especially. The agency is an ever-changing operation, and its need to control costs results in more and more documentation to justify medical procedures. A billing service must therefore maintain an ongoing knowledge of Medicare, not just learn about it once. As you operate your business, be sure to read the Medicare bulletins and attend the Medicare and Medicaid conferences.

Area 2: Computer Software and Hardware Issues

The level of computer knowledge you will need to be successful in medical billing is growing. As in all professions, more and more tasks are computerized, and the future predicts a constant stream of new technology you will need to keep up with. You also need to prove to prospective clients that you are as computer literate as—if not more than—they are. So, if you don't have a technical background in computers and software, you may be at a disadvantage in this field. However, Nancie Cummins, profiled earlier, is proof that you don't need to be a computer wizard; you simply need to master whichever medical billing software package you purchase to the point that you can do what your clients need better than they can.

Here's a brief explanation of some of the issues you need to understand.

HARDWARE In most cases, the level of your hardware knowledge will pertain only to your own computer. You must obviously know how to use and care for your own PC to keep it healthy and running without problems or memory lapses. The worst thing you could do to your business would be to tell clients that your computer is down and their billing will be delayed.

However, because you may also get involved in the "bigger picture" for a client, you may be asked to help the doctor's office update its computer system and/or automate its own procedures. This means that the more you know about hardware, the better. It therefore helps to keep up on the options and prices of new PCs, where to buy equipment (new and used), and other issues such as local area networks, computer-to-computer remote accessing via phone lines, and how to use a modem. Of course, you can subcontract to a computer consultant should the occasion arise when a doctor needs you to consult on hardware issues. For the most part, as an independent billing service, your hardware knowledge goes only to the level of taking care of your own setup.

MEDICAL BILLING SOFTWARE Today's medical billing software has improved to the point that most people can learn what they need to know in a few days. The old days of complex nonintuitive commands and ugly, confusing interfaces are gone. Most billing software does what you want it to do "transparently," meaning that you don't need to get involved in the behind-the-scenes actions the software performs; you can tab through simple menu commands or point with your mouse to an icon to open a file, find a patient record, or post a payment.

It is worthwhile to learn to use your medical billing software before you go into business. In fact, some software companies will give you hypothetical physicians and patients with which you can practice so that you can develop your efficiency in keying in claims. Now is the time to learn your software, not when you are already up and running.

Which software to purchase is covered later in the chapter.

OTHER SOFTWARE. Once you are in business, much of your time is devoted to keying and transmitting claims using your medical billing software. Since many of these software programs are comprehensive, fully integrated practice management software packages, you have little or no need to learn how to use separate stand-alone accounting programs or database programs.

A medical billing service is a business, however, and you may wish to become proficient in using other types of business software, such as word-processing programs or database managers that allow you to create mail-merged letters and to print mailing labels for your marketing materials. Desktop publishing software will also enable you to design and print your own brochures, advertisements, and direct mail marketing pieces. Knowing how to use presentation software can help you prepare charts, graphs, slides, and other printouts when you give presentations to potential clients. Finally, using a bookkeeping or accounting programs is useful to invoice and bill your clients, and contact management programs can help you keep track of your business leads. Each of these categories has dozens of programs available, ranging from simple-to-use inexpensive software to complex and costly programs. To save yourself money and time, consider integrated software programs that combine several of these types of software, such as programs that offer word-processing, database management, and spreadsheet accounting all in one package.

If you have no background in computers, you may start to feel overwhelmed with how much computer work you have in front of you while trying to learn, at the same time, about the medical billing field. Take your time; you can learn it if you have the right attitude. Allow yourself an extra month to get acquainted with your software before you begin your billing service.

My view of the computer hardware and software industry is reminiscent of the ancient Greek mythological king Sisyphus, who was condemned to roll a stone uphill, only to watch it fall again when it reached the top. However, the difference is that our task is not a punishment, but a learning treat! So enjoy your challenge of learning and using new software and hardware. It's only going to get better!

Area 3: Business Knowledge and Skills

Paul and Sarah Edwards wrote in their book *Getting Business to Come to You,* "You are not in business until you **have** business." Their point is especially true in organizing a medical billing business. You can set up the best home office, purchase the most sophisticated software, and study the ICD-9 and CPT books till you have mastered them cold, but unless you have a doctor paying you for services, you are out of business.

Getting clients and keeping them require hard work, knowledge, and business acumen. Nearly everyone I interviewed for this book told me that the first few months of marketing their business were difficult and frustrating. Even worse was closing the first sale. They pointed out many reasons for this:

- Difficulty in getting busy doctors to pay attention to you or allowing you to give a presentation. (Imagine yourself walking into a crowded doctor's office with a waiting room full of ill people and leaning your head over the counter to ask the front office manager, "Excuse me. Is the doctor available?" Do you really think the doctor will interrupt what he or she is doing to meet you?)

- Financial and emotional barriers that prevent many doctors from wanting to hand over their cash flow to anyone. (Imagine a doctor who is already losing income from insurance companies and feeling frightened about his or her future. Will this be a trusting person?)

- Time it takes for doctors and their staff to make a decision to outsource this work. (Imagine a busy doctor trying to make up his or her mind about whether or not to outsource and how much to pay you.

Next imagine the office politics behind the decision to outsource; is anyone threatened?)

■ Concern over the potential for errors when outsourcing this work. (Imagine a doctor's face when her billing clerk tells her that they have $3,000 in unpaid claims; will that doctor believe you can do it better?)

All these barriers add up to a single truth: you must have or be able to develop excellent business skills, especially marketing and sales abilities. Let's examine each of these briefly.

MARKETING Marketing is the skill of letting people know about your products or services, so they can decide whether or not to buy. Marketing is actually a combination of fields and activities: cold calling, direct mail, advertising, premiums, special promotions, and public relations. Each of these requires different talents and skills, and each has its pros and cons. Which of the marketing strategies you use depends on many factors: your personal preferences, your budget, and your audience. Some people are effective at cold calling, while others are not. Some locales are more receptive than others to direct sales. There are many variables, so you must analyze your particular situation and determine what's best for you.

In medical billing, marketing is especially vital because, as just mentioned, getting a doctor to give you responsibility for managing his or her accounts can be quite challenging. Many people I interviewed for this book swear that cold calling works best for them; others stopped cold calling and found success through direct mail campaigns using a persuasive letter or brochure. We'll examine the various techniques in greater detail in the "Getting Started" section of this chapter, but for now, suffice it to say that you cannot succeed in medical billing unless you are willing to market yourself aggressively.

SALES Marketing is useless without sales. You could have the most attractive brochure when you call on the front office manager, or make the most persuasive sales pitch to the doctor, but unless you **close** the deal, you don't have business.

Unfortunately, many people immediately think of sales as a crass profession. They hate the thought of doing sales, and they shudder to think that someday, they might "force" somebody to buy something from them. Indeed, to many people, sales means pressure tactics, deceit, and manipulation. None of these need describe a good salesperson. A more positive way to think of sales is that it is the natural conclusion to a good marketing plan.

Successful selling require three skills:

1. Identifying the customer's motivations. The foremost skill is knowing how to go beneath the surface to identify your customer's true motivations. One of the first rules in sales is making sure you can answer your customer's silent question, "What's in it for me?" Customers know what's in it for you; they need to know how you can help them. According to Jackie Hall, president of the Hall Group, a corporate consulting firm that works with InfoHealth Corporation (the medical billing software company mentioned earlier),

> Salespeople need to ask about the doctor's aspirations and dreams for his or her business. This is the heart of the matter. If you focus on technical jargon about insurance and claims that doctors know nothing about, they will try to ask you questions to test your knowledge and make sure you know more than they do! Instead, ask them about their hopes and dreams for their business.

This advice is sound. In today's healthcare environment, you will likely hear many similar answers from doctors when you ask about their aspirations and dreams. Many will tell you that they want to preserve their independence and income security in the face of managed care. Many will also tell you that they want to practice medicine, not business. They are frustrated by Medicare, Medicaid, and private health insurance rules and regulations. Your ability to sell is therefore strongest when you can address these issues persuasively and convincingly. You need to show your commitment to be a strong advocate for the doctor and to expertly handle his or her practice management problems.

2. Persistence. The second sales skill is persistence. You must be persistent enough to know when you are into a worthwhile negotiation, yet astute enough to know when you are probably wasting your time. Many people who dislike sales actually dislike the idea of having to ask someone (often repeatedly) to buy their service. They also hate rejection. However, thoughtful persistence is needed, because few people buy right away and you cannot afford to lose a potential client by giving up too early.

3. Negotiation skill. The third sales skill is the ability to negotiate for a win/win close. Negotiation is both a skill and an art. You need to know when and how much to compromise, when and how to yield your ground as much as when and how to hold it. Often, people without sales experience dislike negotiating because they believe they must throw themselves at the customer's feet in order to get the business. On the contrary, good negotiation should convey that you respect yourself and expect others to pay you fairly and treat you appropriately. Ask yourself when was the last time you met a doctor who worked for free. If you are like most people, this humorous prodding illustrates how important confident negotiation is to your business success.

Charting Your Challenge

The foregoing sections have presented three areas for you to assess your current knowledge base and skills. Take a moment and reflect on your knowledge of them. How much about medical coding and insurance regulations do you need to learn? How computer literate are you? What is the level of your business skills? If you haven't already, you may now want to complete the chart suggested on page 88, in which you plot your learning curve.

If you are going into business with a spouse or partner, don't forget to examine his or her skills and see if combined, the two of you complement each other. It often happens that one person has one set of skills, such as excellent marketing intuition, while the other has a solid background in another set of skills, such as in computers or medicine. The sidebar on DAPA Medical Billing Services illustrates a husband/wife team whose complementary skills turned their venture into a true success.

Income and Earning Potential

There have been many claims about the potential of a medical billing business, but earning potential is one area to evaluate carefully if you are considering this profession. The difficulty with calculating your earning potential is that until you are in the business, you often can't determine how to charge your clients. Much depends on whether you are able to do claims only or full practice management. Of course, it also depends on how many doctors you have as clients, and how busy they keep you.

In general, there are four methods of pricing in a medical billing business. The following sections explain these methods. I have tried to show each method in an average light, without pretending that medical billing is a get-rich-quick scheme. For most people, it is not. For this reason, I highly recommend that you scrutinize any earnings projections anyone shows you outside of this book. You will frequently find brochures from medical billing opportunity vendors that list income projections, but please take these as strictly hypothetical (and optimistic) projections until you know more about your specific market potential.

Daniel F. Lehmann and Patricia Bartello—DAPA Medical Billing Services

The saying "two heads are better than one" is an apt assessment of the complementary business partnership of these two individuals.

Dan Lehmann entered medical billing after 25 years in management and manufacturing, working into high-tech automotive and robotics industries. He also taught college business courses for a few years, but like many people who grow tired of working for others, Dan yearned for his own business enterprise. His wife, Pat Bartello, had a strong medical background with a master's degree in educational psychology. She had also worked in a hospital in collections and had operated a successful medical transcription business. When they decided to follow their dream, they carefully evaluated many types of businesses and selected medical billing as their best option.

Dan and Pat agree that it takes a combination of skills to be in this business. One skill that Dan contributed was a strong business background. He prepared a business plan for their operation when they first began and does monthly updates to track their progress. Dan was also quite versed in computer hardware and software. As for Pat, she knew medical terminology and was comfortable speaking to doctors and doing presentations. As Pat told me, "Doctors are very suspicious, and so you have to come across credibly. When you first call on them, they may throw out some jargon just to test you, and if you respond accurately, you've got their ear."

Dan and Pat offer complete reimbursement management and they specialize in working with physicians in geriatrics and geriatric psychiatry. Because they live on the borders of Virginia, Maryland, and Washington D.C., they've ended up with clients in all three areas, which complicates their work to some extent. They file a large number of Medicare claims, many of which go to different Medicare carriers. (Note: the Medicare carrier to whom you file claims depends on the location of the doctor's office, not where the patient lives. Pat and Dan have doctors who have multiple offices in different counties, so their claims must be filed to different Medicare carriers.)

Just as with every biller profiled in this chapter, Dan and Pat have noticed a change in the business over the past several years. As Pat told me,

> Things are growing worse. There's a huge increase in managed care today, requiring patients to have authorization to see a specialist. We have many cases where there hasn't been a valid referral, so the claim gets denied. Ultimately, this situation puts a lot of pressure on both doctors and billing offices. Without a valid referral, the doctor doesn't get paid. But it also affects us. We don't want to put effort into filing a claim when there was no authorization, because we don't get paid either. We therefore end up doing a lot of verification to make sure the referral has been made before we file a claim. For example, let's say a patient has been authorized to have ten visits with a psychologist. We plug that information into our computer so that as the patient uses up the visits, our system counts them down.

Dan and Pat believe that medical billing in their area is still an excellent business opportunity, but it has become more competitive. They find doctors more open to outsourcing, but at the same time, more concerned about the costs of doing so:

> Doctors hear that Medicare provides free software, and they think "why should I pay to outsource when I can have my clerk do it more cheaply?" But we show doctors that we can handle their practice with more accuracy and a

better return-on-investment because we do everything: insurance verification for managed care, primary billing, secondary billing, patient statements, and so on. We also do it better, and less expensively than they can do it in their office because we work on volume.

Since I interviewed them for the first edition of this book, Dan and Pat have grown their business to the point at which they can no longer use DOS or Windows-based software. Dan recently invested in an extensive UNIX system for their home office that provides him with many sophisticated features plus simultaneous usage because they have employees who work off-site and need to tie into the system. As Dan told me years ago, "The important thing as a service agency is to respond quickly and accurately." Seems like Dan and Pat are doing just that.

PER CLAIM FEE BASIS In the per claim fee method, you would charge your clients a set fee for each claim you process, whether or not the claim is ultimately paid by the insurance carrier (except if you are at fault for a rejected claim because of a typographical error you committed). The per claim fee varies around the country from $2.00 to $6.00, but the majority of people I interviewed say they are able to charge $3.00 to $4.00 per claim.

Let's use the $4.00 figure to work through an example of a billing service and to calculate its earnings. In this case, let's assume that the billing service uses a clearinghouse that charges a $300.00 annual fee, plus a $50.00 annual setup fee per physician, plus $0.50 per claim. (Note: the per claim clearinghouse fee can range from $0.35 to $0.60, depending on the deal you are able to strike with your clearinghouse.) We will exclude from this projection that some clearinghouses also charge a fee for rejected claims, and a postage fee when they cannot transmit your claim electronically but must "drop it" to paper and mail it.

To be conservative about this projection, assume that you have only two clients for your first two months of operation, and you add a new client every few months, for a total of five physicians over the first year of operation. Each physician sees 3 to 4 patients per hour (some physicians see many more, of course, but some see far fewer). Assume therefore that each doctor averages 15 claims per day for 20 billable days per month. This equals 300 claims per month @ $4.00, hence $1,200 per month per physician. Table 2-9 shows how your income and expense chart would look under this scenario.

From this table, you can see that a "just claims" billing service might generate $47,000 in income with five doctors each supplying 300 claims per month. Remember that this income excludes marketing costs, which could

TABLE 2-9

Income and Expense Projections for a Typical Billing Service Charging on a Per Claim Basis

Month	1st	2nd	3rd	4th	5th	6th	7th	8th	9th	10th	11th	12th	Total
# of clients	2	2	3	3	3	4	4	4	5	5	5	5	5
# of claims @$4.00 per claim	600	600	900	900	900	1200	1200	1200	1500	1500	1500	1500	13,500
Gross Income	$2400	$2400	$3600	$3600	$3600	$4800	$4800	$4800	$6000	$6000	$6000	$6000	$54,000
Expenses @$0.50 per claim + $50.00 per client registration fees	$300 plus $100 new reg. fee	$300	$450 plus $50 new reg. fee	$450	$450	$600 plus $50 new reg. fee	$600	$600	$750 plus $50 new reg. fee	$750	$750	$750	
Total Expenses	$400	$300	$500	$450	$450	$650	$600	$600	$800	$750	$750	$750	$7000
Net Income (Gross less Total expenses)	$2000	$2100	$3100	$3150	$3150	$4150	$4200	$4200	$5200	$5250	$5250	$5250	$47,000

Notes:

1. Excludes income from additional fees such as setup charges or fees for sending patient statements
2. Excludes expenses for marketing, cost of software, and overhead

easily amount to $2,000 or more for brochures, letters, direct mail postage, business cards, stationery, and other items.

On the other hand, this projection does not include additional fees you can charge for setting up new accounts for each physician, or doing any practice management functions such as preparing and mailing patient invoices. Many billing services charge $2.00 or $3.00 per patient when they do the setup. If a doctor has 250 to 500 active patients, this could generate an additional $400 to $1,500. In our hypothetical example, the billing service could increase its net income to $52,000.

A variation on the per unit fee basis is to use a sliding scale, as did one of the people I interviewed. He charges each of his clients according to how many claims per week he receives from them, as shown here:

Claims per Week	Charge per Claim
1—99	$6.00
100—199	$5.00
200—299	$4.50
300—399	$4.00
400—499	$3.50
500 or more	$3.00

The owner chose this method because he had several clients who wanted his services but processed only a limited number of claims per week. Because they needed his services, they agreed to pay a much higher fee per claim to compensate him for the lower volume.

Doing full practice management results in much higher fees. The going rate to send out monthly statements to patients is $2.00 per statement (plus postage). If a physician has 200 active clients to whom he or she must send a monthly statement, you can add another $400.00 per physician per month to your income. That means an additional $3,600 per year per physician × five doctors: an additional $18,000 along with your $47,000 income. As you can readily see, adding services can significantly increase your income potential.

HOURLY BASIS   Another method of charging is to set an hourly fee for your work. However, this method is one of the least used in the medical billing profession. The sidebar on Linda Noel exemplifies one such owner who charges by the hour because she has several clients who process only a small number of claims per week. Charging by the hour, in quarter hour increments, allows Linda to account for the time she spends getting files ready, transmitting them, and doing patient billing and fol-low-up phone calls.

The hourly fee you set will depend on your geographic location, the competition, and whether or not doctors perceive you as a professional biller or just a clerk. If your client is a doctor who has had an in-house billing person for years, there may be an unfortunate tendency to corre-late your work with this hourly paid employee. Beware of this situation.

Try to make your hourly fee as high as you can get it right away, per-haps $20 to $35 per hour, because changing an hourly fee once you sign a contract is difficult. While employees get annual raises, outside services such as free-lancers and consultants usually cannot increase their fees until they have had the contract for several years.

Your annual income based on an hourly fee basis depends on how much you work. If you can work 20 to 30 hours per week at $25.00 per hour × 50 weeks per year, your income will range between $25,000 and $37,500.

PERCENTAGE BASIS   The third method of pricing your service is to charge clients a percentage of every dollar you bring in, including all elec-tronic claims and all patient billing you do. This method of charging is by far the most popular and offers the best potential. Of dozens of people I

Business Profile: Linda Noel

Linda Noel was managing a psychiatric clinic in West Los Angeles when she and her husband decided to start their family. Not wanting to give up her career, she opted for the only logical choice: a home business utilizing her medical experience. Not only did she get the support of her former employer, but he helped her by spread-ing the word to attract other clients who soon signed on with Linda.

Today, Linda has nine clients, enough to keep her working a comfortable 30 hours per week, leaving her time to be with her children. For simplicity, she works only with single physician practices and bills most of them on a straightforward basis of $15 to $21 per hour. For a few, she adds a small percentage fee for collections if the billables are hard to collect. "In my practice," Linda told me, "I do everything from billing to accounts receivable; I function just as someone who works in their office would, including occasionally scheduling appointments. I do transcription and billing (both electronic and paper)."

Linda doesn't believe that you must absolutely have a strong medical background to get into the business, but she knows that working in a physician's office helped her. She points out that the constantly changing Medicare regulations are hard to keep up with, so she seriously recommends taking courses offered by Medicare.

"Running a personalized service is a key to getting and keeping clients," Linda says. "You've got to have doctors who like you and are willing to refer you to others."

interviewed, nearly all were charging from 6 percent to 8 percent of net collectible amounts.

In using the percentage method, note that you need to clarify with your client which items you will get paid on. For example, if a patient pays cash to cover the 20 percent coinsurance or a $15 copayment fee, at the time of the visit will you get a portion of this money? In most cases, no. Most doctors want to pay billers only for the claims and patient statements for which they bill out. However, if you have to update the account, you should rightly get your percentage.

As you might imagine, it is far more difficult to convince a doctor to agree to pay you 6 percent or 8 percent of the practice's total collectibles than it is to charge $3.00 per claim. The key to winning this argument is to show your client the advantages of using your services, particularly that you can significantly increase the "collection efficiency" of the office. This is the level at which the physician is able to collect on billables.

For example, consider a physician who bills $1 million per year and pays 1.5 staff people to do billing in-house at a combined salary of $35,000. Assume this doctor is able to collect at only a 75 percent efficiency (hence, $750,000) because his staff does not have time to follow up on denied claims, rejected claims, lost claims, and patients who don't pay. Contrast that situation with what you can offer: if you commit to collecting on 85 percent of collections (hence, $850,000), the doctor can benefit by more than $50,000. Table 2-10 shows the calculation for this.

TABLE 2-10

Comparison of Collection Efficiency: In-House Staff vs. Outside Service

	Physician Using Salaried In-House Staff	Physician Hiring an Outside Billing Service at 8%
Billables	$1,000,000	$1,000,000
Collection efficiency	×75%	×85%
Collections	$750,000	$850,000
Cost of collections	($35,000)	($68,000)
Net income	$715,000	$782,000

As Dan Lehmann remarked about the percentage method,

> We charge 8 percent or more, but we do everything for the doctors: patient registrations (we even supply the forms), daily charges, electronic filing twice or three times per week, insurance verification. In some cases, we eliminate the need to have an in-office clerk even part time. Their wage plus benefits, which may amount to $20,000 to $30,000, is less than ours, but we can collect far more than they can.

The percentage method is your best choice if you are offering full practice management services. This method compensates you for the efforts you make to follow through on all accounts receivable and make sure they are collected. Of course, any errors or mistakes you make may reduce your income under this method. Doctors will also be much more suspicious if they believe you are doing sloppy work and not collecting as much as you could.

Projecting an annual income under the percentage method is difficult. Whereas with the per claim method, you can estimate how many claims the doctor will have, with the percentage method, you have less control over how much insurance companies will reimburse, how many bad claims you may get stuck with, and what type of patients the doctor may treat. If you are planning to charge a percentage, you need to openly discuss with your client the facts about his or her practice before you commit to this method.

MIXED METHOD   The last method of charging for your services is the mixed method. As the name implies, you can mix any of the methods discussed earlier, depending on your clientele. If you have a client who wants only claims, you will obviously need to charge on a per claim or hourly basis. With another client though, perhaps you might start out on a per claim basis and slowly work your way to percentage as you increase your role in handling full practice management.

Whichever method you choose, don't forget to counterbalance your income projections with an accurate estimate of your expenses, including costs for marketing materials, printing, postage, phone bills, and other overhead (stationery, furniture, mileage, etc.). Projecting your income for a new business in the first year can often be enhanced by making more than one calculation—for example, best-case and worst-case scenarios—and revising your projections as each month of operation passes.

Again, take whatever projections you hear from others with a grain of salt. Your income will depend on your area and on the kind of customers *you* find. While I used 300 claims per month in the earlier example, no one can guarantee that you will achieve any particular number of claims.

Deciding If This Business Is for You

The first part of this chapter presented the background for understanding medical billing services. Armed with this brief sketch, the following checklist can help you decide if this business is for you. Take a moment now to do this 15-question checklist before reading the remainder of the chapter.

- Does the business of medical insurance and computer coding appeal to me?
- Do I have the drive to grasp complex medical terminology and coding matters?
- Can I work comfortably with doctors and their office personnel?
- Do I have enough computer skills and an interest in learning new software?
- Do I enjoy detailed work, such as keying in medical records?
- Can I sell my services face to face and close a deal?
- Do I have the drive and persistence to close several clients?
- Do I understand direct mail marketing and other forms of marketing?
- Do I negotiate well?
- Do I want to assume financial responsibility for ensuring my clients get paid?
- Do I have two to three months to get my business started?
- Do I have from $500 to $7,000 to purchase medical billing software or a business opportunity package that includes training and marketing support?
- Do I have the talents, skills, knowledge, and abilities that can help me succeed in the healthcare business?
- Does my partner (if I have one) provide complementary skills to my own so that we can work together to succeed?
- Do I have a suitable location from which I can conduct this business?

If you answered yes to most of these questions, the next section provides brief guidelines on how to get started in your own medical billing business. The section is organized according to the sequence of steps you need to take: choosing your software and hardware (including whether or not to buy a business opportunity); obtaining training; learning how to price your services; guidelines for marketing your business and getting a first client; and overcoming common start-up problems.

Section II: Getting Started

Choosing Your Software

Many medical billing software firms and business opportunity vendors are competing to sell you software. If you read business magazines such as *Home Office Computing, Entrepreneur, Success,* and others, you'll find a variety of advertisements for medical billing software and/or training. There are literally dozens of companies involved in selling practice management programs; some sell only to doctors' offices, but as the business changes and there is greater recognition of the need for independent medical billing companies, you will find more and more companies eager to sell software and training to entrepreneurs who want to set up their own businesses. (See the next section, "Should I Buy a Business Opportunity.")

How do you decide which software to buy? Unfortunately, there is no one answer to this question. Each person has his or her own needs, and each program has its unique design that creates both advantages and disadvantages. Additionally, software is an ever-changing product, with new bells and whistles constantly added each year. If I were to recommend one software program today or critique another, my recommendations will become flawed quickly because they will be outdated within months or years. Thus, it is impossible to provide specific software recommendations.

Nevertheless, here are some guidelines about what to look for:

1. There are differences in software. Some software programs are DOS-based while others are Windows-based. That choice depends on your preferences and your computer system. Needless to say, the Windows environment has become nearly the dominant software platform in recent years, so most software firms will move their DOS-based software to Windows in the coming years if they haven't already.

2. Most software products are designed to make the medical billing process efficient, but among the products I reviewed, enough signifi-

cant differences exist that I urge you to evaluate for yourself *more than one product*. Don't try out just one software demo copy and make a decision based on that. Judge for yourself which of several software programs makes you feel comfortable and which one is easiest for you to use.

3. Don't buy a software program without seeing a demonstration of how it performs. Most companies are willing to send you a free demo copy, or you can visit someone who uses it.

4. Look for professional features in the software. For example, make sure your software allows you to do the following:

   - True billing service capability. Because you'll probably aim to do full practice management, you want to be sure your software allows you to keep track of many different providers. Some software is intended to handle a single practice only and is not appropriate for a professional billing service.

   - Claims only versus practice management software. Some software allows you to submit electronic claims, but it doesn't contain the accounting operations you need to do full practice management.

   - Open item accounting. Because Medicare and other insurers sometimes approve only some of the charges on a claim, you must be able to record payments and link them to the charges billed. That way, if you need to question a denied claim, or bill the patient for the difference, you can tell which charges were not paid.

   - Multiple fee schedules. With the growth of managed care plans, doctors need to be able to have multiple fee schedules. They are required to accept one set of fees for Medicare patients, another set of fees for patients under HMO Plan A, and another set of fees under PPO Plan B. This means that your software should be able to store up to several dozen fee schedules. As mentioned earlier, some software also has special modules for managed care patients who fall under a capitated plan, because you need to log their reimbursements differently.

   - Pop up windows for common data sets. Some data sets, such as insurance companies, procedure and diagnostic codes, and fees are annoying to have to retype over and over again. To facilitate this, many software products provide pop-up windows that store the data sets, so all you need to do is point and click on the item you want instead of typing it.

▪ Clearinghouse flexibility. Does the software allow you to work with any clearinghouse you want, or must you use the clearinghouse recommended by the software vendor?

The CD-ROM disk accompanying this book includes several samples of medical billing software. These programs are demonstration copies; some are self-running demos and others are real working versions of the software, albeit "disabled" or "limited" in their scope (i.e., don't try to use them to get into business because they won't allow you to input many patients or claims; they are sample copies only). The vendors of these software products invite you to contact them directly or, in the case of Lytec and Medisoft, to contact any of the several business opportunity vendors who resell the software along with training. You can contact InfoHealth and Santiago SDS directly about purchasing their software plus training. See Appendix E for more information.

Should I Buy a Business Opportunity?

Because of the complexity of learning about the medical billing business, many software companies do not offer training to entrepreneurs. They prefer to focus on selling their software directly to medical providers' offices. Other software companies will sell to entrepreneurs, but they don't provide the level of training you need to market and succeed in this field.

As a result, many "business opportunity" companies have appeared that follow the model of software VARs (valued-added resellers). These people package the software from respected medical billing software houses, along with their own materials and training programs. They charge you a much higher fee than you would pay for just buying the software directly from the software company, but in general, they provide far more training and support.

However, because of their nature, business opportunities are regulated by many states almost like franchises, to help prevent consumers from investing in bogus deals. Business opportunities are known as "seller-assisted marketing plans" (SAMPs). They differ from franchises in that you are not required to pay continuing royalties or a percentage of your profits year in and year out. You are also not allowed to use their company name nor do you need to adhere to strict rules about how you run your business, such as franchise laws impose. When you buy a business opportunity, you are simply paying someone to sell you (you hope) good information about what's required to operate the business, often along with software and collateral materials.

If you are considering buying a business opportunity, it is wise to scrutinize the vendors closely to be sure you are dealing with an honest and qualified company that truly knows the business and can train you. Unfortunately, ever since medical billing became a popular business in the 1990s, a number of the business opportunity vendors selling software and training did not truly know the medical profession. Several of these companies enticed hundreds of entrepreneurs to purchase their opportunity, and then these firms went out of business after cashing the checks, leaving their customers with no support. Worse, several of these same companies then reopened under a different name in another state and repeated the ruse. Much to our dismay, several of these companies are still around, preying on people who are seriously exploring new careers and livelihoods. Some of these companies have been charged by the Federal Trade Commission (FTC), which also regulates business opportunities, but they continue to stay in business.

Here are some tips to assess whether you are dealing with a good business opportunity vendor:

1. If you experience high-pressure sales tactics, it is likely not a company with which you want to do business. Many people have called me to complain about high-pressure tactics from companies, such as offering a special price that is "good only if you buy it today." Don't fall for such maneuvers and tactics. If a company offers you a deal to buy today, you can be sure it is not interested in working with you over the long term. It only wants your money.

2. Find out if the vendor has any complaints lodged against it with the attorney general's office in your state. If any prior customers have had difficulty with the unscrupulous vendor, they may have filed a lawsuit or notified the state attorney general's office. If so, you can find out about these complaints. You should also check with the Better Business Bureau in your state as well as with those of surrounding states. If there are numerous complaints about the company, this is certainly a red warning flag for you. Don't underestimate it.

3. Find out if your state is one of those that regulates business opportunities or SAMPs. At this time, the following states have such laws: Alabama, California, Connecticut, Florida, Georgia, Illinois, Indiana, Iowa, Kentucky, Louisiana, Maine, Maryland, Michigan, Minnesota, Nebraska, New Hampshire, North Carolina, Ohio, Oklahoma, South Carolina, South Dakota, Texas, Utah, Virginia, and Washington. Other states may have similar regulatory programs over SAMPs by the time this book comes out. If your state regulates SAMPs, make sure your vendor adheres to the regulations. Request a document from the vendor indicating that it is registered to sell in your state. (The registration must reflect the state in which you live, not the state in which the vendor resides.) If it is not registered, it is up to you to decide whether you want to buy from it. If you do purchase and change your mind or find that you have been seriously shortchanged in the level of support you were promised, you have little chance of getting your money back.

4. Note also that under most SAMP laws, business opportunity vendors are not supposed to make representations about how much income you can earn in medical billing, or if they try to do so, they must report names, addresses, and phone numbers of those people who have made the income level they contend. Watch out for exaggerated income projections, such as people earning $70,000 or $100,000 within one year. It takes time to get this business going, and even the most successful people say that the first year was a financial struggle.

5. Get at least three references from the vendor and check them out. Unfortunately, some vendors use "plants" (also called "singers") who are paid to confirm how wonderful the vendor was; you have no way to know this. However, make every effort to assure yourself that these references are truly in the medical billing business.

6. Be precise in identifying exactly what type of support the vendor is supposed to give you for the price you pay. Does it consist of live training? Phone support? Manuals? Technical training? Marketing training? Several people have told me terrible stories of vendors who spend all day teaching the basics of software, which can be learned from a manual, with no time spent on teaching how to market to doctors. Marketing is the hard part, and if the vendor cannot help you with marketing, you may not be successful in getting a client.

7. In addition, be clear in your own mind how much support you need. If you have experience as a bookkeeper, administrative assistant, or a computer consultant, for example, you might feel that you don't need as much training. However, for all but the most experienced people with medical backgrounds, it is very likely that buying training from a qualified business opportunity vendor can make the difference between success and failure.

LIST OF RECOMMENDED VENDORS OF BUSINESS OPPORTU-NITIES If you agree that it is in your best interest to purchase training and support along with your software, here is a short list of the most reputable and reliable business opportunity vendors that I recommend:

- Medical Management Software—Merry Schiff—800-759-8419
- ClaimTek Systems—Kahil Farhat—800-224-7450 or 503-239-8316
- Santiago SDS Inc.—Tom Banks/Mary Lee Hyatt—800-652-3500
- Electronic Filing Associates—Ed Epstein—800-596-9962

Appendix A contains details about each of these vendors. These business opportunity vendors are all companies that I have come to respect from their track record in this industry for honesty, integrity, and verifiably *high-quality* training and support. You may find other companies to work with on your own, but I am confident that these business opportunity vendors will work with you in an honest, forthright manner. No one can guarantee your success, but these vendors will at least give you the training and support that you expected to get as part of your package.

If you believe that you have the background and work experience to jump right into the medical billing business without special training, you might want to consider purchasing software directly from a software house. I recommend the following: MediSoft, Lytec, and Oxford Medical Systems. You can find details about these software firms in Appendix A.

A Note on Starting Out

Be prepared for a delay in doing electronic claims filing when you first start. If you are working through a clearinghouse, you may need to fill out several agreement forms, one of which can only be done when you get your first client. Your doctors must also sign agreements with the clearinghouse. All this takes a few weeks to complete. The clearinghouse will probably ask you to process 20 or so claims to make sure you know what you are doing. This also adds time. Meanwhile, if you are already taking claims from a client, you will have to print them on HCFA 1500 paper forms for these first few weeks. Don't try to fool your client; be honest and make sure he or she understands that it takes time before the fast results of electronic claims processing can be observed.

Choosing Hardware and Other Equipment

If you don't have a PC yet, you should choose your hardware based on the software you decide to purchase. As indicated earlier, however, most software is moving toward a Windows platform, so purchasing the most cost-effective yet powerful PC you can afford is your goal. In general, this means buying a PC with a Pentium chip with 16 or more Mb of RAM. You can get by with a 486 personal computer and 8 Mb of RAM, but prices are going down so fast that it usually costs little more to buy a Pentium PC now. You may also be able to use a 386 computer, but your software will run much more slowly.

You will need at least a 500 megabyte hard drive. Fortunately, most PCs sold in retail stores or via mail order (such as Gateway, Dell, or Micron) are now sold with hard drives that have ample space; today's new computer generally comes equipped with anywhere from 1.2 to 2.5 gigabytes of hard disk space. Remember that it helps to have this extra disk space to store all the other software you will want to own to perform many general business functions. Software such as desktop publishing or database programs usually require 10 to 20 Mb of hard drive space for the program alone, and your data will usually occupy another 50 Mb. This means that for each program you load into your computer, you probably want to reserve space for 60 to 100 Mb. Five or more programs, including a desktop publishing package, a database, a spreadsheet, and you are approaching ½ gigabyte.

Whether you are purchasing new hardware or upgrading what you already own, I recommend thinking long term. With prices dropping quickly, you can often spend as little as $1,000 to $1,500 to equip yourself with a professional computer system.

As far as other equipment goes, you will need the following:

- *Monitor.* A color monitor (VGA or SVGA) eases strain on your eyes and helps you work more productively. The colors help distinguish menus and screen entry fields. If you can afford it, consider purchasing at least a 15" monitor instead of a 14" model as visual studies have shown that people are more productive when their screen area is larger.

- *Fax machine.* One of the most common ways to conduct your business is to have providers fax you their superbills. As a result, a good fax machine is critical. You need to keep the faxes as your permanent records, so do purchase a plain paper fax rather than a thermal paper machine. Reliable plain paper fax machines cost as little as $400 at office supply stores and through computer/technology catalogues.

Note: you cannot use an internal fax/modem for this purpose. You need a paper copy of faxed superbills to place in your records.

- *Modem.* Most software and clearinghouses support 9,600, 14,400, and 28,800 baud modems. Obviously, the higher the baud rate, the faster your transmission, so 28,800 or higher is your best bet.

- *Backup Devices.* You should be able to keep backups of your files for security purposes. Do not risk a hard drive crash with your client's data. A tape drive backup is less than $200 and well worth the expense. If you prefer, use one of the portable or removable hard drive backup devices, which sell for just slightly more than tape drives.

- *Printer.* Even if you are doing electronic filing, it is worthwhile purchasing a laser or inkjet printer to use for all your other practice management functions, such as patient invoices, reports, and graphs. Having a laser or inkjet printer also allows you to prepare your own marketing materials such as brochures, fliers, and direct mail letters. You can also use a laser printer to print the occasional HCFA 1500 you may need if your clearinghouse does not send to a small insurance company, although these days, the clearinghouse will probably drop it to paper for you.

- *Office Furniture.* Processing claims and setting up patient files is tedious work. To prevent neck and back strain, or problems such as carpal tunnel syndrome in your wrists and fingers, buy yourself an ergonomically designed chair with arm rests.

- *Phone Lines.* As a professional businessperson, you must have a business phone distinct from your family phone. You do not want a client to speak to your child, a relative, or the baby-sitter. You can order either a regular personal phone line or a business line, which costs more. Some phone companies now offer special pricing for home-based businesses. A home-business line or regular business line usually entitles your business to a listing in the *Yellow Pages.* This can be useful for marketing; several medical billing companies have told me they did receive calls from their *Yellow Pages* ads. While the phone company is installing your second line (your home line is the first), consider having a third one installed at the same time to use for your fax machine and modem. A third line allows your clients to fax you at any time instead of having to interrupt you on the second line if you are on the phone. You also do all your electronic transmissions via modem over the third phone line, so you can take business calls on your second line at the same time.

■ *Postage Meter.* If you handle patient statements, it is also well worth the slight expense to lease a postage meter, thus saving many trips to the post office. Meter rentals are not expensive today, particularly if you compare the cost to the time you lose going to the post office and the price of gas.

Resources and Training

Preparing yourself to run a medical billing service is perhaps the most valuable action you can take before starting your business. As indicated throughout the chapter, this business has become a real profession, requiring increasingly sophisticated knowledge and skills. Without adequate training, you will take much longer to get your business under way—or you will become so frustrated that you will quit before you get your first client. Here are some suggestions for educating yourself.

INDUSTRY ASSOCIATIONS   One of the first steps you can take is to contact the association that serves people in the medical billing industry.

NATIONAL ELECTRONIC BILLER'S ALLIANCE (NEBA).   This association was founded by Merry Schiff (owner of Medical Management Software, Inc., one of the software and business opportunity vendors listed earlier). NEBA provides an extensive array of training and marketing support materials, including books, audiotapes, and a newsletter.

If you are interested in learning more about medical billing in a home-study course, NEBA has a comprehensive program that contains details on every aspect of the business. NEBA also offers a certification exam for billers who would like a credential. The organization currently includes several hundred members, ranging from people who are new to medical billing to experienced billers. NEBA also provides a World Wide Web site with information and advice to improve marketing skills and develop expertise of reimbursement issues. You can contact NEBA at 415-577-1190 or fax at 415-577-1290 to request information. The Web site address is www.nebazone.com.

COURSES   Many community college and adult education schools have courses or workshops in medical billing and coding. In some cases, these courses are intended to train people who want to work in the front office of a physician's practice, but other courses are specifically targeted to entrepreneurs. For example, the Learning Annex in Los Angeles has several popular courses on running a home-based medical billing service. If you enjoy a classroom atmosphere, this type of training may be for you. These courses are most often inexpensive, but they are typically quite limited in scope. If you are eager to get your business under way, taking college courses one at a time may prolong the amount of time it takes to learn what you need to know.

As indicated earlier, NEBA has a home-study course that goes into extensive detail on insurance, medical office procedures, coding, and marketing/sales.

Another home-study medical billing course is offered by At-Home Professions, a Colorado-based home-study company that has courses in many disciplines. See Appendix A for more information about its courses.

BOOKS AND NEWSLETTERS   There are many books you can read to learn more about billing, coding, and other aspects of medical billing. Look for a medical bookstore in your city where you can purchase coding manuals and other reference books. One excellent book is *Understanding Medical Insurance: A Step-by-Step Guide* by JoAnn C. Rowell, available in many medical bookstores and from medical suppliers such as Medicode (see following).

The ICD-9 is available from the U.S. Government Printing Office, and the CPT coding book can be purchased directly from the American Medical Association. You can also obtain both these books from several private companies that republish them under license in special easy-to-use formats. One such supplier is Medicode, which offers the most recent CPT edition and a large assortment of medical coding "how-to" guides, including the following titles:

- Reimbursement Manual for the Medical Office: A Comprehensive Guide to Coding, Billing, and Fee Management

- CPT Coding Made Easy!: Technical Guide (2 vols.)
- Insurance Directory
- Coder's Desk Reference
- CPT Billing Guide
- Code It Right!
- Reimbursement Strategies

Medicode can be reached at 800-678-8398 in Salt Lake City, Utah. Ask for Ann Jacobsen. See Appendix A for details about special discounts that Medicode offers readers of this book.

Another source of excellent information on medical billing is Gary Knox, of AQC Resources, a consulting company in San Jose, California. Gary has been studying medical software and business opportunity companies for many years. As Gary has noticed, the field has matured. He says,

> Medical billing today is a better industry than it was a few years ago. There is more acceptance to outsourcing billing now. Unfortunately, many people are not taught the skills to market themselves; even if they get one or two offices, they're not trained well enough and they fail.
>
> I would like people to know that success in this industry is 75 percent marketing. It's no longer a "just claims" business that physicians will consider. If they are going to outsource, they want more than that. They want a full service agency, especially with HMOs dictating to them what to do. They want someone who can help them with eligibility verifications, authorizations, and so on. So you need to have a broad experience today; it isn't "just claims" anymore.

Gary publishes an informative bi-monthly newsletter on the medical billing industry for $59 per year. Gary can be reached at 408-295-4102. See Appendix A for more information on AQC resources.

ONLINE FORUMS   In addition to the Web site for NEBA, there are two public online boards that many people in medical billing find useful.

- **CompuServe.** In the Work from Home forum of CompuServe, there is a subsection for people interested in medical billing. (This section also covers medical transcription.) You will find here "libraries" of files that can assist your research. For example, the forum periodically hosts a "live" chat night in which many people get together to discuss medical billing online, and these written conversations are eventually compiled into a file you can download and read at your leisure. There are also files that other people (including myself) have uploaded for anyone to read and comment on. If you are already a subscriber to CompuServe, just enter the command in the Go menu, "Work from Home" and you will be transferred to that forum. Then go to the Libraries menu, and select "Medical Billing and Transcription." If you are not yet a member of CompuServe, you can easily join by installing its software in your computer and dialing up the pre-arranged number. You can find CompuServe software for free in many computer magazines sold on newsstands, or call 800-487-0453.

- **America Online.** Like CompuServe, there is an area on AOL that serves as a forum for people interested in medical billing. You can find this section by entering the key word "Business Strategies," then go to the "Home Business Message Board." Then enter "New" and "Medical Claims Processing." You can obtain free AOL sign-on software in nearly any computer magazine sold on newsstands, or call AOL at 800-827-3338.

GENERAL BUSINESS TRAINING Because medical billing is very marketing intensive, you may want to expand your entrepreneurial skills with courses in marketing, sales, publicity, and business planning. Many extension schools and local colleges offer courses or workshops on these business topics. You will likely find many kindred souls at such courses, since many people today are interested in learning to run their own home-based business.

There are also dozens of business books that teach the skills of marketing and sales. Browse through your local bookstore for books such as those from Paul and Sarah Edwards: *Working from Home, The Secrets of Self-Employment,* and *Getting Business to Come to You* (co-authored with Laura Clampitt Douglas). Read magazines such as *Home Office Computing* and *Success.* Given the political nature of healthcare in this country, it is also worthwhile to read newspapers such as the *Wall Street Journal,* the *New York Times,* and even *U.S.A. Today,* so you can stay abreast of new legislation affecting the healthcare field as well as profiles of successful businesspeople who might inspire you.

Contact your department of commerce or local chamber of commerce for booklets they publish about starting a business. SCORE (Service Corps of Retired Executives) and other associations of businesspeople and networking organizations can also be helpful. You will be surprised by how many people are willing to share their expertise and knowledge with you. Start by making a chart of people you know, and ask each one if he or she has any friends in the medical field with whom you could chat to get advice and information about your new venture. Many of the successful medical billing owners I interviewed got advice from their own doctors about the business and their marketing ideas.

Whatever you do, make time each week for learning more about medical billing and operating a business as a home-based entrepreneur. Chapter 5 addresses general business self-improvement issues in more detail.

Tips for Pricing Your Service

Choosing your pricing strategy is always a difficult task. If you price too low, you will not maximize your earnings, and you may even lose money. For example, one medical billing service I interviewed that was doing "just claims" began its pricing at $2.00 per claim and quickly found that it had no profits. On the other hand, if you price your service too high, you may drive away potential clients, or lose them quickly to lower priced competitors. Because this is a service business, your prices need to reflect the quality and level of service you are delivering. Will you process 50, 100, or 150 claims a week for a given doctor? Will you also do regular patient invoicing? Send out late notices? Key in checks and cash payments to complete accounts receivable? Will you be providing your clients with monthly reports such as aged balances and practice activity analysis graphs?

In short, you cannot price your service until you know your clients' needs. It is advisable not to put any printed notice showing your fees in your advertising or direct mail brochures. You need first to find out about each practice that expresses an interest in your services, so you can return later with an accurate proposal reflecting what you can do for it. Only when you know what services you will provide can you decide how much to charge. Some guidelines for all these decisions follow.

LOCATION   Location is always an important consideration in pricing. Living costs are greater in large metropolitan areas than in small cities and towns in most parts of the country. You need to get some sense of the fee structures in your community. If you are doing just claims, you might be able to charge $4.00 to $6.00 per claim in some cities. However, in many smaller areas, you'll be limited to $2.50 or less. If you are handling full practice management, you may be able to charge from 8 percent to 12 percent of all collections if there is a lot of overhead work for you to do, such as many secondary claims, appeals, patient statements, and soft collections. However, in other locations, you may be able to get only 6 percent at best. Whatever your fee, negotiate for the highest rate you can right at the outset, because it is difficult to raise your rates after you have started. If you go back in six months to ask for a higher fee, you risk losing your customer(s).

ESTIMATE OVERALL AMOUNT OF WORK Like any business, doctors have good days and bad days, so try to estimate how much work and how many claims your client has in one month. Use a full month as your measure of business, not a day or week. Set your fee structure at a higher rate if you will be handling fewer claims per month, and lower your rate if the client will be giving you many claims. This will give your clients the sense that you discount your fees for volume work. Alternatively, you could offer a sliding fee schedule for each month, depending on how many claims and/or patient statements are ultimately processed.

COMPARE PER CLAIM METHOD WITH PERCENTAGE METHOD
To compare these two measures, you need to have a frank discussion with your client to learn how many claims per month are filed versus their dollar value. Many doctors will not want to divulge such personal financial information to you. However, if you can focus the doctor on how well you will increase his or her collection efficiency, you may be able to obtain a ballpark figure that allows you to estimate the doctor's annual income. You can then do your own comparison of per claim versus percentage methods to see which way you come out ahead. In general, most people who do full practice management find that charging according to the percentage method generates the higher income.

BE REASONABLE When you set your fees, don't think that doctors make so much money that they have enough to share generously with you. As discussed earlier, today's doctors are feeling many cutbacks in income because of managed care. You will encounter doctors who want to penny pinch everything you do. Nancie Cummins suggests a good line to use when you find yourself in this position. Tell the doctor that you will not nickel and dime him or her when you do your work; you will not charge for long distance phone calls or for special trips to their office to pick up superbills, and so on. In return, tell the client that you believe you deserve not to be nickled and dimed either. As Nancie says, "Let the doctor know you are worth that extra 1 percent and that you take pride in what you can do for his or her practice." In addition, remember that each practice you service doesn't need to know about your other clients or what you charge them.

Marketing Guidelines

Nearly every person I interviewed for this book told me, "Getting clients is the hardest part of this business." *Do not forget this* and certainly don't think that it won't be true for you. Although many other people or vendors may tell you that medical billing is a great business opportunity in which you can become "rich" quickly, remember that you *will* have difficulty getting customers unless you can convince doctors that you have the skills and expertise to get their claims filed more quickly, increase their cash flow, and help them manage their practice.

One reason for doctors' reluctance to outsource billing is that this portion of client contact has traditionally been thought of as easy and unimportant. In a doctor's eyes, the emphasis has always been on treating the patient. Filling out claims was a secretarial function.

But as indicated throughout this chapter, today's healthcare environment has completely changed this perspective. Cost is now as important as treatment. Doctors and insurance companies are no longer simply on opposite sides of the fence; they are on opposite sides of the universe! For the most part, their financial interests are diametrically opposed. Doctors would prefer to do and spend whatever it takes to keep their patients alive and healthy; insurance companies would prefer to spend as little as possible, regardless of what happens to the patient. Doctors also believe they should be paid commensurate with their extensive educational background and the risks they take. Insurance companies believe doctors' incomes should be pared way down.

Despite the new environment, you will face an uphill battle convincing doctors to (a) hire an outside billing service to take care of their accounts and (b) hire *your* billing service as opposed to someone else's. This means that you must apply nearly all of your initial efforts to marketing and sales. Many doctors are still adverse to outsourcing their billing and practice management; they believe that their staff can handle these functions, or they are simply reluctant to make a change.

Here are some tips for conducting a successful marketing campaign. Note that there is simply not enough room in this book to provide a comprehensive medical billing marketing course that ensures that you will get some clients. If you do not have a background in marketing or feel anxious about selling to doctors and other healthcare providers, I recommend that you purchase a business opportunity from one of the vendors listed in Appendix A, who can provide the extensive training and support in marketing that you truly need. Also contact the two associations already mentioned, NEBA and NACAP; each one has a library of specific marketing materials, such as sample direct mail letters and brochures, presentation materials, and audiotapes that provide in-depth guidance in this complicated subject.

SPECIALIZE YOUR SERVICE Several successful medical billing owners I interviewed ended up focusing their business on doctors in a certain specialty. In some cases, it happened by chance, such as Nancie Lee Cummins, who found herself working largely with psychologists, social workers, and mental health clinics. Dan Lehmann and Pat Bartello work extensively with physicians in areas related to gerontology. The value of specializing your business is that you become as much an expert in that field as the doctors, at least when it comes to coding and insurance reimbursement. Through practice, you start to master the ICD-9 and CPT coding, and you know even the uncommon situations. You also become familiar with the fee schedules in that field, and if you have several clients in a specialty, you can compare how they each run their businesses. In short, specializing often adds a dimension to your knowledge that impresses potential new clients, so you can build your business faster.

Table 2-11 shows a list of medical specialties you might want to consider.

DETERMINE WHICH MARKETING TECHNIQUES YOU ARE MOST COMFORTABLE USING The best way to approach marketing is to first determine your own special talents and interests. After all, there is no point pursuing a marketing approach that you cannot bring yourself to do.

Start by examining yourself. Each of us has some natural marketing talent that simply needs to be discovered. Consider your previous business experience and see what marketing tools you've already developed Ask yourself, "Have I done direct mail? Have I written catalogue copy or product specifications? Called on clients, patients, or doctors and put them at ease during a first meeting?" Perhaps you have a flair for design and copywriting, so developing a powerfully persuasive flier or brochure will be your lead into the office. Or perhaps you have the gift of a charming personality and easy conversation that enables you to approach the most abrasive receptionist and quickly smooth over relations.

If you feel uncomfortable about your ability to do marketing, take a course at a local college or business school, and read some books about it. You will need to learn about "marketing mix" (the proportion of the four major marketing methods you can use: advertising, public relations, direct

TABLE 2-11

Medical Specialties in Medical Billing

- acupuncturists*
- allergists
- ambulance services
- anesthesiologists
- cardiovascular physicians
- chiropractors
- dentists and dental hygienists***
- dermatologists
- durable medical equipment suppliers (DMEs)**
- endocrinologists
- gastroenterologists
- general practice doctors
- general surgeons
- geriatric doctors

- gynecologists
- hematologists
- immunologists
- internal medicine physicians
- medical laboratories
- nephrologists
- neurologists
- obstetric physicians
- occupational therapists
- oncologists
- ophthalmologists
- optometrists
- oral surgeons***
- orthodontics specialists**
- orthopedic surgeons

- osteopaths
- pathologists
- pediatricians
- physical therapists
- plastic surgeons
- podiatrists
- proctologists
- psychiatrists
- psychologists
- radiation therapists
- radiologists
- rehabilitation specialists
- rheumatologists
- thoracic surgeons
- urologists

Notes:

*Medicare will not accept claims electronically or on paper.

**Claims may require a special format of the HCFA 1500.

***Requires American Dental Association format and dental software for some procedures not billable on an HCFA 1500 form.

---

selling, and sales promotions), direct mail campaigns, copywriting, market segmentation, niche marketing, and a host of other topics.

If you prefer, hire a marketing consultant to help you in those areas with which you are unfamiliar if you are willing to pay for help. Specialists can sometimes make the difference between success and failure.

Note: Some business opportunity vendors will promise to do cold calling and other marketing on your behalf to set up appointments with providers. While this may seem useful, unless you are ultimately willing to do marketing on your own, such promises of getting you appointments are hollow. You must be able to do some portion of your own marketing and you must be able to give a good presentation (unless you intend to work with a partner who can do the sales presentations for you).

LET PEOPLE KNOW YOU ARE IN BUSINESS You cannot simply take an ad out in the *Yellow Pages* and wait for customers to come to you. That is unrealistic. You must do one or more marketing activities, such as networking, direct mail, cold calling, publicity, or workshops, to let people know you are in business. In other words, you must take action in one form or another. In general, most billers seem to be the most successful using networking, cold calling, and direct mail (followed up with calls).

On the other hand, I have received reports of people who purchased their medical billing software and made a few phone calls to doctors, thinking that this was "marketing." When they were rejected after two or three "not interested responses," they gave up and concluded that they were never going to succeed. Such trivial first steps do not make a marketing campaign. You must be willing to follow through with a well-thought-out and continuous attack for several months.

KEEP YOUR DIRECT MAIL SIMPLE Direct mail letters or solicitations were one of the most common marketing techniques among people I have interviewed. Direct mail is useful because it reaches a large audience of doctors to announce your business and seek appointments.

When you write and design your first direct mail letter, remember that a busy doctor has little time to read. Keep your letter short, succinct, and to the point. See the sample direct mail letters shown in Figures 2-18 and 2-19. (Note: these are intended to be samples only; it is recommended that you adapt and customize them to your market, depending on whether you are doing just claims or full practice management.)

Mailing out a few hundred letters per week is expensive, so be sure to allocate enough of your financial resources for this type of marketing, at least for the first few months. Many new billing professionals mail out 25 to 50 letters to healthcare providers in their area each week. Of course, they also follow up on letters sent out in previous weeks too. Direct mail is not useful without follow-through.

Another popular direct mail piece is a three-fold brochure. Brochures give you more space to write about the merits of your electronic claims processing, and your expertise in practice management. However, they are more expensive to produce, so you may want to use brochures only for your most important prospective clients.

Where do you get names for your mailings? Some business opportunity vendors will supply you with a list of 1,000 names of doctors who do not bill electronically. Such lists are often generated through Medicare. NEBA can also supply you with such lists; see Appendix A.

Figure 2-18
Sample Direct Mail
Letter #1

Your Letterhead Stationery
Address
City, State, Zip

Date

Dear Dr. (insert name),

Are you dissatisfied with the amount of time it takes your insurance claims to be processed? Are you waiting 60 or more days to obtain reimbursements?

If so, my company can significantly improve your claim-to-check turnaround time. We can literally cut in half the amount of time it takes you to receive insurance reimbursements.

We are also experts in helping doctors in your specialty manage their practice, from improving your patient reimbursement ratio to working with you to develop effective business strategies in today's managed care environment.

I will call your office within the next few days to arrange an appointment during which I would like to personally show you the specifics on how my company can benefit you. I look forward to speaking with you then.

Sincerely,

(Your Name)
(Your Title)

One problem with direct mail is that you must send out a generic letter to a large client base, but you do not know what their specific problems are. One physician may be more concerned with staff turnover, while another is worried about lost claims. This is why you must follow up on each mailing you do and try to speak directly with the physician so you can learn the specifics of his or her situation.

DEVELOP A PROFESSIONAL APPEARANCE Yes, a good marketing campaign costs money, but you can't expect to compete or attract attention without high-quality brochures, business cards, stationery, and a company logo. I'm not suggesting that you must buy the services of the best professional designers and printers in your area, but simply that you not be penny wise and pound foolish. Your marketing materials announce that you are a professional businessperson.

If your printer tells you to use a higher quality business card stock that costs an extra $30.00 per thousand, it may well make the difference in a

Figure 2-19
Sample Direct Mail
Letter #2

Your Letterhead Stationery
Address
City, State, Zip

Dear Dr. (insert name),
Try out our electronic claims processing and billing service for two weeks free!

The only way to know whether or not something is right for your practice is to try it out. We are so convinced that our medical billing service will reduce your office paperwork, eliminate suspended claims, and reduce delays in insurance reimbursement that we'd like to make it easy for you to try us out.

We know that you and your staff would rather concentrate your efforts on caring for your patients than worrying about insurance payments and denied claims. We at (*Your Company Name*) are experts in electronic claims filing and physician practice management.

Your claims will be processed faster, and you'll notice an immediate reduction in rejections. Your billing costs will be lowered, and your billing headaches will disappear.

Now is the time to take advantage of our expertise. In today's managed care environment of greater cost containment, we can help you regain control of your practice and your income security.

This is a risk-free, no-obligation opportunity. If at the end of the two-week trial period, you are not completely satisfied, you owe nothing. So take the first step and call us at 444-1234 today to ask whatever questions you have and arrange for us to start.

Sincerely,

Your Name
Your Title

prospect keeping your card and calling you a few months later. For example, Nancie Cummins had her stationery letterhead printed in silver foil; she used this stationery to write a direct mail letter that she sent to just 25 prospects. One of them was so impressed with her letter that he hired her right away, so she actually landed her first client within weeks of starting out.

Spending time on developing your marketing materials is important too. Don't rush through the writing process as you compose direct mail letters and brochures. Once you've written a draft, let it sit for a few days, and then review your writing to see if you might find a better way to convey your message. Be detailed oriented in all your correspondence and written materials. I have seen cover letters with grammatical errors and misspellings, suggesting that they were written by a person who did not pay attention to details. Would a doctor hire that person? Certainly not.

In addition, get feedback from others on your marketing materials. Ask the opinion of your spouse, business partners, friends, and even a few doctors on any letters or brochures you produce. You may find what you have written to be perfect, but don't be defensive if someone suggests different wording. If you are in doubt, hire a professional copywriter to revise your brochures and direct mail pieces.

FOCUS ON SERVICE AND BENEFITS   In all your marketing materials, focus on the benefits to the customer you can provide, such as improving cash flow, increasing the reimbursement ratio, and stabilizing the physician's income security. Avoid wasting words touting your credentials or on details about the technology of electronic claims. Aim to answer the doctor's question, "How does this person make operating my healthcare practice better?"

If you are doing just claims, let the client know that you can simplify the claims filing process, reduce office paperwork, accelerate the speed at which he or she is reimbursed, and increase collection efficiency. If you offer full practice management services, add to the list that you can improve the doctor's income by thoroughly tracking and collecting on all accounts receivable.

THE PROS AND CONS OF COLD CALLING   The verdict on the effectiveness of cold calling is still out. I interviewed many people who told me that cold calling was a complete waste of their time. They indicated that they were never able to see a doctor or set up an appointment by just visiting a doctor's office off the street. However, other people told me that cold calling worked for them, and even that they made cold calling their #1 marketing strategy. Ultimately, the use of cold calling always seemed to reflect more the individual's special talents in this area than a true indication of an easy marketing technique. So, try cold calling if you feel comfortable doing it; otherwise, don't bother.

However, if you use cold calling, here are some tips to improve it:

■ Don't aim to make a sale during the first cold call. Most people indicated that cold calling works best when your objective is simply to make an appointment to come in and see the prospective client to make a larger, more coherent presentation. You can either make a cold phone call or visit the doctor's office, but don't expect to be invited right then and there to close the deal.

- Send printed materials in advance of cold calling. Send out a direct mail piece first, so that when you cold call, it's really more of a warm call. The doctor or office manager may recognize your name from the mailing you recently sent.

- Make use of any networking contacts you have before you make a cold call. Remember, doctors have a constant stream of sales representatives calling on them day in and day out from pharmaceutical companies, equipment manufacturers, office supply people, and temporary agencies. Your business may be important to you, but to a busy front office person, you are just another salesperson.

- Be prepared for rejections, but don't let them interfere with your professionalism. Always leave your name and business card—and leave on good terms. You never know when a staff billing person might quit, or when the doctor realizes that it is time-consuming to train a new person every few months. Several successful billers told me that they heard back from a doctor months after their initial call—and the doctor eventually became their client.

GET TO THE DECISION MAKER Medical practices vary greatly in terms of who is actually in a position to give you their business. In some practices, the doctor is the only one who can make a decision, but in others, it may be the physician's spouse, or an office manager, or a staff billing person. You need to find out who might be involved in the decision making to do billing offsite, and then convince that person that you can benefit the office in many ways. You may also find that a staff person feels threatened by you and believes you will eliminate his or her job. However, as indicated earlier, many billing service owners I interviewed, such as Mary Vandegrift, told me that staff people often feel relieved when they are no longer assigned to do the billing. There are usually many other tasks they can do around the office.

Whoever the decision maker is, your goal is to find that person and get a face-to-face interview for at least 20 minutes during which you should have a well-prepared presentation. Many professionals use flip charts or have a self-running computer demo that uses graphics to help them cover the issues.

Note: Several business opportunity vendors and others sell a software program you can use during your presentation to compare how much it costs a doctor to file paper claims versus electronic claims. The software lets you key in salary information for office personnel, overhead costs, claim rejection rates, and so on. From this information, the program calculates the cost per paper claim and contrasts this cost with how much an electronic claim will cost to process. From all reports, the software is generally impressive and effective. You can purchase this software, *ClaimsWizard*, from NEBA. See Appendix A for information.

If you have an opportunity to do a presentation, aim to make personal contact with the doctor to find out what problems he or she is experiencing in the office—and how he or she is impacted by managed care in your area. Explore as deeply as you can what the physician's situation is: Has his or her income been falling? Has he or she been at odds with HMOs and PPOs that have put pressure on him or her to join? Seek to get the doctor to feel that you are trustworthy. Trust is perhaps the most essential element in your relationship with a medical practice that is handing you its financial survival.

After your presentation, ask for details about the number of patients, claims, and billables that allow you to prepare a proposal to present at a follow-up meeting within a week. In general, don't negotiate for closure that day; let the doctor know that you would like his or her business and that you need time to create a truly customized bid that reflects how your service can help that office.

Once you get to the second appointment, seek out any objections and try to answer them one by one that day. Look for a way to begin closure: Is the doctor showing approval of your ideas? Does he or she admit to having a falling income? Is he or she asking you more and more questions? These are often clues that you can begin to funnel your discussion down to brass tacks, such as when you might begin the work.

OFFER A FREE TRIAL PERIOD   One of the most effective ways to boost the closing process is to offer a free trial period so you can show the physician how your service can help. This advantage of a trial period is that it provides you with a way to get your foot in the door. You can then size up the practice, determine how many claims it may get per week, and modify your bid accordingly. For instance, the average family practice doctor has about 400 claims per month. (He or she sees approximately 30 patients each day, with 10 paying cash and 20 having insurance claims to file. Hence, 20 claims per day times 20 working days per month = 400 claims.) This also means that when you work with a family practice doctor, you will probably need to pick up the superbills daily or have them faxed to you for processing once per day or at least every other day. This increases your time. On the other hand, the number of claims you receive from many specialists may be small, so that you need to pick up superbills only once a week. This reduces your commuting time, and perhaps your processing time.

In sum, you get a chance to evaluate the complexity of your work when you offer a free trial period. You can decide if this practice requires extra time, if the staff is well organized and efficient, giving you complete data immediately, or if the work is going to be chaotic. Each practice's claim volume will differ as well, affecting how you retrieve the superbills.

A free trial period is also valuable because you can increase your knowledge of many different practices. For example, some specialties such as chiropractors, psychologists, and physical therapists have many repeat patient visits, so it is easy for you to do the claims. In contrast, surgical offices usually do not have repeat patients, so the amount of work you need to do for such offices is greater. Similarly, some practices, including psychologists, record several office visits on one claim form, so this work is easy. Other practices want only one office visit per claim, so again, you will have a lot of keyboarding to do.

Some billing agencies offer to do a trial period limited to one week or a specific number of claims such as 50, while charging for anything above that number. This strategy allows them to sign a contract immediately for a period of one or two months, because you convince the doctor that he or she can save money by taking some free claims right now in exchange for signing a longer-term contract that can be canceled if he or she is dissatisfied. As in many types of businesses, people tend not to annul contracts once they are written.

Overcoming Common Start-up Problems

It isn't surprising that every business has some common start-up problems that can prevent you from succeeding if you don't resolve them within six months. Following is a brief review of those problems that seem to plague medical billing businesses. By reading about them now, before you are in business, you can take steps to avoid them lest they happen to you.

COMPUTER GLITCHES AND SOFTWARE PROBLEMS Don't wait until you are in business to discover computer or software problems. Make sure you know what you are doing before a doctor is relying on you to process claims and track his or her accounts receivable. However, don't focus on learning your medical software to get into the business; you must also learn the medical industry basics and marketing principles discussed in this chapter. Knowing how to use software doesn't get you clients.

LOW DIRECT MAIL RESPONSE RATES   Many people have high expectations when they send out direct mail, but typically a 1 percent to 3 percent response rate is about all you can expect. This means if you send out 500 letters, don't expect more than about 15 call-backs. However, if you get fewer responses, consider redesigning your brochure or letter. Get someone to help you, and test it before another mailing by showing it to at least six people for reactions.

SLOW BUILD-UP OF CLIENTELE   Many of the billing services I spoke with told me that getting their first client took as many as six months, but after signing their first doctor, they quickly signed another few and more over time. You should definitely have enough savings to keep going at least 12 months. As this chapter has warned, marketing is the toughest part of this business.

MARKET RESISTANCE   You may find resistance to your services for a variety of reasons. If so, assess if you have tried a wide enough variety of doctors, and are you doing everything you can to build trust with your customers?

One point of resistance is that doctors may tell you that they already have computers in house; if you hear this response, don't fail to ask, "Yes, but are you doing electronic billing, including Medicare and commercial carriers?" Also ask whether the prospective client has a high turnover rate among staff so that he or she is training people frequently and losing money on lost claims. These questions point to issues frequently neglected by physicians—and they help reinforce the service you can provide.

As you can see, you should be prepared to allay many concerns that physicians read about and hear every day from colleagues. Convincing a physician to use your outside service is possible if you focus on the four Cs:

- **Complexity.** Since insurance reimbursement and medical coding change frequently, why burden a staff person with keeping up on this never-ending struggle when *you* are an expert in it? You can stay abreast of changes and reduce errors and mistakes.

- **Cost.** In the long run, it almost always costs more to have a salaried worker do billing than an outside expert agency that can increase reimbursement efficiency.

- **Consistency.** You can provide round-the-clock coverage in a more consistent manner than a staff that is subject to constant turnover or is occupied with other office duties.

■ **Competition.** In today's competitive managed care world, everyone in the medical profession is feeling the pinch. Because of your expertise, you can help doctors compete more effectively against HMOs and other arrangements that are cutting physician salaries and independence.

If you take the four Cs and put them together with the four Ps of marketing (price, product, place, and promotion), you get the four PCs, a good mnemonic device to remember the basic guidelines in marketing for a medical billing business.

LOW PROFITABILITY   If low profitability is your problem, you may not have done enough homework to calculate your fees in your favor. As mentioned earlier, it is better not to face this problem, but if you do have it, you need to find new clients immediately, with whom you can charge a higher rate. Although getting your first client by offering a low rate may have worked at that time, you cannot make a living by charging too little.

Alternatively, try to sign these current clients into purchasing additional services from you at higher fees, such as having you work into full practice management so you can move into charging on a percentage basis.

TURNOVER IN CLIENTELE   It is wise to ask clients to sign a contract with you for a year at a time. This minimizes client turnover and gives you 12 months to prove yourself. Even if you make one mistake, you have time to correct it, apologize, and perhaps do something special for the client to convey that you value his or her business and want to keep it.

Building Your Business

Several business opportunity companies I interviewed told me that they see many people purchase the medical billing software package and months later, they have done nothing with it. For such people, the idea of purchasing a business venture was promising, but they did not have the motivation and knowledge to get the business off the ground.

Remember this as you consider medical billing. As in romance, there is a thrill in the chase, but if you spend the time and money to get into the business, you should be prepared to live with your business for a few years. One common mistake made by too many entrepreneurs is thinking and acting for the short term.

Medical billing services are here to stay, though the business may change as new technologies come to fruition and as new managed care arrangements and Medicare regulations move the industry in increasingly cost-saving directions. But if you are getting into this business, stay abreast of these changes and look to a bright future!

CHAPTER 3

Claims Assistance Professional

Do you believe in helping the little guy? Does your hair stand on end when you hear about undue and unfair hardships and corporate injustice? Do you enjoy verbal sparring with a worthy opponent? Do you like to nitpick and find mistakes? Do you feel drawn to helping others fight "the system"?

If your answer is Yes to these questions, then being a medical claims assistance professional (CAP) may be the right career for you. As mentioned earlier, claims assistance professionals work for people (not doctors) who are consumers of medical services. Their primary role is to help people organize, file, and negotiate health claims of all kinds. Like tax assistants or personal business consultants, their job is to ensure that the consumers get the maximum benefits and the best possible services from their medical providers and from their insurance companies.

This chapter explores the business of a claims professional, explains the necessary background and preparation for this career, and details the many ways you can conduct and market this valuable service. (Note: if you didn't read Chapter 2 on medical billing, it may be useful to do so now, since that chapter covers many basic issues that are pertinent here, especially the sections on the health insurance industry, Medicare, and Medicaid.)

Section I: Background

What Is a Claims Assistance Professional?

Anyone who has ever read a health insurance policy or who has waited months for a reimbursement check to come through knows firsthand the frustration and confusion that can overwhelm even the brightest individual when it comes to dealing with our complex healthcare system. With thousands of different health insurance carriers in the United States offering nearly 10,000 different types of plans, it's easy to see how consumers can feel totally baffled whenever they have to deal with health insurance claims.

Today's world is especially complicated when it comes to healthcare. First, there are millions of people who have joined or been assigned to a managed care program, but they cannot figure out how much to pay and to whom to pay it. There are many cases of spouses who both work but each has a different health plan. There are situations in which one spouse is retired and on Medicare while the other still works and is covered by an employer health plan. These scenarios depict the complexity of health coverage for millions of people when it comes to filing health insurance claims.

Enter, however, the claims assistance professional who knows health insurance rules and policies inside out, who has the exact phone numbers for all the local Medicare and insurance company offices right at the tip of his or her tongue or Rolodex, and who fears not when it comes to arguing with doctors or insurance claims adjusters. Such people are, in effect, a combination of professional consultant, personal advisor and representative, and hard-core negotiator, wearing each of these hats in turn as they help ordinary mortals through the thick and thin of dealing with their health insurance nightmares.

The CAP profession seems to have actually come into its maturity just in the past few years. Much of the impetus for its rise is due to the burgeoning enrollments in Medicare and the growing complexity of the program, as you saw in Chapter 1. A major indication of the growth of the CAP career is the fact that a national association was formed in 1991 to formalize the profession and give it some respect and clout. Called the National Association of Claims Assistance Professionals, Inc. (NACAP), the organization helped to solidify the industry and bring together over 1000 claims assistance professionals from across the country. Unfortunately, just as this new edition of this book was going to press, the two leaders of this private association withdrew and it went out of business until new leadership emerges. At this time, Lori A. Donnelly, a CAP in Bethlehem, Pennsylvania, has agreed to help develop a new association from interested parties. You will find information on contacting her later in this chapter.

Despite the temporary loss of an official NACAP organization, the CAP profession still stands strong. As the former NACAP National Director Norma Border told me, the need for claims assistance professionals doesn't appear to be changing.

The success of NACAP speaks strongly for the growing importance of this profession. Border pointed out, for example, that insurance regulations are constantly changing, and so some part of her job is to stay abreast of the political happenings in Washington, D.C., so that the association can keep tabs on congressional hearings dealing with the insurance industry—and even lobby when necessary to support its interests. In addition, one might surmise that the growth of the profession reflects serious social and political healthcare policy issues in this country, because so much is at stake when it comes to health insurance. For example, at this writing, Congress and President Clinton were implementing the new legislation that will take effect in 1997 that allows for "portability" of health insurance to protect people who change jobs.

Border completely supported the idea presented in Chapter 2 that today's managed care environment is changing a great deal in the healthcare industry, not just for doctors, but for consumers, too. She told me,

> The newest thing for CAPs is managed care. Some CAPs ask me, "If we are moving to a managed care environment, or what seems to be a claimless environment, is there anything left for a CAP to do?" The answer is most definitely *yes*. Anytime the insurance industry establishes a gatekeeper and sets up procedures for consumers to get care, there's a need for CAPs. The consumer needs an advocate to make sure that the paperwork is processed properly and that the physician services are provided at an optimal level.

Border added, for example, that her mother recently had a knee replacement, and her orthopedic surgeon never completed the insurance form, leaving her mother with a bill for $16,000. This is the type of situation that calls for a CAP.

It is now absolutely certain that becoming a claims assistance professional is a viable career. As Harvey Matoren, owner of Claims Security of America (formerly Health Claims of Jacksonville, Inc.) and, ironically, a former insurance company senior executive himself, explained to me,

> Nobody is out there to fend for the average [health insurance] consumer. There are lots of people to protect the interests of the insurance companies, hospitals, physicians, and other healthcare providers, but when it comes to recovering what is due to the average person, most people can't maximize their reimbursements and so they live under tremendous frustration and stress.

Let's turn our attention now to see how the claims assistance professional can help, and what people in this profession do day by day.

Whom Do CAPs Help?

CAPs may help anyone and everyone who has health insurance and files claims. As Chapter 1 pointed out, this means that your client base includes more than 220 million people who are covered by private or public health insurance. More important, each one of these people sees a doctor an average of six times per year. In fact, in 1993 (the latest statistic available) there were more than 1.6 billion physician contacts in the United States. Go back and review Table 1-3 on page 7, which breaks down physician contacts by age and sex. Notice that women see doctors more frequently than men in most age categories, except over age 65, when men—probably because they failed to see doctors more often at younger ages—surpass women!

Another interesting set of statistics is shown in Table 3-1. While the data are from 1991 and are the most recent available, the table demonstrates the huge number of office visits that Americans make to physicians each year: a total of nearly 670 million.

But why does this cause a need for claims assistance professionals? The answer is, processing health insurance claims is prone to a significantly high error rate. Errors can be made at the insurance company, at the doctor's office, or at the hospital—and these errors create havoc for consumers. Claims to insurance companies can be erroneously denied, delayed, or underpaid, leaving the consumer with an incorrect balance due the physi-

TABLE 3-1

Number of Office Visits by Physician Specialty—1991

Specialty	Number of Visits (in millions)
All visits	669,689
General and family practice	164,857
Internal medicine	102,923
Pediatrics	74,646
Obstetrics and gynecology	56,834
Ophthalmology	41,207
Orthopedic surgery	35,932
Dermatology	29,659
General surgery	21,285
Otolaryngology	19,101
Psychiatry	15,720
Urological surgery	12,758
Cardiovascular diseases	11,629
Neurology	6,798
All other specialties	76,341

Source: U.S. Department of Health and Human Services, National Center for Health Statistics, Advance Data, 1993.

cian. Although they write the policies and program the computers, insurance companies often make mistakes in the amount of a patient's deductible, copayments, or stop-loss limit. Physicians too make mistakes. They may bill patients for amounts that the primary insurance carrier should have paid. They may bill patients for amounts that secondary insurance coverage should have paid. They may even double bill patients for amounts that a primary or secondary insurance carrier already paid. As a result, consumers must be ever-watchful of each and every claim they generate.

There are also many people who want nothing to do with their insurance claims. Such people know they cannot possibly keep up with the "fine print" in their health insurance policy. They hire CAPs to avoid the dirty work of checking claims and arguing with doctors, insurance adjusters, and hospital administrative staff.

To categorize the types of people or situations a CAP can help, I have developed the following profiles.

THE LAZY SELF-FILER   Many doctors simply refuse to file non-Medicare claims, and so millions of patients end up filing themselves—after they've paid their doctor or dentist—using traditional paper forms and receipts. When they sit down to do this though, many people are simply put off by the technicality of the work and would prefer to have someone do it for them. Particularly if they have an extended illness and end up with many bills over time, these people suddenly realize that they have paid hundreds or thousands of dollars out-of-pocket, and so they look to a claims assistance professional to get them out of the jam.

THE MANAGED CARE PATIENT   A growing problem in today's managed care environment is that many HMOs are newly established, and they literally don't know what they are doing. According to Lori Donnelly, a CAP in Pennsylvania, many HMOs are so new that they haven't worked through their own procedures and are not able to provide the consumer with consistent explanations of what's approved and what's not. Remember also that an HMO or PPO may be comprised of many affiliated doctors, and the coverages can vary from policy to policy. In short, despite its supposed simplicity, managed care generates its share of billing mistakes.

THE "NOT-AUTHORIZED" CLAIM   Sarah Bissel went to her primary care physician for a stomach problem. He recommended that she see a gastrointestinal specialist if her pain persisted for more than another day. However, Sarah forgot to call the primary care physician to approve the referral when she went to the specialist the next day. When the claim was filed, the insurance company refused to pay it, claiming that approval had not been given. Sarah hired a CAP who was able to straighten out the situation with a few phone calls.

THE SHIRKING DOCTOR PASSES THE BUCK   Kyle Assad recently saw his physician for a strep culture. The physician's billing clerk told Kyle that his office would handle the insurance claim. However, two weeks later, Kyle received a bill in the mail. He called the doctor's office and they assured him they would take care of the insurance claim. A few more weeks went by, and Kyle received another bill. Finally, he contacted his CAP who called the doctor's office and reminded them that they had agreed to take responsibility for processing the claim. Kyle was finally left in peace.

THE FLUSTERED VICTIM OF LEGALESE   Roberta Stevenson can't stand paperwork. Give her a contract or any document with legal jargon and her mind turns right off. It's not that Roberta isn't bright; she simply can't follow the formal legal terminology and sentence structure typically used in insurance documents. Roberta would simply prefer to hand over her claims to a CAP, who has the expertise needed to understand the policy and know what is and is not covered.

THE BUSY FAMILY   John and Jane Adams and their two teenagers never have any leisure time. The Adamses, who both work, come home from the office early in the evening and immediately get involved in dozens of projects, from shuttling the kids to ballet rehearsals and baseball games to fixing the kitchen sink and planting the spring garden. The result of their busy lifestyle is that whenever a member of the family visits the doctor, Mr. and Mrs. Adams have no time left to fill in the claims and file them. When there is a problem on a claim, they also don't have a moment to spare to make phone calls back and forth to their doctor's office and insurance company to clarify the issue. For many families like the Adamses, paying a small fee to have a professional handle claims work simply makes life more enjoyable.

THE MIXED INSURANCE FAMILY   Al Smith works for a local manufacturer and has a family health insurance policy through his employer. His wife Sally also works, and her health insurance plan, which acts as her secondary coverage, is supposed to pay any copayments she owes after her husband's family plan pays out the primary benefits. However, some recent medical bills have totally confused the family about which insurance company is going to pay for what—and why neither wants to pay one of the charges. The mixed insurance family is an excellent candidate for a claims assistance professional.

THE MULTIPLE INSURANCE INDIVIDUAL   Arnold Pimler believes in health insurance. Over the years, he has collected and/or purchased five different policies. When he finally became ill with cancer and had an extended hospitalization, he left it to a CAP to figure out who should pay what to whom.

THE RETIRED LIFERS   Jack and Bobbie Mormin recently retired to a Sun Belt state to enjoy some peace and quiet, and a bit of golf. While they do not have any major medical ailments, they prefer to spend not a drop of their time thinking about their health insurance policies. So they hire a CAP service to handle whatever comes their way each year for a small fee.

THE CHILD OF AN AGING PARENT   Maggie O'Brien's 78-year old mother recently had surgery and required several thousands of dollars in follow-up treatment and physical therapy. Little did the mother know that her Medicare and Medigap insurance policies did not cover all the procedures, and now Maggie is stuck with trying to figure out how to maximize their reimbursements and minimize their out-of-pocket payments. Unfortunately, Maggie works at a demanding job and has little time to make phone calls to the insurance company or to Medicare. She loves her mother but does not really want this problem dumped in her lap, so she hires a claims assistance professional.

THE CRISIS FAMILY   Tragically, 52-year-old Alan Roberts has a terminal illness, and his family is spending every waking minute trying to comfort their loved one through the ordeal. Meanwhile, the medical bills keep mounting, and some health claims sent to Mr. Roberts's insurance company are being denied or rejected for unexplained reasons. This family realizes that there are more important things in life at the moment, and so they hear through word of mouth about a claims assistance professional in their area who can handle their problems. The family can now live in peace and be with their loved one, while the CAP ensures they get what they deserve from their insurance policy.

THE CAUGHT-IN-THE-MIDDLE SITUATION   Mike Loring recently went to his doctor twice in one week for a bad cold, and while he was there, he also received a chest X-ray and blood test from the lab next door. He paid all four charges (two doctors' visits and two tests) in cash, since the physician and lab preferred to have the money immediately and insisted that Mike deal with his own insurance company. However, when Mike filed the claims amounting to $300, his insurance company said that the diagnostic codes were missing from his receipts, and that the procedures didn't match. Mike started to make the phone calls to straighten out the situation, but eventually he became fed up with the runaround he was getting; he simply wanted his 80 percent of $300 back. He called a local CAP and signed up immediately to have the claims pursued on his behalf.

THE MEDICARE SQUEEZE   Norman Fields, a 72-year-old retired teacher, recently fell off a ladder while painting his house one summer day. He suffered a broken arm and numerous minor injuries that required a brief hospitalization followed by repeated physical therapy treatments. Unfortunately, his slew of claims was only partially paid by Medicare, with many claims being downcoded from what the doctors had billed. He also began receiving invoices from his doctor for amounts of money that he thought were greater than the allowable amounts. When Norman contacted a CAP, he learned that the doctor was erroneously billing him for amounts beyond the "allowable"—amounts that he was not supposed to charge patients.

THE COBRA LURCH (COBRA is a nationally mandated law that became effective in 1986 to cover certain qualified people who had group insurance but lost their coverage through job loss, divorce, death of a spouse, unemployment, or reduction in working hours. When such situations occur, a qualified person is allowed to convert his or her group insurance into an individual policy, paying monthly premiums for up to 18 months. This situation, however, sometimes engenders the following circumstance.)

Rochelle Williams was covered by a COBRA policy. She dutifully mailed her monthly premium check to the insurance company so that her account would remain current. One month, however, after she had seen her doctor, she began receiving calls from the doctor's office to pay the bill because her insurance had been rejected. After hiring a CAP to check the situation for her, it turned out that the insurance company was taking several weeks to credit her COBRA insurance with her monthly checks. It refused to pay Rochelle's claims because the computer showed her as being canceled from the group policy and delinquent in her COBRA payments. The problem was entirely the fault of the insurance company.

THE EXPERIMENTAL PROCEDURE CLAIM Ruth Kress was diagnosed with a rare blood disease in the early part of the year. Fortunately, her best friend recommended a wonderful doctor who was using a somewhat new treatment for this blood disease; this treatment was, however, an accepted treatment for another disease. Ruth was miraculously cured, but now her insurance company denied the $25,000 in claims, claiming that the treatments were "experimental" and were therefore not covered under her policy. Ruth used a CAP to negotiate the case and was able to get the majority of the claims paid.

THE BUREAUCRATIC RUNAROUND Glenda Peterson incurred $30,000 in medical bills over the past year due to a serious illness. They were all rejected by her insurance company, and in frustration she hired a claims assistance company to work on her behalf. When the company took over, it learned that several simple errors had been made and that by resubmitting the claims with new diagnostic codes, the claims would be paid. The problem was that no one at the insurance company had the courtesy to tell Glenda that all she had to do was to reprocess the claims with the errors corrected.

THE INTIMIDATED VICTIM   Randy Bern hates to argue. Although he knows that his insurance company made a simple and obvious mistake on a recently submitted claim for $860, he feels that he must "convince" the person with whom he spoke about this error. Unfortunately, Randy was speaking with a supervisor, who growled and howled at him. The supervisor insisted that "Mr. Bern doesn't understand company policy." Mr. Bern felt burned, and so he contacted a claims professional who wasn't afraid to put the supervisor into her proper place.

Saving Your Clients More Than Just Money

The preceding scenarios are indicative of the kinds of situations people get into when dealing with our health insurance system. In each case, an experienced, knowledgeable, efficient medical claims assistance professional can provide valuable services. Foremost is getting the reimbursement money from the insurance company for fees the client may have already paid to a doctor, or which the client owes the doctor who graciously awaits the reimbursement. But more than this financial role, claims assistance professionals also provide the following important services:

■ **Eliminate stress.** CAPs remove a tremendous amount of stress most people experience when dealing with intimidating bureaucratic organizations. From the lunch-hour calls when the insurance clerk puts you on hold for 20 minutes, to the frantic trips to the doctor's office to get your claim form signed, most people feel like they are unwitting victims in a Kafka-esque nightmare over which they have no control. And worse, the stress can be unhealthy for some people, particularly the elderly. As Mary Ellen Fitzgibbons, a CAP in Chicago related to me, "I have one client who says she feels like she's going to have a heart attack whenever she speaks with her insurance company. She gets so emotionally upset, she just can't do it by herself."

- **Save people money.** Many people mistakenly pay providers before Medicare or their insurance company reimburses the provider, and so the burden is on the patient to recover his or her money, which can take weeks. Even when a physician or hospital provides assistance to patients for their health claims, it is a self-interested service, usually limited in scope to reviewing claims for services only it has provided. For example, some hospitals offer clinics to senior citizens to teach them how to handle their own health insurance claims, but these people are often too old or too sick to handle the balance of the required work.

- **Save people time.** The average consumer knows little about navigating through the channels of the insurance industry and can spend hours and hours to take care of a situation that a claims professional could handle in 30 minutes. But time is money today; many people would rather pay someone $20 or $50 if it saves them a few hundred dollars and their valuable time.

- **Save people embarrassment.** When a foul-up occurs, many doctors' offices will turn a bill over to a collection agency. Suddenly, the consumer finds himself or herself getting dunning notices, and perhaps even has a negative report made to his or her credit record. I had this happen to my family recently. My wife had a series of about six charges, each for $80.00, for blood tests from a laboratory to which she was sent by her allergy clinic. We thought we had paid all 6 bills; none ever came in the mail. One day, we started getting dunning notices from a collection agency for $80.00. We called the lab and were told everything was paid. Eventually though, as we continued to get dunning notices, we discovered that one of the payments was erroneously recorded to another doctor in the allergy clinic, and that the laboratory had also misdated the invoice, calling it a "post-test" result instead of a "pre-test" result, thereby confusing two claims. In the end, I had no way of knowing that all the confusion was happening behind the scenes, and that we did owe one bill for $80.00, but my credit received a black mark. I would have gladly handed this problem over to a claims professional!

- **Help people in time of crisis.** CAPs preserve family priorities and help people in times of need and crisis. Many families today find themselves responsible for the healthcare of their aging parents. For them, spending a few dollars is much less important than being with their family and being sure they can devote their attention where it is most needed. CAP Lori Donnelly also notes that many times people going through a divorce utilize a claims professional to avoid seeing the ex-spouse and to help deal with the sticky financial arrangements that their divorce engendered.

■ **Maximize investment in health insurance.** The majority of people don't know what to expect when it comes to health insurance reimbursements. Consequently, they have no protection against mistakes, errors, delays, and even intentional malfeasance on the part of an insurance company. In fact, among health insurance insiders, few doubt that most insurance companies intentionally delay claims payments, or give people the runaround when they don't want to pay a claim to preserve their own cash flow. Every CAP I spoke with had quite a few horror stories to tell about people who had lost money because of a minor error or a simple mistake on their claims. Harvey Matoren of Claims Security of America had one client who had more than $60,000 of bills rejected by her insurance company. When Harvey looked into it, he discovered that the claims had been submitted under the wrong component of her insurance policy, but no one at the insurance office had bothered to tell the woman to send the claims in the name of the other component—Major Medical—under which they would have been accepted and paid. Harvey easily got 90 percent ($54,000) back for the client. As ludicrous as this sounds, Harvey and many others I spoke to indicated that such intentional mistakes happen all the time.

■ **Advise about health insurance matters.** CAPs often informally consult with people to help them decide which health insurance policies to purchase, especially when it comes to Medigap policies. Note: in some states, this will be considered insurance brokering, and since claims professionals are not technically allowed to do this, you need to be careful about how you phrase your recommendations. Many CAPs therefore discuss insurance with their clients only by offering to give a "personal opinion" rather than a "professional" one. But their suggestions do help the average consumer understand health insurance.

■ **Provide a service to physicians and hospitals.** Many CAPs help doctors and hospitals in a very concrete way. This occurs when a patient owes money to a physician or hospital, but the person expects it to be magically paid by the insurance company, forgetting that he or she also owes a copayment or a deductible. The CAP can therefore clarify the billing for such patients, allowing doctors and hospital billing departments to get their money faster.

Business Profile: Barbara Melman

Barbara Melman is perhaps one of the originators of the CAP business. Her company Claim Relief, Inc., in Chicago has been operating since 1984. Barbara spent many years as an insurance adjuster and noticed the need for this service in the early 1980s when she realized that people did not know how to submit claims to her company.

Since that time, Barbara has turned her CAP business into a well-known Chicago story. She writes a weekly Sunday column for the *Chicago Sun-Times* to answer questions people send her about their health insurance problems. (See Figure 3-1 for a sample column.) Barbara believes that the health insurance problems of yesteryear pale in comparison to today's problems. As she sarcastically points out,

> Before, you could submit a claim and if it was done correctly, an insurance company would pay. Today, however, even if a claim is correct, you have to argue about everything with insurers. In my view, insurance companies simply do not want to pay most claims, especially those that are expensive or are ongoing.

Barbara gave an example. She was working with the family of a four-year-old child who was born with many birth defects. She was hired because the insurance company stopped paying the child's claims. In the child's early years, the insurer paid most of the child's therapies; one day, however, it simply stopped paying the claims, demanding more documentation as if the situation were a new one. The family became annoyed: the more details that were sent in, the more the insurer demanded. That's when the family contacted Barbara, who was able to straighten out the situation and get the claims paid again.

Because of Barbara's reputation, most of her clients come from word of mouth, although she also maintains good relations with financial advisors who hire her on behalf of their clients. Barbara now has hundreds of active clients, and she can count total clients in the thousands. She employs two people to help her with the claims. Nevertheless, Barbara is still home-based. She charges clients on an hourly basis (currently $45 per hour) but she bills in half-hour increments. Much of her work is focused on appeals of denied claims, but she also handles the filing of many secondary claims that are not done electronically, and claims for catastrophic coverage. Her clientele is mixed, although Barbara sees it changing. It used to be mostly seniors but she now has more and more people with private insurance who she says have it the worst because commercial insurers are not paying.

Barbara's advice for people thinking about the CAP business is: "You need a good grounding in insurance and how it works. You also need to be willing to do whatever it takes to get claims paid that are being denied."

Figure 3-1

Sample newspaper column for a CAP by Barbara Melman. Reproduced with permission.

HEALTH & FITNESS

Insurance Co. Claims It Just Doesn't Get It

Q. *I have submitted my insurance claim two times to my insurance company and for the second time they have told me they do not have it. What should I do at this point to get my claims paid?*

A. Unfortunately this happens all too often. Let me give you a couple of options. Call your insurance company and ask for a supervisor and explain the situation. Ask if you can fax or send the claims directly to him or her marked "personal and confidential." Another option is to send your claims via registered mail with a return receipt requested. Always make copies of your claims.

Q. *I will be turning 65 shortly and have been flooded with Medicare supplement information. How can I be sure I am making the right decision when all the plans appear to be the same?*

A. It is very confusing because all of the companies must offer you the same plans (A through J). However, not all companies offer all of the plans to you. If you want a prescription drug benefit, you must choose the companies that make this benefit available (plans H, I or J). If you do not think you need a drug benefit, look at plans A thru G and choose the company with the most affordable premium, as the benefits are all the same. Also, be aware that if you are unsatisfied or next year another company offers a lower premium you can switch with no penalty of any kind.

Q. *My father passed away in January, and his insurance was paid up until March. Do I have to wait until all of his bills are paid before we can advise the company of his death?*

A. Your father's insurance was active until the date of his death. You are entitled to a premium refund for any premium paid after that date. Send the insurance company a copy of the death certificate and a short note advising where to return the excess premium. All of his claims will continue to be processed until they are concluded.

Q. *I am three months pregnant with my first child, and some* of my friends tell me their medical insurance covers their well baby care, and others have said theirs does not. Can you explain the discrepancy?

A. I have never understood why insurance carriers would not cover well baby care when it makes sense to protect against a condition before it starts. It certainly would seem cost-efficient. Many companies cover these services, many still do not. If you will be obtaining new insurance after the baby's birth, try to find a plan that does provide this benefit as check-

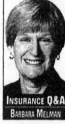

INSURANCE Q&A
BARBARA MELMAN

ups and shots can be very costly. Check with your current carrier to see if this is a benefit of the plan you now carry.

Q. *I am very upset over a denial of a medically necessary surgical procedure I had done a few months ago. I have submitted additional information to my company, but they denied the claim again. What recourse, if any, do I have?*

A. You sound like a fighter, and that's a very important factor. Write the insurance commission of your state (in Illinois the address is Illinois Department of Insurance, 320 W. Washington, Springfield, Ill. 62767) and send it all the data pertaining to your claim and the denial. The commission will conduct a review with your insurance company and contact you.

An exception is if your coverage is carried through a self-insured group; then you would go directly to your employer for the review.

Barbara Melman is president of Claim Relief, a Chicago company that helps people with health insurance problems. Write to her at the Chicago Sun-Times, Sunday Health & Fitness, 401 N. Wabash, Suite 400, Chicago 60611.

The Life of a CAP

The day-to-day life of many CAPs I interviewed was invariably hectic. These claims assistance professionals operated full time and indicated that they had 300 or more active customers (i.e., people who contacted them at least once over the course of a year). It was not surprising to hear of 10-hour days, spent doing the following:

Typical Duties	Time Spent (hours)
Taking phone calls or in-person meetings from current customers	3.5
Making phone calls to insurance carriers and doctors	1.5
Filling out claims forms and writing appeals	2
Reading professional materials and insurance policies	1
Marketing (phone calls or in-person meetings with potential new clients)	1
Opening mail and filing	1

As you can see, much of the time is taken up by phone calls or in-person contact with clients and insurance companies.

For simplicity, the actual claims work a CAP performs can be divided into five common types of activities:

- Filing primary claims to insurers
- Filing secondary claims to insurers
- Reviewing Explanation of Benefits (EOBs) letters for clients
- Filing appeals of disputed or denied claims to insurers
- Filing appeals of disputed bills to a doctor's office

FILING PRIMARY CLAIMS Because many patients must file their own claims, the CAP obtains a copy of the superbill or receipt that the patient has from the doctor's office, indicating the diagnosis and the fees charged. The CAP must then fill out a paper HCFA 1500 claim form, photocopy the superbill, and send it via mail to the insurer. If all works well, the claim will be paid by the insurer.

FILING SECONDARY CLAIMS Many people purchase a private secondary insurance policy to pay their deductibles, copayments, and any noncovered healthcare services. However, most such private secondary insurance claims must be filed on paper because the secondary insurer needs to see a copy of the EOB showing how much the primary carrier paid. (This is becoming less true for Medigap secondary insurance, which is increasingly handled electronically directly from Medicare after the primary Medicare claim is filed and paid. However, in general, it is still common for private secondary insurance not to be processed electronically; a paper claim is generally required.)

In such secondary situations, the CAP must therefore obtain from the patient a copy of the original superbill plus the primary insurer's EOB. The CAP must then file a paper HCFA 1500 via mail to the secondary insurance company along with the photocopies. If all works well, the claim will be paid by the insurer.

REVIEWING EOBs For each claim filed, Medicare or the private insurance carrier issues an EOB to the patient listing the amount charged by the doctor, the amount approved, and the amount paid. Despite computerization, a CAP reviews all the EOBs for each client to make sure that the claim was processed correctly and contains no errors that can cost the patient.

FILING APPEALS This step derives directly from the review of EOBs. As indicated earlier, insurance companies and Medicare process many claims incorrectly, resulting in a mistake that can cost the patient. The claim may be denied, underpaid, overpaid, or delayed. A large portion of a CAP business therefore involves detecting the errors and filing an appeal to the insurer to get the claim reconsidered and paid.

FILING APPEALS TO DOCTORS Errors can also occur in bills that patients receive from their doctors. A CAP must therefore review every doctor's bill and make sure that any amounts charged match up with real charges as well as any payments that have been made. It often happens that a doctor's bill has not credited the patient for an insurance payment made, or has double billed the patient although the insurance company has paid.

We'll review more details about how to detect errors in EOBs and file appeals later in the chapter.

Business Profile: Tom and Nancy Koehler

When Nancy Koehler, a social worker with a variety of work experiences, met a woman in 1986 who was doing medical claims assistance, she was curious about the profession but didn't do anything about it. A year later, when her friend showed up one morning, excited about her upcoming retirement, but worried about the capabilities of the person to whom she was thinking of selling her business, Nancy suddenly realized that an opportunity was knocking at her door. Her friend agreed to cancel the other sale, and Nancy found herself with a new venture in life: In Home Medical Claims, of Poway, California.

Business was slow at first, but Nancy loved the job and the feeling of helping others. Her enthusiasm was so unbounding, in fact, that her husband Tom, a former Navy fighter pilot for 20 years, came home one day and decided to quit his job as a project manager for a Defense Department manufacturer of navigation systems. Never imagining that one day they would find themselves working together, Tom and Nancy slowly recognized they had the perfect complement of skills to make their business work. With her medical background, Nancy brings a solid understanding of Medicare and the claims business, which Tom has now learned too. With his project management background, Tom takes charge of their business planning and handles what he aptly calls the P&L responsibility for their business. He uses a Casio digital diary to keep track of their daily appointments, and an "oldish" personal computer with various programs such as *Timeslips* to keep track of their clients and do their monthly invoicing.

In business now for 10 years, Nancy and Tom have several hundred clients for whom they regularly handle medical claims assistance, mostly focusing on the elderly Medicare subscribers who live in their upper-middle-class southern California region. Tom and Nancy were fortunate to get their first client at a large apartment complex. That person then referred many others to them, and today, nearly every one of their clients comes from referrals. Tom and Nancy do practically no marketing, except for occasional speaking engagements Nancy takes on as a noted Medicare expert.

Tom admits,

> What makes our business great is the demographics here. But we also did our homework. We took several workshops from the Small Business Administration (SBA) on marketing and business planning, and Nancy also went to SCORE (Service Corps of Retired Executives) for some advice and managed to get a former Blue Cross executive from Michigan who had retired here as her mentor. Our operation is sophisticated but simple. We limit the number of clients we cover so we can maintain a quality service and trust, which is one of the most important aspects of this business.

There are two factors that distinguish their CAP business from most others, however. First, as the name of their company, In Home Medical Claims, implies, Tom and Nancy go to their clients, not the other way around. This is a major factor for them, since many of their clients cannot leave their homes easily. Second, Tom and Nancy have naturally evolved their business into handling many financial and personal matters for their elderly clients. The level of trust that their clients have come to place in Tom and Nancy is so great that they have accepted whatever tasks are

(Continued)

Business Profile: Tom and Nancy Koehler (*Continued*)

required, including balancing checkbooks, paying bills, making appointments with lawyers and doctors, and even assuming power of attorney for a few clients who could no longer act in their own behalf.

Because of her expertise in insurance, and the increasing conflicts between Medicare HMOs and patients, Nancy also gets pulled in occasionally to attend meetings on behalf of her elderly clients to protest many new types of healthcare service problems. When I recently met them for an interview, Nancy recounted several long stories about complications that regularly occur among Medicare HMO patients who are denied coverage for services to which they are entitled. In one angry meeting with Medicare officials, Nancy pulled in several professional colleagues to argue in favor of a 90-year-old man who was being threatened with loss of insurance because his doctor wanted him to move to a facility closer to his practice. Nancy helped win the argument, probably preserving the man's life for several years.

Tom and Nancy have become well known in the CAP field and are active members of NACAP. They are excellent models for anyone interested in this profession. Meeting them in person leaves no doubt that here is a couple who have truly found their niche in life: helping other people in any and every way they can.

Knowledge and Skills Needed

Like medical billing services, a CAP deals in depth with the complex rules, vocabulary, and procedures of the health insurance industry and doctors' offices. Also, like medical billers, a CAP must spend enormous time and energy setting up the business and getting clients. Many of the same skills and knowledge base therefore apply to this profession as well. The next part of the chapter is therefore divided into the following five sections:

- Knowledge of health insurance and the claims process
- Knowledge of EOBs and appeals
- Organizational skills
- Knowledge of business, including marketing and sales
- Knowledge of computers and business software

As with medical billing, the more experience you have in any of these areas, particularly in the insurance industry, the easier building your business will be if you are just starting out. For example, if you have worked in a physician's office doing billing, or as an adjuster in a health insurance company, or in a corporate personnel department doing benefits, you will probably have a much easier time getting your business off the ground.

All of the needed skills are learnable, however. The novice will simply need more time or a different entry path into the business, such as working first in a medical office or with an established claims service to build up your background. After reading the following sections and exploring these areas in detail, you might want to do the activity suggested in the previous chapter in which you informally plot your learning curve across the three principal areas of this business: insurance industry knowledge, business skills, and computer literacy. See Chapter 2 for more information about this planning activity.

Knowledge of Insurance and the Claims Process

First and foremost, a claims professional must have a complete understanding of the health insurance business—who the players are; how doctors, hospitals, and insurance companies interact; how claims are processed; and how to read EOBs. Without a sound grounding in these areas, one simply cannot be a "professional." As Tom Koehler of In Home Medical Claims characterizes it, "This profession requires integrative skills; you have to look at EOBs, at the physician's bill, and at all the insurance policies a client has, and put it all together to come out with one conclusion: did the person get paid the right amount?"

As a result, you need to know about items such as the following:

- How to read a health insurance policy (see the sidebar, "Reading an Insurance Policy")

- The terminology commonly used in the health insurance business, such as deductible, out-of-pocket limit, stop-loss limit, coinsurance, allowable amount, limiting charge, excess charge, and so on

- The differences among types of healthcare coverage offered (i.e., basic, major medical, wraparound, catastrophic, cancer)

- The specialized rules covering coordination of benefits (i.e., when a subscriber has more than one policy, such as two working spouses with policies, or children of divorced parents. When this occurs, you must know which policy is considered primary and which is secondary. It depends on whether the insurance company follows the *gender rule* or the *birthday rule*).

- The rules and regulations governing Medicare Parts A and B and Medigap policies

- The major-medical coding systems: ICD-9-CM, CPT, HCPCS, and so on

- The procedures followed by doctors' offices and other types of healthcare providers in billing and accounting for patient charges

- The trends toward managed care and Medicare HMOs, and how they affect consumers

- The various types of fee schedules used to pay physicians, including UCR, capitation, and RBRVS

Much of this information was presented in Chapter 2, so if you have not read it by now, you may wish to review that chapter, particularly the sections on health insurance and Medicare.

Please note especially that understanding medical coding is almost as important for a claims professional as it is for a medical billing service. A claims professional must have an excellent command of these codes (although you won't need to memorize them, since there are thousands) because many claims are rejected or downcoded (i.e., reimbursed at a lower amount) because of incorrect coding, missing modifiers, and wrong location codes. This means that your client may not be reimbursed, or may receive a lower amount than he or she deserves. As you may recall from the previous chapter, there is little doubt that insurance companies, which have a vested interest in minimizing their payouts, are not bending over backward to make sure the patient is properly paid. In short, if you don't know your coding, you cannot protect the interests of your clients.

In addition, staying abreast of Medicare rules and regulations is vital, since a large number of your clients will be the elderly. For example, Medicare has specific exclusions for certain procedures, as well as many limitations on payments. Many Medicare subscribers don't even understand the basic difference between a PAR and NON-PAR provider, so the CAP may need to explain this to help them avoid going to a more expensive doctor or overpaying a disallowed fee. You also need to know the rules to follow when Medicare is not the primary insurance carrier, even for an elderly person. This situation is referred to as MSP—Medicare as Secondary Payer—and can occur when a person over 65 is still working and has an employer group insurance plan. (It can also occur if the person's spouse is still working and the family is covered by that employer, or if the medical services were related to a work injury or automobile accident, in which case Medicare will not pay as primary insurance.) You must also know the changes in Medicare fees each year: the amount of the deductible and copayments for Part A and Part B, as well as the dollar limitations placed on certain services and hospitalizations. And finally, you must also understand the somewhat complex realm of Medigap insurance policies, which many consumers are still confused about, despite the recent federal government regulation that limits them to 10 standard policies.

As you can see, there is quite an extensive array of insurance industry knowledge and inside information that a claims professional must have under his or her belt. If you approach the field as if it were a puzzle though, you will feel challenged by learning it all, rather than frustrated and confused. One piece at a time does it!

Reading an Insurance Policy

As a CAP, you need to become familiar with reading commercial (private) insurance policies. The typical outline for these policies is as shown in Figure 3-2.

Because of space limitations, it is not possible to reproduce a full policy in this book. It is highly recommended that you examine your own policy or one belonging to a friend or relative to gain experience in reading such documents.

Figure 3-2
Outline of a Typical
Insurance Policy

OUTLINE OF A TYPICAL INSURANCE POLICY

I. Schedule of Benefits

II. Eligibility Requirements

    A. Dependent requirements

    B. Termination of coverage

III. Definitions

IV. Covered Expenses

    A. Hospital Expenses

        1. Precertification requirements

    B. Major Medical Expenses

V. Limitations and Exclusions

VI. Coordination of Benefits

    A. Effect of Other Coverage

    B. Effect of Medicare

    C. Effect of Automobile coverage

VII. Continuation of Coverage

    A. COBRA

    B. Conversion

VIII. Claiming Benefits

    A. Time to File Limitations

    B. How to Appeal

    C. ERISA Rights

Knowledge of EOBs and Appeals

Another key skill of a CAP is the ability to look at an EOB (or an EOMB from Medicare) and determine if it contains any errors. Figures 3-3 through 3-6 show samples of a commercial EOB and the three types of Medicare EOMBs.

The fact is, simple errors and screwups occur constantly, and if you are unable to detect them, you cannot do your job.

The types of errors made are truly amazing and include errors due to

- Miscoding of physician services
- Missing information
- Incorrect policy numbers
- Incorrect allowable amounts
- Services never rendered
- Services rendered but not charged
- Downcoding of services
- Denied payments due to lack of authorization

Most people are simply not aware of the errors that may be contained in their EOBs. For example, in researching this book, one elderly woman in a senior center related to me that she once received from Medicare an EOMB indicating that her account was being charged for a hip operation—but she had never had one! It seemed that the wrong Medicare ID number had been used.

Nancy and Tom Koehler related many stories affirming the simplest of errors:

We've seen all types of mistakes. One hospital in this area billed a client for outpatient services, and when we called to ask if it had billed Medicare first, it turned out it hadn't. Another client received a bill for the copayment amount on a Medicare Part B outpatient service, but because he had neglected to tell the hospital that he had supplemental (secondary) insurance, he thought he had to pay the bill himself. We simply told the hospital to forward the bill to the secondary insurance, and it was taken care of. In another case, the doctor billed both our client and the secondary insurance company, and so we made sure the doctor didn't get paid twice. We also have a client who retired from a company in Tennessee that was self-insured, and for some reason, the hospital didn't want to send the bill there. So we helped the client get it taken care of: he paid the 20 percent copayment, and then we made sure the company received the bill and paid it. The client was happy and it saved him a lot of time and stress.

Some situations are much more complex. CAP Mary Ellen Fitzgibbons of Chicago recounted one incident to me in which a hospital made several serious errors in billing Medicare for services rendered for a woman. The problem was, the woman had died, and the secondary insurance

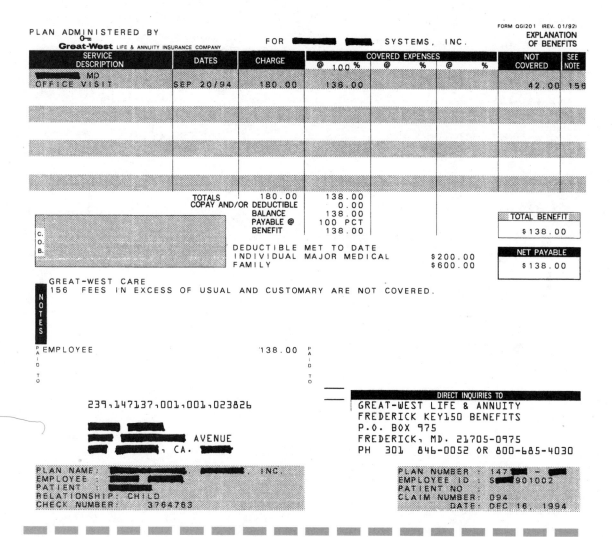

Figure 3-3 A Typical EOB from a Commercial Insurance Company. The doctor's charge was $180, but the insurance company determined that the usual and customary fee should be only $138. That leaves $42 not covered. In this case, the insurance company paid 100% of $138.

U.S DEPARTMENT OF HEALTH AND HUMAN SERVICES/HEALTH CARE FINANCING ADMINISTRATION

MEDICARE BENEFIT NOTICE

DATE 06/24/96

HEALTH INSURANCE CLAIM NUMBER

Always use this number
when writing about your claim

This notice shows what benefits were used by you and the covered services not paid by Medicare for the period shown in item 1. See other side of this form for additional information which may apply to your claim.

1	**SERVICES FURNISHED BY**	**DATE(S)**	**BENEFITS USED**
	HOSPITAL	05/24/96 THRU 06/04/96	11 INPATIENT

2 PAYMENT STATUS

$736.00 WAS APPLIED TO YOUR INPATIENT DEDUCTIBLE.

MEDICARE PAID ALL COVERED SERVICES EXCEPT:
    $736.00 FOR THE INPATIENT DEDUCTIBLE.

IF NO-FAULT INSURANCE, LIABILITY INSURANCE, WORKERS' COMPENSATION, DEPARTMENT OF VETERANS AFFAIRS, OR, IN SOME CASES, A GROUP HEALTH PLAN FOR EMPLOYEES ALSO COVERS THESE SERVICES, A REFUND MAY BE DUE THE MEDICARE PROGRAM. PLEASE CONTACT US IF YOU ARE COVERED BY ANY OF THESE SOURCES. YOU DO NOT HAVE TO CONTACT US TO REPORT A MEDI – CARE SUPPLEMENTAL (MEDIGAP) POLICY.

BLUE CROSS OF CALIFORNIA - MEDICARE
P. O. BOX 70000
VAN NUYS   CA   91470
                        (818)-593-2006

If you have any questions
about this record, call
or write

TELEPHONE NUMBER

FORM HCFA-1533 (3-92)

Figure 3-4 A Medicare Part A EOMB

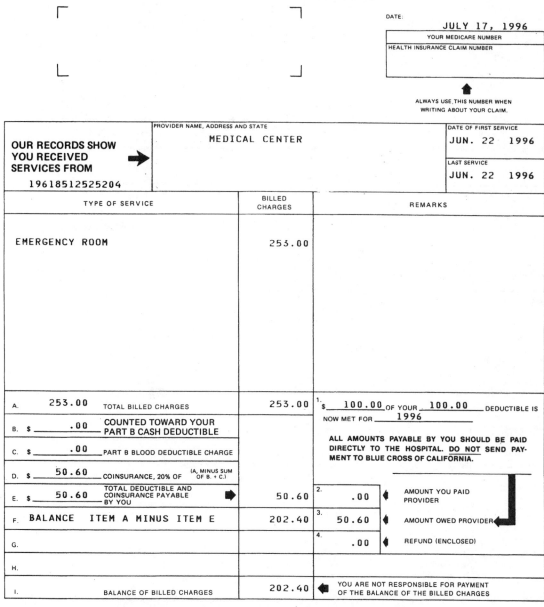

PLEASE READ OTHER SIDE OF THIS NOTICE FOR IMPORTANT INFORMATION

THIS IS NOT A BILL

DATE:
JULY 17, 1996

YOUR MEDICARE NUMBER

HEALTH INSURANCE CLAIM NUMBER

ALWAYS USE THIS NUMBER WHEN
WRITING ABOUT YOUR CLAIM.

OUR RECORDS SHOW YOU RECEIVED SERVICES FROM
19618512525204

PROVIDER NAME, ADDRESS AND STATE
MEDICAL CENTER

DATE OF FIRST SERVICE
JUN. 22 1996

LAST SERVICE
JUN. 22 1996

TYPE OF SERVICE	BILLED CHARGES	REMARKS
EMERGENCY ROOM	253.00	

A. 253.00 TOTAL BILLED CHARGES	253.00	1. $ 100.00 OF YOUR 100.00 DEDUCTIBLE IS NOW MET FOR 1996		
B. $ .00 COUNTED TOWARD YOUR PART B CASH DEDUCTIBLE		ALL AMOUNTS PAYABLE BY YOU SHOULD BE PAID DIRECTLY TO THE HOSPITAL. DO NOT SEND PAYMENT TO BLUE CROSS OF CALIFORNIA.		
C. $ .00 PART B BLOOD DEDUCTIBLE CHARGE				
D. $ 50.60 COINSURANCE, 20% OF (A, MINUS SUM OF B. + C.)				
E. $ 50.60 TOTAL DEDUCTIBLE AND COINSURANCE PAYABLE BY YOU	50.60	2. .00	AMOUNT YOU PAID PROVIDER	
F. BALANCE ITEM A MINUS ITEM E	202.40	3. 50.60	AMOUNT OWED PROVIDER	
G.		4. .00	REFUND (ENCLOSED)	
H.				
I. BALANCE OF BILLED CHARGES	202.40	YOU ARE NOT RESPONSIBLE FOR PAYMENT OF THE BALANCE OF THE BILLED CHARGES		

556 6/95

PLEASE READ OTHER SIDE OF THIS NOTICE FOR IMPORTANT INFORMATION.

Figure 3-5 Medicare Part B, Hospital EOMB

THIS IS NOT A BILL
Explanation of Your Medicare **Part B** Benefits

Summary of this notice dated **February 2, 1996**		
Total charges:	$	72.00
Total Medicare approved:	$	53.81
We paid your provider:	$	0.00
Your total responsibility:	$	53.81

ll.l....l.l...ll.l.ll.l..l.l.ll.....ll..l.l..ll...lll...ll

Your Medicare Number is:

YOUR PROVIDER ACCEPTED ASSIGNMENT

Details about this notice (See the back for more information.)

BILL SUBMITTED BY: MED CORP

Mailing address:

Dates	Services and Service Codes Control Number 96017-4139-12-000	Charges	Medicare Approved	See Notes Below
Jan. 2, 1996	1 Office/outpatient visit, est (99214)	$ 72.00	$ 53.81	a

Notes:

a   The approved amount is based on the fee schedule.

Here's an explanation of this notice:

Of the total charges, Medicare approved	$	53.81	The provider agreed to accept this amount. See #4 on the back.
Less the deductible applied	–	53.81	**You have now met $53.81 of your $100.00 deductible for 1996.**
Medicare pays 80% of this total	$	0.00	
Medicare owes	$	0.00	
We are paying the provider	$	0.00	
Of the approved amount	$	53.81	
Your total responsibility	$	53.81	The provider may bill you for this amount. If you have other insurance, the other insurance may pay this amount.

IMPORTANT: If you have questions about this notice, call us at 1-800-675-2266. If you reside in area codes 213 or parts of 310 or 818, call 213-748-2311. Or visit us at 1149 S. Broadway, Los Angeles. Please have this notice with you.

To appeal our decision, you must WRITE to us before AUG. 2, 1996 at Transamerica Occidental Life Insurance Co., P.O. Box 30540, Los Angeles, CA 90030. See 2 on the back.   (000-0467641)

Figure 3-6   Medicare Part B, Provider EOMB

company wouldn't figure out the difference between the Medicare allowable amounts and the amounts paid because of the mistakes made by the hospital. Meanwhile, the family was being held liable by the hospital for the deceased woman's bill of $20,000. The family was receiving collection notices, although the hospital refused to correct its own mistakes. As Mary Ellen said, "The average person pays the collection notices without question, but in many cases there's been a serious misunderstanding or error made that must get rectified."

Figures 3-7 and 3-8 illustrate one situation that contained an error. Figure 3-7 shows the actual EOB from Pennsylvania Blue Shield dated 3/11/95 and Figure 3-8 shows the doctor's bill sent to the patient on 4/17/95. See if you can guess what is wrong, then read the caption. (These are real EOBs; the names of the patients and doctors involved have been deleted to protect their privacy.)

This case is just a sample of what you need to learn as a CAP. Unfortunately, space limitations preclude showing you more practice EOBs here.

EXPLANATION OF BENEFITS

Pennsylvania BlueShield
An Independent Licensee of the Blue Cross and Blue Shield Association

Camp Hill, PA 17089

KEEP FOR YOUR RECORDS

PENNSYLVANIA BLUE SHIELD
CUSTOMER SERVICE
PO BOX 890036
CAMP HILL PA 17089-0036

Subscriber: ELIZABETH ▒▒▒▒▒
Patient: ELIZABETH ▒▒▒▒▒
Provider: UNIVERSITY OF ▒▒▒▒▒▒
        (000▒▒038)

ID Number: ▒▒470
Claim Number: 65065033550

Page: 1 of 1
Date: 03/11/▒

PROCEDURE DESCRIPTION PROCEDURE CODE (NUMBER OF SERVICES)		SERVICE DATE(S)	PROVIDER'S CHARGE	ALLOWANCE	AMOUNT PAID	AMOUNT NOT PAID	REMARKS
DIAGNOSTIC TEST/EEG 95816	(001)	02/03/95	180.00	84.00	84.00	96.00	Q1010
		TOTALS	180.00	84.00	84.00		

Q1010   These services were provided by a Pennsylvania Blue Shield Participating Provider. Blue Shield's ALLOWANCE will be accepted by the provider as full payment for covered services. You do not owe the Provider any balances for the covered services listed above.

Pennsylvania Blue Shield has paid the Provider the amount shown in the AMOUNT PAID column.

Figure 3-7   Example of EOB from a commercial insurer. Note that the doctor's original charge was $180, but the allowable amount was only $84. The doctor must write off the $96 excess. The statement printed on the EOB specifically says that this amount is supposed to be "full payment." Now look at Figure 3-8.

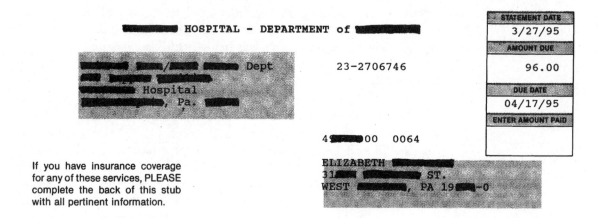

Figure 3-8 Example of a Doctor's statement to a patient containing an error. In Figure 3-7, the EOB indicated that the doctor must accept $84 as the full payment and write off $96. However, this invoice was erroneously sent to patient a few weeks later, demanding the remaining $96. A trained CAP will catch errors of this type and save their clients money.

Obviously, when errors are found, the CAP must take action to rectify them. A claims professional must therefore know the protocol for appealing claims. In some cases, the CAP can try a quick phone call to get the claim reviewed by either the physician or the insurance company, without sending anything in writing. However, in most cases, the first level of a formal appeal will involve writing a letter to the insurance company, Medicare, or the doctor's office pointing out the mistake and how it needs to be corrected. Medicare has an official form to be used—Form 1964—but most CAPs indicate that they write all their appeal letters, even those to Medicare, on their company letterhead without problems. Similarly, when the mistake has been made at the doctor's office, the CAP must phone or send a letter with copies of any necessary documents, such as the EOB.

For any appeal, knowing whom to contact via phone or by mail can be critical. As Tom Koehler points out, "Knowing exactly the right person to call or write is often what makes the difference between falling into claims limbo or getting action." Some CAPs even resort to having a friend who works at one doctor's office call another physician's office to discuss the situation "from the inside."

Figures 3-9 and 3-10 show simple template forms that CAP Lori Donnelly uses to submit appeals for her clients. As you can see, all that is needed is to write in clear English the errors you have discovered, why they are mistakes, and how they should be corrected.

Getting Authorized to Represent Your Client

Because the CAP profession is still relatively new, many doctor's offices and insurance companies are not familiar with the fact that a third party can call or write them to discuss the status of a patient's claims. Medical information and claims are often considered private and confidential information that no one but the patient has a right to know. If a CAP finds an error on a physician's bill and calls the insurance company or doctor's office to query the matter, he or she often gets the following response: "Who did you say you are? Are you related to the patient? Oh, no, we can't discuss such information with anyone but the patient himself (herself)."

To get around this, some CAPs simply tell insurance adjusters and doctors that they are a "friend" of the patient, or that they are related to the patient, or that they are "helping" the patient straighten out the problem. One CAP told me that she can usually get around the situation by simply saying, "I'm a friend of Mr. (Mrs.) So and So," and then moving on quickly to the issue without giving the person time to react.

However, to avoid the appearance of unethical behavior, many CAPs now have resorted to asking all clients to sign a formal document that authorizes them to act on the client's behalf in related healthcare matters, such as reviewing doctor's bills, insurance claims, and filing appeals. In general, this document appears to work in most cases, even with Medicare. Figure 3-11 shows an example of this type of authorization document.

(Print on your Letterhead)

REQUEST FOR REVIEW

Date: _____

Appeal #_____

Please be advised that we request a review of your denial of
claim # _____ , based on the information stated below.
Please advise us of the result of this review as soon as
possible.

_____

_____

_____

_____

_____

_____

_____

Patient _____Service Date _____
Provider _____Total Charge _____

Please note that this company, {name of your company}, is
acting on behalf of your insured with regard to the submission
and payment of all medical claims. All inquiries should be made
to {name of your company}. The insured's written authorization
is attached.

Figure 3-9   Insurance Appeal Letter

(Print on your Letterhead)
Your Name
Your Address
Today's Date

Doctor's Name
Doctor's Address

Dear Dr. {......},

I am a claims assistance professional representing {*name of client*}. I am authorized to act on behalf of Mr./Ms./Mrs. {name} with regard to the submission and payment of all claims. The insured's written authorization is attached.

My client recently received your bill for {*amount*} for {*name of service provided*} which you rendered on {*date of service*}.

As you can see from the enclosed copy of my client's Explanation of Benefits, the insurance company {Medicare} has
- rejected the claim because {*enter the reason in your own words*}

  _____

  _____

- indicated that the allowable fee is only _____
- {other} _____

  _____

We therefore respectfully submit that you review and/or correct the charges as follows:

_____

_____

Sincerely,

{*Your name*}

Figure 3-10   *Provider Appeal Letter*

[Print on Your Company Letterhead]

AUTHORIZATION TO REPRESENT

I hereby appoint {*name of your company*} as my agent to file all claims for benefits on my behalf, for myself, and all dependents covered under my benefit plan(s).

I authorize my insurance carrier(s) to speak to or correspond with an agent of {*name of your company*} in connection with claims filed by them on my behalf.

I hereby authorize any Physician, Dentist, Hospital, Pharmacy, Insurance Company, Employer, Third Party Administrator, or Organization to release any information regarding the medical, dental, mental, alcohol or disability or employment related information concerning this claim to {*name of your company*} for the purpose of validating and determining the benefit(s) payable in connection with this claim. A copy of this signature will be valid.

    Insured's Signature _____

    Spouse's Signature _____

    Date _____

Figure 3-11 Authorization to Represent

Organizational Skills

Although Chapter 2 pointed out the growing computerization of claims processing between doctors' offices and insurance companies, at the consumer level, claims are still a paper-intensive business. This means that a CAP must have excellent organizational skills, including the ability to categorize priorities, organize paperwork, remember to make copies, and color code the filing system.

For instance, assume you have 100 clients, and each client has 20 EOBs and 20 doctor bills for you to review over the course of 2 months. That equals 4,000 pieces of paper that will likely pass by your desk at least once in 60 days! Since most claims take several days to settle, it is actually more likely that you will need to look at each document two or three times, which means that those 4,000 pieces of paper go by your eyes more like 8,000 or 12,000 times. So if you are the type of person who stacks paper in random piles on a desk, this job is not for you (or if you insist it is, your clients will probably fire you for losing their paperwork).

In short, being a CAP requires that you have an intuitive sense of organizing information. While a personal computer will help you do this, much of the business is not yet highly computerized, because of the sheer number of paper documents (EOBs, doctor's invoices, appeals letters) that must be physically generated and stored. I will address the growing use of computers in the CAP business in greater detail later, but for now, suffice it to say that the mountain of paperwork you will get in this job is far more than most people realize. Many CAPs have not computerized extensively, preferring to develop a fool-proof tracking scheme that they can use for each client.

For example, some CAPs adhere to a multifolder system such as a 3-level color-coded folder system for each client. This might be something like red = active claims, yellow = recently completed claims, and blue = old claims. If a client has active claims being filed or appealed, his or her red folder is kept on your desktop as a reminder of what needs to be done. Any time a completed claim or appeal is mailed out, a copy is made and stored in the red folder. Then, when claims are eventually settled, the corresponding documents are moved to the yellow folder. The yellow folder is occasionally cleaned out and older documents are shifted to the blue folder. And so on.

To make sure that proper records are kept, CAP Lori Donnelly uses a one-page "tracking form" in each client's red folder. This tracking form, shown in Figure 3-12, gives her the ability to log the status of each claim when it is first filed. If a claim must be appealed, she then has a separate appeals tracking form for each client (this form is not shown; it looks similar to the tracking form in Figure 3-12).

Of course, CAPs also have to generate invoices for their clients, so that's even more paperwork! As you can see, this is not a career for the type of person who stacks tax documents in a shoe box and expects to find everything at the end of the year.

Knowledge of Business

Earlier in the chapter, I mentioned that the claims professionals I spoke with indicated that they had 200 to 300 clients and more. As you might

CLAIMS TRACKING FORM -- PRIMARY INSURERS

Client: Client #:

Patient: Batch #:

Sent to: Date:

1	2	3	4	5	6a	6b	6c	7
Date of Service	Identify Service	Provider (name of doctor)	Actual Charge	Allowable Fee per Insurer or Medicare	Payment made	Date	Balance due	Appealed? (if appealed, mark Appeals Tracking Form #)

Figure 3-12 Claims Tracking Form. 1) Fill in top portion. 2) Fill in columns 1-4 on submission of original claim. 3) Fill in columns 5-6a, 6b, and 6c after the EOB is received. 4) Indicate in column 7 if claim needs to be appealed.

imagine, it takes time to build up such a large clientele, and marketing and selling your services are critical skills if you want to stay in business. Although you might think that many of the same marketing concepts discussed in Chapter 2 apply here, remember that the CAP profession deals with the public at large as its potential customers, not with doctors. This means that getting customers is accomplished very differently.

MARKETING Unlike medical billing services, your market is broad, unfocused, and seldom knows about the CAP profession. In general, consumers have little comprehension of what you can do for them. Doctors at least know about medical billing and electronic claims, so they are often a much easier target for the entrepreneur seeking a business.

In contrast, a CAP must have a good sense of how to market "services" to the general public. Because your audience is so vast, cold calling as the primary method of getting customers is useless. It would be highly unproductive to spend your time knocking on doors or making dozens of phone calls to find one client at a time.

In the CAP business, your best bet for marketing is to learn how to get people to come to you. You need to learn about *marketing mix*, that is, how to select from four major marketing methods to bring clients to you: advertising, public relations, direct mail, and sales promotions.

ADVERTISING. Some CAPS advertise in local newspapers, or on a midday talk show on the local radio, or even on the back of cash register receipts. To do this, you must understand advertising rates and how to design effective print and/or spoken advertising. You will need to calculate your budget and what the payoff might be in comparison to the costs of such advertising. You might consider local newspapers and other less expensive or free sources for advertising. You may also want to design unique brochures to leave at bus stops, stores, or parking lots, or any number of methods that are used when you need to reach thousands of people. This all means that your copywriting and graphic design capabilities need to be developed.

PUBLIC RELATIONS. Every claims professional I spoke with indicated that public relations was one of the best forms of marketing. Writing articles or getting them written about you and your business is an extremely cost-effective method of getting your company name in front of tens of thousands of people. See the sidebar on Harvey Matoren, whose company Claims Security of America has been written up in numerous newspapers including the prestigious *Kiplinger's Personal Finance Magazine*, for an example of the value of PR.

DIRECT MAIL. The third area of your promotional mix, direct mail, is of course a major undertaking and probably worth studying if you are inexperienced at it. It costs money and takes time to print thousands of letters, find a good mailing list, and get your mail out properly. Learning from others or simply hiring a direct mail consultant could prove useful. Visit a bookstore and find some books on doing direct mail, such as *Direct Mail Copy that Sells* by Herschell Gordon Lewis (Prentice Hall).

SALES PROMOTIONS. This fourth aspect of your marketing mix can actually be quite valuable. Because people don't often know about the

Business Profile: Harvey Matoren

How would you like to have your company written up, at no expense to you, and paraded in front of millions of people who are your potential customers? Sound too good to be true? It's not, and that's exactly what happened to Harvey Matoren and his wife Carol. Their company (formerly called Health Claims of Jacksonville, Inc., but now titled Claims Security of America to reflect their growing nationwide clientele) was covered in a variety of local Florida newspapers and in the prestigious *Kiplinger's Personal Finance Magazine* as well as in *Business Week, Cosmopolitan,* and *Working Woman* magazines a few years ago—and from that point on, their business has skyrocketed.

Ironically, Harvey and Carol left excellent positions in the insurance industry in Florida to start their own business as claims assistance professionals from their home in 1989. Harvey had been a senior vice president with Blue Cross and Blue Shield, and president of its HMO subsidiary. Carol was a senior health industry analyst and a registered nurse. But they had dreams of forming their own business, and they felt drawn toward helping the average person navigate through what they knew firsthand was a tough world in the insurance business. As Harvey told me, "We were already in our middle years and we looked at this as an opportunity to grow a business that had lots of potential and that we felt was much needed in our country. We know how difficult it is for the average person to get through the insurance system, and we wanted to make a difference."

After eight years in business, Harvey is more than upbeat about the future of the profession. As he told me,

> My feeling is that we have hardly scratched the surface of clients for this business. Anyone and everyone needs this type of service, from Medicare recipients to individuals, couples, and families who just don't have time. Even with healthcare reform, we see that there is a continuing need for claims assistance with all the paperwork that has to get done.

Harvey continued, buoyant about the need for qualified CAPs,

> In fact, regardless of what happens with healthcare reform—or shall I say, even more so *because* of it—with more managed care, there is an even greater need for CAPs. Anytime there is a change, people have trouble. For instance, there are a lot of issues in managed care to contend with right here in Florida. We have many patients who have joined managed care programs, but they don't understand the rules of the game. When their claims are denied, they encounter lines like, "Sorry we're not going to cover this because you went out of the network." This is why my business exists.

Harvey then related a specific incident in which he took part,

> We had a client in a managed care system. The gentleman went to his closest emergency room one night at 3 A.M. suffering from chest pains. Fortunately, he did not have a heart attack, just chest pains. But it turned out that this hospital was not his HMO hospital, so the HMO denied payment, saying it was not an emergency since he didn't actually have a heart attack. This has turned out to be a major issue in healthcare: HMOs are making decisions based on "diagnosis," not "symptoms presented." The problem has gotten so bad that in some states, they have made laws that HMOs must base their decisions on symptoms.

Harvey believes that the key to success in the CAP business is to make it an intervention business. He points out that some CAPs just file a claim and make sure it gets submitted; on the other hand, he points out, "My company goes the extra mile to maximize the reimbursement and make sure the client pays only those bills he has to pay."

While Harvey isn't sure how many clients he's received from publicity over the years, there's no doubt that the PR has contributed to his prestige and credibility in the public's eye. Thanks to hard work, exceptional knowledge of the insurance industry, and lots of publicity, Harvey and Carol now have a large suite in an office complex, several employees, and clients stretching all across the country.

Harvey is willing to speak with prospective CAPs and conducts workshops and training seminars. He is also distributing a CAP business opportunity for those unable to attend the workshops. Harvey also has specialized software for your CAP business. For details on his training, business opportunity package, and software, contact him at 904-733-2525, or by writing to Claims Security of America, 3926 San Jose Park Drive, Jacksonville, FL 32217.

CAP business, you could offer a special promotion such as working on one claim for each new client for free, or reducing your fee by one-half to every new client in the month of June. Special promotions are often helpful to get new customers to sign up with you; many people can be enticed to try out your service and then will stay if they like it.

One additional aspect of any marketing campaign—no matter what the business—is networking and getting word-of-mouth referrals. Nearly every CAP I interviewed said that getting current customers to recommend you to other clients is the surest way to generate new business. Whether it's relatives, professionals you know, or current clients, you want to encourage everyone in your sphere of daily contacts to talk about your business with others and spread the word. Many entrepreneurs assume that their customers know that referrals are appreciated, but they don't end up with new business. It therefore helps to let your friends and clients know that you would like referrals. You might even offer a discount to those clients who refer new customers to you.

To learn more about all these areas of marketing, one of the best books is *Getting Business to Come to You* by Paul and Sarah Edwards (Jeremy P. Tarcher). I also recommend *Selling Your Services* by Robert W. Bly (Holt), but you can find literally dozens of other titles in bookstores. This is a business area in which you can easily build a library, consulting it regularly for ideas, tips, and brainstorming tools.

SALES As a claims assistance professional, you will deal extensively with the general public. This means that you must remember that each person is different and that the customer is always right. Whoever your clients are, you need to think in terms of preserving your integrity and reputation in the business, as Tom and Nancy Koehler have done.

Also keep in mind that many people may not fully understand what you do and so getting your first clients to sign on with you is often frustrating and time-consuming. I interviewed one CAP in the Los Angeles area who had tried for six months to get clients, but unfortunately she could not even sign a single individual, despite what appeared to be reasonably good marketing literature.

Being a CAP was unanimously described as a people-oriented business, in which you are like a public defender protecting the innocent victims of our nightmarish health system against the penurious corporate giants of the insurance industry. All of the individuals I spoke with loved their work, especially the thrill of winning a claim for their clients. As Rikki Horne, founder of Medical Claims Management in Newbury Park, California, proudly announced, "I like providing a real service. People come to me and they are vulnerable. You need to care about the people you work for. When your client gets a check for $1,200, you feel as if you did it for yourself."

Knowledge of Computers and Software

The claims assistance professional does not work with electronic claims; these can be filed only on behalf of physicians and healthcare providers to insurance companies. A CAP therefore does not need to purchase medical billing and electronic claims software, such as those described in Chapter 2.

In addition, as mentioned earlier, most CAPs continue to do their work manually, without a heavy usage of computers and software to record the claims they file on behalf of their clients or to track the appeals they may submit. A few CAPs use a standard off-the-shelf database program to create records for each client and each claim, but most simply record these tasks using paper documents and standard office filing procedures. When a CAP uses a computer, it is simply to word process letters and appeals.

Nevertheless, it is expected that we will see an increasing computerization of the field in the future. NACAP reported to me that it was aware of several developers who were creating CAP software. As indicated in the sidebar on page 174, Harvey Matoren has also created specialized CAP software for his own company and is considering making it available for the general market. If you are interested in examining such programs, contact NACAP and Harvey Matoren.

As with any business though, you will still find that computerizing your general business functions will add to your efficiency. For example, since you will likely deal with hundreds of people, you can benefit by using contact management software to track the status of your marketing efforts and record your appointments and daily schedule. Like many sales-people, you may find software such as Symantec's *ACT!, Lotus Organizer,* or *The Maximizer* to improve your efficiency and productivity. Be sure to get a program that matches your hardware capability, as some of the programs are DOS-based while others are Windows 3.x or Windows 95. Visit a retail software store such as CompUSA where you can usually try out hundreds of software programs to see if one appeals to you.

If you are not familiar with such programs, you should not fear their highly technical-sounding names, as they are really only software versions of filing cabinets and Rolodex indexes, although they are much more powerful and can help you organize more information quickly. Database software and contact management software are merging into the same product, in that both serve what is often called a *personal information management* function. These programs contain electronic record-keeping systems in which you get either preformatted screens or ones that you design yourself to keep track of your contacts. Each screen contains fill-in "fields," such as name, address, phone number, fax number, date of last meeting, action plan, and so on. Each screen (or perhaps two tied together) is called a record and is similar to an index card or file you might keep on a person or company you wanted to track. A group of records composes a database. The advantage of this software is that you can browse through a database very quickly to find the information you want. Even better, you can have multiple databases, such as one for all your insurance companies, and another for your clients, one for your prospects, one for your daily appointments, and so on. The power of the database is that you can link records in an interrelated fashion (called a relational database) so that you can jump from one record in one database to another record in another database.

Database management programs effectively allow you to keep tabs on all your clients, which claims you've filed for them, how often you see them, how much time you spent on their project, and what results you achieved. Most also let you produce weekly schedule listings and customizable calendars.

Other programs, such as *Timeslips* from Timeslips Corporation, consistently a best-seller, allow you to accurately track your time if you bill clients on a per hour basis. The software, available in both Windows and DOS versions, automatically logs the time you spend on a project and then allows you to generate reports and invoices that incorporate any of several fee schedules you have stored. For example, you can bill one client at $50/hour, and another at $35/hour if you so desire. (You can use this software even if you charge on a flat-fee basis. By keeping track of your time, the software allows you to compare how many hours you have spent on a project so you can judge if you have been charging too little or too much.)

Database and contact management programs are quite powerful, but they generally require time to learn to use. However, such productivity software can assist you enormously by making you more efficient. Given the number of programs on the market, be sure to experiment and read reviews so that you can find the right software program for your needs.

Income and Earning Potential

Projecting your potential income in a CAP business is difficult. First, every claims professional I spoke to mentioned that it took at least half a year to a year to build up his or her business to a level that could even be classified as income. Second, CAPs use four different methods of pricing their service. As a result, the best way to discuss income potential is to evaluate the four basic pricing strategies and extrapolate from there.

FLAT-FEE PRICING   Using the flat-fee method, the claims service simply charges a single annual fee to a client for however many claims that person has during the year. One business, Claims Security of America, charges $250 per year for a single person, $450 per year for a couple, and $550 per year for a family of four, plus a one-time registration fee of $35 to set up the account for an individual or $70 for a family. For these prices, Matoren and his staff will work on as many current claims as a client has. (They also charge additional fees based on a percentage of what they recover for any old claims that they take over and appeal.)

The advantage of this method is that you can obtain your money up front (or in a few installments); the disadvantage is that you could end up with some clients who have far more claims than the average person, and for whom you could spend dozens of hours working while getting a very low payback. In general, claims professionals who use this method told me that they felt it all averaged out, because many people who pay the one-time fee have only a few claims per year.

To illustrate earning potential, Table 3-2 shows what your income might look like over one year with the following assumptions: you are just starting out; and over the course of the year, you get 144 clients joining your

TABLE 3-2

Income Projections for a Claims Service Charging on a Flat Annual Fee Basis

Month	1st	2nd	3rd	4th	5th	6th	7th	8th	9th	10th	11th	12th	Total
Number of Single Clients @ $200 per Year	5	5	5	5	5	5	5	5	5	5	5	5	60
Income	$1000	$1000	$1000	$1000	$1000	$1000	$1000	$1000	$1000	$1000	$1000	$1000	$12,000
Number of Couples @ $350 per Year	4	4	4	4	4	4	4	4	4	4	4	4	48
Income	$1400	$1400	$1400	$1400	$1400	$1400	$1400	$1400	$1400	$1400	$1400	$1400	$16,800
Number of families @ $450 per Year	3	3	3	3	3	3	3	3	3	3	3	3	36
Income	$1350	$1350	$1350	$1350	$1350	$1350	$1350	$1350	$1350	$1350	$1350	$1350	$16,200
Total Number of Clients	12	12	12	12	12	12	12	12	12	12	12	12	144
Plus $35 Registration Fee for Each Client or Family	$420	$420	$420	$420	$420	$420	$420	$420	$420	$420	$420	$420	$5,040
Total Monthly Income	$4170	$4170	$4170	$4170	$4170	$4170	$4170	$4170	$4170	$4170	$4170	$4170	$50,040

service at the hypothetical rate of 5 singles, 4 couples, and 3 families per month. To be conservative vs. the rates charged by Claims Security of America, assume your clients pay $200, $350, and $450 respectively for their annual fees, plus a $35 registration fee.

As you can see, this scenario can lead to more than $50,000 in gross income in a year. Remember though that this is based on an optimistic estimate; it is only a projection and your monthly growth in paying customers may be much lower, depending on how successful your marketing is and the size of your client base. You could end up with only 50 or 75 clients in the first year, rather than 144, and so your earnings would be much lower. This projection also does not account for any expenses, such as marketing, phone service, gas, overhead—which could consume up to 40 percent of your income in that first year. Be sure also to calculate your overhead and direct expenses. If you work from home for a while, you can probably keep your overhead low, spending only a few thousand dollars for brochures, business cards, stationery, and computer supplies, without paying for office space or secretarial help.

HOURLY PRICING   Several of the companies I interviewed tried the flat-fee structure and decided they weren't earning enough for their needs so they switched to an hourly fee basis. As one owner said to me, "I think an hourly fee is more fair to the client, and they know what they are getting." On the other hand, one company thought that charging an hourly fee made the public compare the CAP to an attorney or a tax accountant, but that the CAP didn't deserve to make as much as those professionals.

Nevertheless, in many areas, an hourly fee makes sense. It might be difficult to get people to pay a flat fee up front, because they are not sure whether they want to use you for an entire year. People are often more willing to pay a small amount until they know you can handle their needs.

As you might guess though, there was no uniformity among the hourly fee charged. It depends on location, clientele, and competition. The lowest rate I found was $24 per hour, with $40 being an average rate, and $80 being the highest. Note that even if you charge an hourly rate, you still should always bill in at least 10- or 15-minute increments, just as lawyers or accountants do. This is fair to you because you might spend 15 minutes on a few phone calls and still want to get paid. It is also fair to the client who wouldn't want to pay you for two hours work when you put in only 1.5 hours.

Table 3-3 illustrates one income projection based on billing at $40.00 per hour and starting out very slowly. In this conservative scenario, you bill

TABLE 3-3

Income Projection for a Claims Service Using a $40.00 Hourly Fee

Month	1st	2nd	3rd	4th	5th	6th	7th	8th	9th	10th	11th	12th	Total
Number of Billable Hours per Month @ $40/hour	20	25	30	40	50	60	70	80	90	100	110	120	795 hours
Income	$800	$1000	$1200	$1600	$2000	$2400	$2800	$3200	$3600	$4000	$4400	$4800	$31,800

only 20 hours in your entire first month of operation, then build up your monthly billing hours every consecutive month by adding an additional 5 or 10 hours.

As you can see, even under conservative circumstances, if you build your business slowly over 8 or 10 months, you can still arrive at a reasonable $30,000+ income per year. If you begin your business more quickly, you can easily outpace this projection. Don't forget that handling one claim may not take an hour's work, so in this scenario of 795 billable hours over the course of a year, you actually need several hundred clients to bill at this monthly work rate (and even more to bill at a higher work rate).

THE PERCENTAGE METHOD   Few companies use the percentage method, but it was implemented by at least one firm. In this method, you take a percentage of any claim you appeal for your clients. The percentage varied, starting at 10 percent of any reimbursement greater than $300 to 15 percent of any reimbursement less than $300.

Estimating annual income under this method is by far the hardest to do. Without any experience in the field, you have no way of knowing how many claims you might handle, or how much they might be worth. Even with experience, you cannot count on getting claims with high-dollar values. You also need to track your claims in great detail, probably using a computer.

On the other hand, this method probably has the greatest potential earnings. All you need are a few hospital claims, for example, in which you find errors worth $10,000 or more.

As you can see, this method is geared toward handling appeals and counts on finding large errors. This method is often used in a business related to CAP work, hospital bill auditing. See the sidebar on page 183 for more information about this related profession.

Business Profile: Rikki Horne

Rikki Horne got into CAP work from a mixed background as a reference librarian at Northwestern University Medical School and a professional career in marketing for a greeting card company after she got her M.B.A. Never one to sit still, Rikki decided that she wanted to have her own business, but which one?

The answer came providentially. With her own mother sick, Rikki ended up handling all the claims that were generated from the illness. When a friend commented that Rikki was quite gifted in ferreting out the errors on her mother's claims, her business was born. Her company officially started in Chicago in 1983, and her first niche was Medicare patients (because they had to file all their own claims until the 1990 law required doctors to file for them). Rikki also discovered an excellent source of clients: trust departments of banks that supervised the estates of wealthy individuals. Rikki got a couple of big banks in Chicago to give her the claims for these clients.

Rikki eventually moved to Los Angeles, but her clientele was so enamored of her work that they continued using her services, despite the distance. To continue building her business, Rikki made another smart move. She did a direct mailing to all people in a high-income zip code area and one letter fell on wise ears. The recipient was a wealthy individual, who took Rikki's letter to his personal business manager. That manager also turned out to work for a variety of Hollywood celebrities, and soon Rikki was invited to handle the claims and appeals for an assortment of stars. As she told me, "This turned out to be a great pitch letter. From one lead, I ended up with 20 or 30 clients." She also explained why she was hired: "The business managers don't have the expertise to review claims, and they have other priorities. I or my staff go to the agent's office about once a week, or perhaps twice a month. The only problem with this is that confidentiality is an important issue for them; and only recently have they started letting me bring some of the paperwork back to my office."

Since moving to L.A. in the late 1980s, Rikki has built a solid business. She currently has two full-time employees to handle hundreds of clients. Rikki charges by the hour at a rate of $60/ hour; and she bills in 10ths of an hour. She says that most of their work is straightforward bookkeeping; they keep track of payments and make sure that the insurance companies are paying correctly. In addition to her "celebs," she also has other clients, such as retired schoolteachers and middle-class working families.

Rikki agrees that CAP work continues to be needed. She pointed to one area that seems to be growing: appealing denied claims for private nursing at home. Many insurance companies are now refusing to pay for home care, although the policy covers it. The insurers are turning around and claiming that the home care was not "medically necessary." As Rikki says, "There's ways around this. You have to know how to read an insurance policy; there are a lot of gray areas in which a good CAP can help a client."

THE MIXED METHOD The last pricing structure involves mixing and matching the methods according to your risk tolerance, clientele, location, and needs. You might, for example, charge a lower annual fee for up to 10 claims per person, and then an hourly rate for additional claims. Or you might charge a flat fee for new claims, and an hourly rate or a percentage for old claims that a client brings in when they first sign up.

The mixed method makes predicting your income difficult, and it may confuse clients—especially the elderly—if your fee schedule has too many scenarios. Nevertheless, the mixed method can be a good way to start your business and make people feel that you are offering a special promotion. For example, you might offer a low annual fee for the first year to cover a client's first 10 claims, followed by an additional fee or

Hospital Bill Auditing

A closely related business to CAP work is hospital bill auditing. Many experienced CAPs, such as Harvey Matoren, include hospital bill auditing in their services without any special distinction from doctor bills and EOB auditing, but some people consider hospital bill auditing as more specialized. One reason for this is that hospital bills can be much more complex than bills for outpatient physician services and office visits. Hospital bills may include charges for supplies, equipment, lab tests, doctor's visits, room fees, and an assortment of items that can go on for pages. In addition, most hospital billing is done according to entirely different fee structures than those a CAP sees for physician billing. For example, under Medicare rules, hospitals usually bill according to DRGs (diagnosis-related groups) rather than individual procedures and supplies. A DRG might be compared to a "price fixed menu" in that it includes everything. For instance, rather than billing separately for all procedures and supplies needed for a gall bladder surgery, only one inclusive charge is billed. Medicare implemented DRGs in an effort to curtail excessive billing, and many commercial insurance companies and managed care organizations are now contracting with hospitals to use such grouped fees as well.

It is often stated that hospital bills contain far more errors than standard outpatient physician bills, and that these errors can amount to large sums of money. In *Understanding Your Hospital Bill,* an independent nurse auditor hired by authors Nancy Collins and Jan Sedoris did 1,144 audits of hospital bills between 1992 and 1994. She found 859 bills with overcharges, totaling nearly $900,000. In other words, 75 percent of the bills audited contained errors.

The complexity of hospital billing and the chance for errors explain why some people have taken to specializing in hospital bill auditing. Such entrepreneurs typically seek clients with large hospital bills, such as people who have had surgeries or extended care. Some auditors even obtain contracts with insurance companies and large companies who want to be sure they are not being overcharged for hospital services. In exchange for their auditing services, many hospital bill auditors expect to receive 50 percent of any errors they find that result in a refund.

If you decide to enter the CAP business, you may wish to learn more about this specialized area of hospital bill auditing. One company, Healthcare Data Management, Inc., operated by William Conlan, sells software and a training package for this profession. (A self-running presentation demo of the business opportunity is included in the CD-ROM that accompanies this book. Note: this presentation does not include an actual demonstration of the Windows-based software Mr. Conlan includes in his business opportunity package; be sure to ask him for a copy.) Mr. Conlan can be contacted at 800-859-5119 or 610-341-8608 or at his Web site http://www.healthserve.com. See Appendix B for more information about Healthcare Data Management.

hourly rate or percentage commission for all claims thereafter. Then in the second year of each client's term with your service, you might simplify the rate and offer an hourly fee or annual charge.

Estimating Your Expenses

The start-up costs for becoming a CAP are generally low compared to most businesses. Most CAPs I interviewed began by working out of their home, although some like Rikki Horne and Harvey Matoren eventually moved to a small office in an effort to enhance their credibility and increase their storage space.

Your investment in office equipment (computer, printer, phones) and supplies is fairly minimal, from $2,000 to $5,000 on average, and you might even get by with less if you already have a computer, a furnished home office, and other general business equipment. Your expenses might amount to

Office equipment (computer, printer, software)	$1,500—$3,500
Business cards, letterhead, envelopes	200— 500
Brochure	500— 1,000
Office furniture	600— 1,000
Photocopier	400— 1,000
Phone (including installation)	300— 500
TOTAL	$3,500—$7,500

Deciding If This Is for You

Now that you've reviewed the first part of this chapter about the claims profession in general, you may be ready to decide if this is a business for you. The following checklist will help with your decision or prompt you to think about the conclusions you may have already drawn. Take a moment now to do this 15-question checklist before reading the remainder of the chapter.

- Am I organized, logical, punctilious, attentive, and patient? _____

- Can I track many projects at a time without getting confused or forgetful? _____

- Do I have a business background or medical background that can serve me in this business? _____

- Do I enjoy working with the public? _____

- Do I enjoy office work, filling in paper forms, filing, and managing information? _____

- Do I enjoy or am I willing to spend much of the day inside an office on the phone? _____

- Do I enjoy being a detective and working with numbers and details? _____

- Do I understand or am I willing to learn about health insurance procedures and claims? _____

- Do I find it easy to read a long, legalese document, such as an insurance policy, and understand what it says? _____

- Can I tolerate the bureaucratic snafus and snarls that invariably happen in this business? Will I persist when necessary, such as calling Medicare eight times if I have to help one of my clients? _____

- Am I articulate and able to convince other people to listen to my argument? _____

- Do I feel comfortable disagreeing and negotiating with intimidating people in positions of authority at insurance companies or Medicare? _____

- Do I enjoy marketing, networking, and putting my face out in the public in order to drum up business? _____

- Do I like working with elderly people who may be a large percentage of my clientele? _____

- Are people drawn to me because I give them a feeling that I am trustworthy and confident? _____

If you answered the majority of these questions affirmatively, or if you have any doubts but want to proceed, the next section provides brief guidelines for how to get started in your business. The section is organized according to a sequence of steps you might wish to take: setting up your office; resources for training and learning; tips for pricing your service; marketing your business; and overcoming common start-up problems.

Section II: Getting Started

Setting Up Shop

One of the first items of business in getting started is to make sure you can legally practice as a CAP in your state. Norma Border of NACAP reminds anyone who is contemplating this business that in at least 14 states, a claims assistance professional must be licensed and/or bonded in ways similar to insurance brokers or what are called "public adjusters." These states include

■ Alabama	■ Minnesota
■ Alaska	■ Nebraska
■ Arizona	■ New Hampshire
■ Connecticut	■ New Mexico
■ Florida	■ Oregon
■ Hawaii	■ Rhode Island
■ Kentucky	■ Vermont

This list may change, so Border suggests that you check with your state's insurance commissioner to make sure you are adhering to any licensing requirements that have occurred since the publication of this book.

If your state is one that requires a license, contact your state's insurance commissioner to find out about the appropriate rules and requirements. You may need to take an exam. If so, the commissioner will likely have a manual to help you prepare for the exam, such as the Florida Adjuster's Study Manual that contains general information about health insurance, types of policies, Medicare information, and so on. Even if you don't live in a state that requires an exam, you might ask a friend who lives in an exam state to request a study manual for you. This will improve your general knowledge.

The purpose of licensing is to protect consumers. Claims professionals deal with the public and must be knowledgeable and skilled; they cannot mislead people or unknowingly advise them about insurance matters. As you might guess, such regulations suggest that the states and insurance companies have a great deal of influence over the average consumer of health insurance.

Setting Up Your Office

Most CAPs begin their business in their home, and only over time and with a growing practice do they move into an office. A home office will obviously save you much money in overhead expenses, but you will need to make sure you set up a professional home office where clients can meet you and spend time reviewing their health claims and discussing their needs.

You must carefully evaluate your home office situation. Do you have a separate location away from the rest of your house? Is it soundproof, so that you will be undisturbed by children, pets, and neighborhood noises? Can you make a separate entryway so that clients will not disturb your family? Will people need to climb stairs to get to it (not a good idea if your clients are elderly people)? Do you have a professional-looking desk and comfortable chairs for yourself and your clients? Do you have enough space in this area for at least three people to sit comfortably (many couples may visit you)?

First, consider all of these issues in designing your space, or hire a space planner or an interior designer to help you make the best use of the space you have. Look into the modern office designs that are frequently described in computer and home business magazines, and check out ergonomic furniture at office stores. Furniture products from companies such as Herman Miller and Steelcase have received good reviews for comfort and health. Plan ahead so that your filing systems, in-boxes, and wall charts all work together.

Second, as pointed out earlier in the chapter, it is not an absolute requirement that you computerize your office in this business, but you will greatly enhance your image and your productivity if you have a computer and the right software, such as a contact management program and a time-keeping and invoicing program. The right software will allow you to do your own project management, word processing, and graphic design, saving money on marketing, typesetting, bookkeeping, and other traditional business expenses.

If you intend to purchase a computer, or if you are upgrading the hardware you own, consider the long-term consequences of your purchase. If you can afford it, splurge and buy a high-quality personal computer (Pentium or above) system that gives you faster speeds and more computing power.

If you intend to offer your services at your clients' homes, as Tom and Nancy Koehler do, it is useful to purchase a laptop computer that you can take with you on appointments. This will allow you to take notes and examine your computerized records. A laptop may actually be a worthwhile investment if many of your clients will expect you to come to them.

For software, find a database manager or contact management program that fits your computer experience and budget. Many programs are available in a wide array of prices. Another choice is to use an integrated program that includes word processing, a spreadsheet, and a database, such as *Microsoft Office*.

HARDWARE

- Printer. A laser printer will give you clean, crisp documents that enhance your professional image on letters you write to clients, doctors, and insurance companies. Laser printers can be purchased for very little today and will make the difference in having your company perceived as a professional business.

- Label printer and postage meter. Since you will do extensive correspondence via mail, you might wish to invest in a dedicated label printer, a special narrow gauge printer that handles a long line of stick-on mailing labels. Similarly, a postage meter can be rented for a small amount, saving you many trips to the post office.

- Phone system. Much of your business is done by phone, so spending your money on the best equipment you can buy makes sense. Invest in a business phone that is separate from your family phone; consider also the use of a two- or three-line phone so that you can take more than one business call at a time, rather than using call waiting. If you find yourself spending many hours on the line, get a headphone set to alleviate the strain on your neck and arms.

  Be sure to have a high-quality answering machine or voice mail, so that you never risk losing messages. Finally, you may wish to pay the extra fee to your phone company to categorize your phone calls and organize them on your bills according to phone numbers. This will facilitate tracking your calls if you want to bill your clients for long-distance charges.

- Car phone. With the rapid decrease in the price of a car phone, consider investing in one, particularly if you travel to your clients' homes. You can use the phone to take other calls, do business while you drive, or let clients know you are on the way.

- Modem. You will probably not need a modem, except for logging on to online services and the Internet. Norma Border of NACAP indicates, however, that in the near future claims assistance professionals may be able to access their clients' records through a network or clearinghouse connected with the Medicare carriers, so stay abreast of this situation.

- Photocopier. A personal copier will be a time-saving and valuable investment in this business. In general, you must make copies of anything you mail out to insurance companies and doctors' offices. Keeping good records of your clients' claim forms, receipts, and correspondence is critical to this job, so get the best personal copy machine you can afford.

- Fax machine. Faxes are becoming more and more useful in any business. Some CAPs receive copies of EOBs from their clients by fax, so consider this piece of equipment as a necessary purchase.

Resources and Training

ASSOCIATIONS As indicated earlier, the old NACAP organization folded just as this new edition of this book was going to press. Several former members of NACAP are eagerly working to establish a new organization, which will include individuals who have been practicing CAPs for many years as well as any people new to the industry who are seeking assistance in getting their business off the ground. At this time, CAP Lori Donnelly from Bethlehem, Pennsylvania, is willing to hear from anyone interested in developing a new association for CAPs. As Lori states, "there is a clear need for an organization in this field where members can help each other with difficult cases, exchange information and marketing ideas, and even meet on an annual basis to renew their friendships and professional credentials."

One of the items that a new association might undertake, similar to the old NACAP, is a certification process that provides members with a credential to use in their marketing. The certification shows the public that, as a CAP, you understand the insurance industry and all its details, and that you are qualified to represent clients and handle their claims.

Lori Donnelly can be contacted by e-mail at dbclad@aol.com or by fax at 610-974-8271. She will be pleased to hear from people who are new to the CAP business and would like to participate in developing a new association for professionals. The new association will offer many opportunities for networking, training, and marketing support.

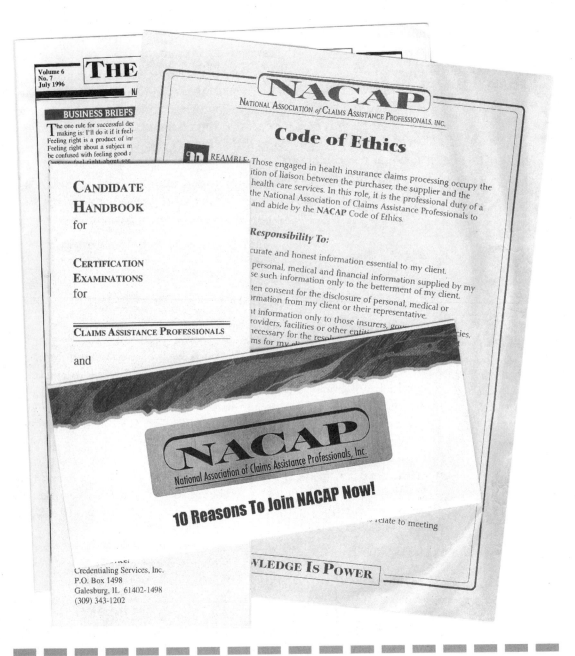

Credentialing Services, Inc.
P.O. Box 1498
Galesburg, IL 61402-1498
(309) 343-1202

Figure 3-13   Brochures and Newsletters from NACAP

COURSES/TRAINING MATERIALS Here are a few additional ways to prepare for becoming a CAP.

- Contact the Institute of Consulting Careers (ICC) at 800-829-9473. This company publishes an extensive CAP training course developed by CAP Lori Donnelly and myself. The course includes two manuals, two videos, and a diskette. See Appendix B for more information about ICC.

- Contact Harvey Matoren of Claims Security of America. Mr. Matoren provides workshops and seminars to train new CAPs. For information, call 904-733-2525 or 800-400-4066.

- Take a course in medical billing and health insurance in a community college or extension school. Such courses can help you develop some of the background you need in medical coding and various kinds of insurance regulations and policies.

BOOKS To begin, you must have a copy of the current annual edition of the *Medicare Handbook*. This guide is invaluable in helping you understand Medicare's complex policies, the yearly amounts for deductibles and copayments, and the health coverage provided under Parts A and B. The book is updated each year, so be sure to get a current copy from your local Medicare office. You can download the annual *Handbook* from the Medicare Web site: www.hcfa.gov. See Appendix B for more details.

You can also browse a Government Printing Office (GPO) store; there's one located in 21 cities or call the order desk at the Superintendent of Documents in Washington, DC., at 202-783-3238. The GPO publishes additional information on Medicare as well as on various congressional hearings and laws regarding the insurance industry and other topics of interest to people in the medical professions. Your public library may also have a copy of the GPO Monthly Catalog and GPO Sales Publications Reference File.

For information on medical coding books, contact a medical supply company such as Medicode or go to a medical book store in your area. As indicated in Chapter 2, Medicode sells a full supply of health industry reference books, such as the ICD-9 and CPT coding books, the *Insurance Industry Directory*, the *DRG Guide*, and many other titles. Medicode can be reached at 800-678-TEXT.

GENERAL BUSINESS DEVELOPMENT Many local chapters of the Small Business Administration offer courses on starting a new enterprise, business planning, and marketing. The Service Corps of Retired Executives (SCORE) likewise can prove valuable. When she was starting her new business, CAP Nancy Koehler contacted SCORE and was assigned a mentor who by chance was a former executive with Blue Cross. This helped her gain a strong knowledge of the insurance industry.

For improving your knowledge of marketing, consulting, sales, or running your own business, browse your local bookstores for the latest books on entrepreneuring and running a home-based business. You should definitely read three books from Paul and Sarah Edwards, *Working from Home, The Secrets of Self-Employment,* and *Getting Business to Come to You* (all published by Jeremy P. Tarcher/Putnam). Try also *Selling Your Services* and *How to Promote Your Own Business* by Robert W. Bly (Holt).

If you find yourself with little time to read, I recommend subscribing to a few business magazines and high-quality business newspapers. In this way, you can read shorter articles and still manage to get good information about new software and new business ideas. You may also wish to subscribe to *Medical Economics,* a magazine for the medical profession that covers matters of financial interest to doctors and healthcare providers. The magazine can be reached at 201-358-7200.

Pricing Your Service

You can choose from among four methods to price your service, but you need to consider several factors to determine which method makes the most amount of sense (and cents) for you. Your choice will be influenced by the following:

- *Your clientele.* If you expect to serve a largely elderly population, consider that some may balk at paying a flat fee if they do not know you or your service. They may be more willing to pay an hourly fee. On the other hand, those with many claims may prefer a flat rate, because they will think they are saving money. If you expect to sign up many families and younger couples, you may find that they prefer a fixed rate, because they may not want to pay a high-priced hourly fee.

- *Your competition.* There may be competing services in your area, so do find out how much they charge and by which method. Another agency charging a lower price doesn't prevent you from charging whatever you want, but it is usually difficult to price higher than competitors because consumers today are price sensitive. You should also give some thought to future competitors. If you start at a high price and a competitor opens up a few months after you, you need to protect your territory.

■ *Your locale.* Major metropolitan areas may tolerate a $300 per year annual fee or $60 per hour, but many other areas with a lower cost of living will force you to charge much lower annual or hourly fees. If you intend to charge an hourly fee, it helps to know the going rate for similar professionals in your area, such as accountants.

■ *Your reputation and experience.* It may be difficult charging $60 per hour if you have little experience in this field, but if you have a background in the insurance industry, many people will think you are a professional and would be willing to pay your fees. On the other hand, if you have very little experience, you do not want to be in the position of defending your fees if a client wonders why it took you three hours to do something that an experienced person would have accomplished in one hour.

■ *Your cash flow needs.* Some people have to start out using borrowed money to finance their venture. If that is true for you, the annual membership fee method allows you to bring in large amounts of money more quickly to pay back your debt. However, you need to remember that once you receive up-front money from clients, you must spend a year working on their claims without further payment for your time. As the months go by, you must remain as courteous and helpful to those clients as you are to new ones.

■ *Your other policies.* Are you going to charge for phone calls, postage, or mileage? In determining your pricing, don't forget to allocate enough to cover your direct expenses per client. If you intend to charge $25.00 per hour, you may want to see if you can get $28 or $30 to be sure you cover your expenses.

■ *Your projected number of clients and claims.* You may believe that your area has great potential and that given your contacts and reputation, you will be able to bring in many clients quickly. If so, you might want to charge on a percentage basis, since this method is by far the most lucrative.

■ *Your perception of value.* You have probably heard that when you charge too little, many people don't think you're offering a service of value. This suggests that it is important to be careful that you don't underprice your service.

In sum, your best plan of action is to spend some time with a spreadsheet and calculate a number of different scenarios. Compare and contrast your income opportunity using the flat-fee method, an hourly method, and the percentage method. Be as specific as possible: have your plan estimate income for each week of your first year, showing your growth in clients multiplied by billable hours, annual fees, or percentage. Then examine which method maximizes your income while offering the most reasonable pricing terms for your location, competition, clientele, and reputation/experience. If you find that you can earn the most with an annual fee, you may nevertheless need to operate on an hourly basis if a sizable portion of your potential clients would balk at paying you $200 to $400 all at once. (Note that offering clients the choice of paying an annual fee on a monthly basis through their credit card is often more acceptable to them.)

Whichever pricing method you choose, the CAPs I interviewed suggest that you also charge a registration fee in the first year for each client. It takes time to set up accounts, call insurance companies to obtain information about policies, set up files, and take care of all the initial prep work. Many CAPs charge from $30 to $50 as a registration fee.

In addition, consider if you are going to offer other services, such as those performed by Nancy and Tom Koehler of In Home Medical Claims, who pay bills for their clients, keep financial records, and make appointments with attorneys and accountants for their elderly clients during tax season. If so, you need to either add a surcharge to your annual fee or choose to go by the hourly method. Above all, keep your pricing simple and clear so that your clients can understand what they are paying for.

Finally, consider the reality of this business that many CAPs remark on: whichever pricing method you use, you need to account for losing some number of clients each year. People do die, and if you have an elderly clientele, you might lose from 5 percent to 10 percent or more of your clients each year.

Marketing Tips

The biggest challenge facing CAPs is to let the public know about the business. Your start-up efforts must be directed at informing the public about both the profession in general and your new business in particular. Most Americans still don't believe that they need a professional to help them with their health insurance, because they don't realize that so many errors are made. As Norma Border of NACAP phrased it,

> People with no acute or chronic illness don't need a CAP, but as soon as you
> have a chronic illness or a traumatic incident such as an accident, con-
> sumers need a CAP to make sure they get full coverage. People also don't

realize that many insurance programs have been upgraded, such that their insurance may cover specialized services they didn't know about. That's the value of using a CAP.

If you intend to operate your claims service full time, remember that this is business in which the size of your customer base is critical. Unlike an accountant or attorney who might have some clients from whom they can earn tremendous amounts of money, you will need many clients to generate enough income. Your goal is growth; you need to increase your client base and never let up. Most claims professionals have 200, 300, or more clients, and some serve over 1,000 clients coast to coast. If your marketing is so successful that you get too many clients to handle yourself, hire an employee to do the filing, typing, invoicing, and other administrative tasks, or find a partner to share in both CAP work and the perpetual marketing.

Nearly every CAP agrees that this business can be slow to start. You therefore need to be prepared for a few months of intensive marketing. The following guidelines address what you can do to respond to your challenges.

KNOW YOUR MARKET Get the demographic data on the area in which you intend to conduct your business. Know how many citizens in each age group and sex there are, where they live, and what their income levels are. After all, you are a service business catering to the general public, so being sure you know your clientele is vital. It helps to live in an area with a heavy concentration of elderly people, mixed with professional families with two working spouses and working singles.

USE WORD-OF-MOUTH POWER Word of mouth is by far the most important marketing method in this business. Because people are putting their faith in your service, you want customers who can trust you with their personal medical information and financial situation and will then refer you to others. Just as people frequently obtain their accountant, tax preparer, or attorney based on recommendations from others, you want to have clients who can recommend the quality of your work to others.

Begin by making a contact tree of everyone you know: friends, relatives, former colleagues, employers, neighbors, and so on. Send everyone of them a flier with a personal note to make sure they know you are now in the CAP business. Ask them to sign up with you for a year, and to tell their friends about you. If every client generates 10 leads for you, you could move from zero to 100 clients in just a few months. The sidebar on Fitzgibbons & Associates illustrates the power of word-of-mouth.

Business Profile: Mary Ellen Fitzgibbons

Mary Ellen Fitzgibbons of Fitzgibbons & Associates runs her claims practice about 20 hours a week, without doing a shred of marketing. Each and every one of her clients comes to her through word of mouth. Some of her clients are elderly people who have seen Mary Ellen save them thousands of dollars and so refer their friends to her. Other clients come from Mary Ellen's own friends. She even once had an attorney who heard of her and subcontracted to her for a problematic case he was handling. As Mary Ellen says, "I am not just a claims submitter: I am a heath claims management service. Clients send me their paperwork, and I clean up all the problems they have had."

Mary Ellen got into the business from a varied background that included working in the personnel department of a major food manufacturer, a nursing degree with experience in a hospital, and working as an insurance administrator for a consulting company where she monitored insurance claims to protect the retired employees of the company. She says,

> This job demands toughness and negotiation skills. Sometime people at the insurance companies tell you, "Oh this is not possible," so you need to ask to speak to the manager or someone higher up in the organization. Otherwise you can't get the job done. Trust is also really essential. You want people to know how you do the job, so that they trust you and don't think you're a maverick.

Mary Ellen believes that her success speaks for itself. She adds, "I've never had a case where I didn't find a mistake, and in a few cases, I've found mistakes as high as $40,000."

USE FLYERS AND BROCHURES To get your information to the public, don't be surprised by the recommendation that you print 5,000, 10,000, even 20,000 one-sided, one-page flyers to put in stores or on cars in parking lots or even going door to door in high-density neighborhoods. Keep the flyers simple, clear, and to the point, focusing on the benefits you can provide. Include wording that shows how anyone can gain from your services, not just elderly or people with health problems. To heighten the effect of the flyer, get an artist to do a small illustration that dramatizes the issue, such as showing a concerned looking couple eyeing their doctor's bill, or a perplexed looking person with a stack of bills next to him. Quote testimonials from some of your clients indicating how much money, stress, and time you saved them. In your flier, offer a promotion, such as a free consultation, and include your business phone number.

Regarding brochures, you may wish to print 500 to 1,000 copies of a trial brochure because these are more expensive. Choose a high-quality paper stock and print in two colors. To increase its power, hire a designer to work on the brochure with you, or use your laser printer and desktop publishing program to design one yourself. This brochure should be an $8^{1}/_{2} \times 11$ sheet of paper, single or double folded to end up with four or six surfaces on which to present your message. The folds add drama to the brochure. Figure 3-14 shows the brochures used by Claims Security of America (Harvey Matoren), In Home Medical Claims (Tom and Nancy Koehler), and a brochure produced by NACAP that you can purchase and customize with your business name. You might make one page of your brochure into a business reply return card that the reader can mail back to you for more information, as does the brochure from Claims Security of America in which the righthand fold is a perforated tear-off card. Give out your brochures wisely, because they are expensive. Bring them with you to meetings and public speaking engagements or put them into stores, such as pharmacies, that agree to let you exhibit them.

OFFER A PROMOTION   When you are just starting out, consider offering a promotion to induce people to join your service. Everyone likes to feel that he or she is getting a good bargain, so offer 10 percent to 15 percent off the first year's fees if you charge on the annual basis, or one hour of free claims consulting if you charge on an hourly basis. The key is get people to call you, giving you an opportunity to explain how much you can help them so you can close the sale. Once they sign on with you, you have a good chance that they will become repeat business over the years. In a service business, especially when people don't think they need your service, a promotion is often the single most powerful draw to get people to make up their minds.

GET PUBLICITY   Make your goal the following: each month or week, inform thousands of potential clients about your business. You can try to get publicity in local newspapers, community bulletin boards, cable television, local radio shows—wherever you can find it. You are performing an intriguing service and many reporters and radio show hosts would love to have you relate some of your most interesting successes for the public. After all, consumers always enjoy a moralistic victory in which the little guy defeats the corporate giant and proves that persistence pays off. Once you get a story into the media, you can use copies of it in a press kit to generate more interviews with other writers or shows.

USE SELECTIVE ADVERTISING   Most CAPs I interviewed indicated that display advertising did not help them get clients. Although some

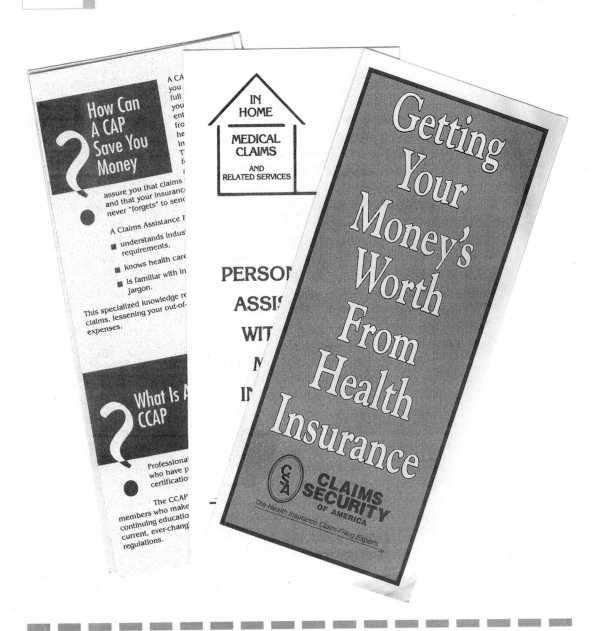

Figure 3-14 Examples of brochures for a CAP business

CAPs advertise in the Yellow Pages, most people aren't aware that they can look up this profession in the phone book. The ads in newspapers are usually too expensive for the results they generate. Spending a few hundred or thousand dollars for a week-long advertisement that brings you only one or two customers is money wasted.

The most successful ads were those in media targeted to the elderly, such as local community newspapers. CAP Lori Donnelly found that advertising on the placemats at a popular restaurant that is frequented by seniors was effective for her.

DIRECT MAIL   Direct mail is not generally used by CAPs, although Rikki Horne had tremendous success using a targeted direct mail piece to residents in a high-class zip code area (Beverly Hills, California). Her direct mail paid off because one of the recipients showed it to a business manager for celebrities, and that manager hired her to handle the claims for all his clients.

You may wish to experiment with a short mailing list of targeted individuals in a certain area of your town, or of a certain age range or income bracket. Another option is "card decks," groups of small direct response cards you receive in the mail. In many communities, you can find publishers of these card decks or coupon books whose prices may allow you to try a few test ads.

NETWORKING   While many people believe that networking is glad-handing or being immodest about themselves, it is really a highly appropriate and successful way to get business. At any meeting you attend, let people know what you do. You will be surprised at how many people respond with a horror story about a relative or friend who just experienced difficulty with a claim. Remember, errors and mistakes on claims happen far more than you might think. Be sure to bring your business cards to such meetings.

Look also to meet other people in the health professions: nurses, home care agency staffs, nursing registry members, and hospital and retirement home personnel. Each of these contacts may be able to refer business directly to you, or at least refer you to other people who can help you find customers. Some hospitals have volunteers who provide advice about claims to patients, but these people cannot handle complex or difficult claims. If you can befriend the staff at a local hospital, you may find yourself with plenty of referrals.

Another venue for networking are accountants, lawyers, and corporate executives in your area who understand that their clients or their company may not be getting the best treatment from an insurance carrier. You may find that you can get yourself hired to work on claims for their clients or employees on a contract basis to be sure that both the firm and the individuals get the proper reimbursements on their medical policies. Several CAPs spoke to me about getting contracts from the trust department at banks to handle the claims for their customers.

PUBLIC SPEAKING As part of your informational campaign, an important aspect of your marketing is to conduct workshops about the business. Find opportunities to speak to groups, associations, or boards containing senior citizens. Go to senior centers, retirement living homes, and community centers where you can offer to give a talk about the health insurance industry, Medicare, and errors on medical claims. Use any previous expertise you have to develop an interesting, informative talk that people will enjoy. Try out different approaches to see which works best, such as a professional and serious title such as "Maximizing Your Returns on Health Insurance" or a controversial approach such as "Are You Being Cheated by Your Insurance Company?"

Be sure that any time you speak to a group, you are allowed to hand out your brochures or leave them for people on a back table.

Overcoming Common Start-Up Problems

Although a medical claims business is a great entrepreneurial opportunity for people who have the right mix of personal experience, medical and business knowledge, and a love for this kind of work, take the advice of those already in the business, "It takes time to build the business." You will encounter start-up problems, from getting clients, to developing the right contacts at insurance companies, to figuring out your fees.

This is one reason why for some people, it is wise to start this business as only a part-time venture initially. Without leaving the security of your paycheck, you can learn the ropes of the business and move cautiously to build up a clientele through word of mouth and networking. Remember that this business depends on being available during the day to see clients and especially to make phone calls, so avoid having your other job interfere with your ability to follow such a schedule.

Here are a few additional guidelines on common start-up problems.

NOT ENOUGH CLIENTS Determine why you may not have enough clients, or fewer than you expected. Are you spending enough time marketing (60 percent or more in the beginning of a new business)? When you tell people what you do, are they aware of your business? Are you generating leads but not closing them? Do you have competition from another business that is doing well?

Each one of these reasons calls for a different response. If you are spending only a few hours per week marketing, you probably need to get out and generate more leads. Get your publicity campaign in gear; print up more flyers and distribute them in new locations; give some talks to a few groups and get feedback on how you present. If after some publicity in your area, you find that people are still not aware of your business, you need to continue educating the public about your service. Step up your publicity campaign, and do more networking. If you are getting people to call you but they don't sign, examine your communication style and sales pitch to see if you are alienating them. Are your prices too steep for your area? If you have a competitor who is doing well, you probably need to change something in your pricing or service.

CASH FLOW   If you feel you cannot change your price, perhaps you can offer more services, such as in-home assistance on paying bills, organizing, and errands. Your own organized personality could prove useful to your clients. More services mean more money for you.

In addition, consider running a medical billing service because it taps into the same background and skills as being a CAP. Lori Donnelly of Donnelly Benefits Consulting offers both services to maximize her expertise and her cash flow.

FEW REFERRALS   People often don't know whether a business wants referrals, or they don't stop to think about it. It is perfectly acceptable to let people know that you appreciate any referrals they can make for you, without badgering them. Most services provide a "reward" for referrals, such as a discount on next year's fees or a free one-time consultation. You might even print on your flyer or business card something like "We appreciate your referring us to your friends" and mention what you will offer in return for the courtesy.

Building Your Business

Developing an ongoing CAP business is done client by client. Few businesses get off the ground without hard work, overtime hours, and tight times. But as every CAP confirmed, you need not worry about the future of this profession. Unfortunately, it appears that America will always have a need for claims professionals, even if we move to a national healthcare system. Our country's medical preferences seem to demand flexibility and choice in healthcare providers and insurance policies—both of which mean that we will continue to have a confused, even chaotic claims system in which mistakes are inevitable.

Medical Transcription Services

A medical transcription service may seem easy to describe. A transcriptionist types up dictated reports and documents for healthcare professionals of all kinds (including doctors, nurses, counselors, physical therapists, and psychologists). The transcribed reports are then stored either in the patient files of private physicians or in hospital medical records departments.

Although this simple definition captures the essence of the job, it only scratches the surface in portraying the importance and value that medical transcriptionists play in our healthcare system. Medical transcription is actually a vital occupation that is highly underrated and in great demand. The shortage of transcriptionists is one reason some American hospitals send their transcription work overseas (another reason is to take advantage of inexpensive labor). Nevertheless, the demand for new transcriptionists is predicted to remain high. In fact, the Bureau of Labor projected a 51 percent increase in the need for medical transcriptionists by the year 2000.

In this chapter, I'll cover the complex skills that are needed to become a medical transcriptionist, the day-to-day work issues faced by people in the profession, and the best methods by which you can enter the business. You will read about the emerging digital technology that is changing the profession. By the end of the chapter, you will have a clear idea of the advantages and disadvantages of this profession, and how you can enter this career if you decide it is for you.

Section I: Background

What a Medical Transcriptionist Does

Each day, healthcare providers in hospitals, clinics, and private offices dictate literally tens of thousands of reports about their patients that range from a few paragraphs to a dozen pages. Dictations must be done for every hospitalization admission or discharge (more than 30 million each year), for every physical exam or radiological study, for every surgical operation performed, and for dozens of other procedures. Dictations include why the patient was seen, what examinations and procedures the healthcare provider performed, and the provider's diagnosis and recommended treatment. These dictations are useless unless they are transcribed into documents that can be read by any physician who might see the patient at a later stage. Dictations may be permanently filed in a patient's private record at the physician's office, or they may be sent to an insurance company or be stored in the hospital's medical records department.

The medical transcriptionist is thus the link between the healthcare provider and the printed report. It is estimated that medical transcriptionists transcribe billions of lines of dictations each year. Table 4-1 lists the numbers and types of operations performed in the United States in a typical year, just one indication of the number of transcriptions that are made. (Note: the table reflects 1991 data, the latest available because of the time lag in collecting information and preparing it for publication.)

Transcriptions are actually medical-legal documents and are important for many reasons:

■ They become part of the medical history for a patient who may later need continued treatment.

■ They are an important source of information for any healthcare provider to whom the patient may be referred for additional treatment.

- They are increasingly required in managed care settings, where primary physicians control patient treatment and must obtain approvals for patients to see specialists. The specialists must also send their reports back to primary care physicians and managed care boards.
- They are frequently required for the payment of insurance claims, because Medicare and commercial insurance companies need to verify procedures and may sometimes dispute fees.
- Statistical information from medical reports is critical in medical research to track diseases and provide clues in understanding symptoms and illnesses.
- Medical reports are often required by lawyers and insurance companies whenever litigation occurs between two parties following an accident, a work injury, a crime, or a medical malpractice case.
- Reports are required in many states for Medicaid and other state-funded health insurance programs.

The role of medical transcriptionists throughout the country is thus pivotal in our healthcare system. Without high-quality transcription, reports can be inaccurate, leading to poor decisions by an attending physician or to an unfair settlement in an insurance dispute. Transcriptionists are the major link between healthcare providers and hospitals and insurance companies, effectively protecting everyone involved from mistakes, lost money, and even the loss of life.

In the past, transcriptionists have been perceived as being glorified typists, but today more and more transcriptionists are taking up the banner and fighting for increased respect and pay. As Linda C. Campbell, CMT, Director of Product Development for Health Professions Institute, told me, "Transcription is moving to the forefront; the need has always been there, but people's awareness of it is finally increasing." Like court reporters, transcriptionists perceive themselves as "language" specialists, not as typists, and today they are aggressively fighting to have the medical community recognize this distinction. For support, they point to a significant factor behind their work: transcriptionists must have a broad education and knowledge of medical terminology and procedures. Transcription work requires highly specialized education and preparation. In short, medical transcriptionists should be considered professionals.

Most people don't examine the training required to understand the typical physician's report. Stop for a moment and think what it takes to transcribe the words of a cardiologist who has performed an operation, or

TABLE 4-1

Procedures Undergone by Patients Discharged from Short-Stay Hospitals by Sex and Age (1991)
(numbers in thousands)

	Sex			Age			
Procedure	Total	Male	Female	Under 15	15—44	45—64	over 65
All procedures	43,922	17,264	26,658	2,235	17,090	9,524	15,073
Operations on the nervous system	970	500	470	236	328	196	210
On the endocrine system	103	28	75	NA	41	22	25
On the eye	399	189	210	25	65	85	224
On the ear	129	75	54	66	36	15	13
On the respiratory system	956	561	396	60	173	290	433
On the cardiovascular system	4,123	2,383	1,740	148	477	176	2,022
On the hemic and lymphatic systems	392	212	180	20	77	110	185
On the digestive system	5,559	2,319	3,241	221	1,571	1,400	2,367
On the urinary system	1,558	884	674	47	376	386	750
On the male genital organs	584	584	NA	46	40	116	382
On the female genital organs	2,308	NA	2,308	8	1,624	445	231
Obstetrical procedures	6,867	NA	6,867	24	6,839	NA	NA
On the musculo-skeletal system	3,323	1,710	1,614	208	1,323	798	994
On the integumentary system	1,324	552	773	75	488	330	431

Note: Details may not add to total due to rounding.

Source: National Center for Health Statistics, Advance Data (reported in 1993).

the medical text of a doctor involved in a worker's compensation case in which the patient was paralyzed, or the autopsy report of a coroner. For instance, get someone right now to read the following passage aloud to you, while you close your eyes, and imagine yourself hearing the text dictated by a Pakistani doctor who is eating lunch as he talks rapidly:

Procedure in Detail: With the patient in the dorsal supine position, a thorough prep and drape of the face and neck was done. The vibrissae were shaved, the nose infiltrated with 0.75percent Marcaine with 1:100,000 adrenaline and the airways were packed with cotton moistened with 4 percent cocaine.

Initial incision in the patient's left nasal sill. The entire face was draped with a sterile plastic sheet with gauze over the eyes to protect the eyelashes. A sterile 4 × 4 was placed over the exposed parts to protect my gloves from touching the skin.

The initial incision was made in the patient's left nasal sill and carried anteriorly along the columella for 4—5 mm. A Joseph elevator was used to dissect tissue away from the nasal spine going laterally past the alar facial grooves bilaterally. A Cottle periosteal elevator was then used to make certain all soft tissues were dissected away from the site. A 3-mm roll of Marlex mesh saturated with Ancef was placed in the pocket, making certain that the marked center of the implant was over the maxillary spine....

Well, that should suffice for now (and that wasn't even the good part!). If you can imagine yourself listening to such dictations on tape, then you know what it would be like to be a medical transcriptionist. If, however, you feel turned off by this poetic passage, this may not be the profession for you.

Note though that there are many types of dictations, just as there are many kinds of physicians. Some dictation is clearly harder than others, and there is a major difference between hospital and office medical dictation. Some transcriptionists handle office work that is typically focused on physical exams, consultations, and referral letters, while others do transcription for hospitals that requires a much deeper knowledge of surgery, radiology, and various medical specialties.

In general, medical transcriptionists must have the skills and experience commensurate with the tasks. They must know at least several of the following subject areas, depending on their area of specialization: anatomy, physiology, biology, chemistry, pharmacology, psychology, neurology, cardiology, pediatrics, surgical procedures, and medical technology. They also must know the special formats used for transcribing medical reports so that headings stand out and readers can find information easily. They must know correct English grammar, punctuation, and patterns of capitalization and abbreviation. And finally, they must be able to type fast enough to make it worth their own time, if not their employer's (usually 60 to 80 words per minute or higher). We'll look at these requirements in more detail shortly.

Let's turn our attention now to the nitty-gritty truth behind medical transcription: what does a medical transcriptionist do while on the job, and how does he or she cope with the pressures of the work?

Transcriptionists' Work Styles

A transcriptionist might have three different work styles:

1. *Employee.* Many transcriptionists are employed by hospitals, clinics, or managed care facilities, where they work onsite transcribing dictations from the many practitioners in the facility. Transcriptionists are also employed by large transcription services that obtain contracts from hospitals and private physicians to do transcription for them; such transcriptionists work onsite at the service.

2. *Telecommuters.* In recent years, communications technology has allowed many hospitals and healthcare facilities to take advantage of using offsite transcriptionists rather than requiring them to come in and take up office space. Telecommuting transcriptionists are still employees, but they have the flexibility to work from their own homes.

3. *Independent.* This is perhaps the fastest growing segment of transcriptionists, those who are independent and may be home based or work out of an office. One reason for the growth of independent transcriptionists is the downsizing of many hospitals and even services. Staff transcriptionists have been laid off because of the savings achieved by outsourcing the work to independent contractors. The independent home-based transcriptionist is self-employed and has the flexibility to choose his or her own schedule and clients.

In general, telecommuting and independent transcriptionists may work in any of three ways:

1. They may pick up cassettes from hospitals and private medical offices and do the work at home.

2. Doctors may call them directly and dictate over the phone into specialized dictation/transcription machines located in their office or home.

3. They may call a recording station located at a hospital, service, or private office into which physicians have dictated; once they are connected to this central "server," they may transcribe while listening to the dictation over the phone line, or they may have specialized equipment that downloads the dictations into their home-based transcriber or computer.

We'll examine more details about the technologies for each of these arrangements later.

Note: this chapter is oriented toward describing the independent transcriptionist, although most of the information also pertains to telecommuters.

The Types of Transcription

The type of work performed by transcriptionists depends greatly on whether they are doing hospital or doctor's office transcription. Each setting generates its own types of reports, and there are many distinctions among them.

Hospital transcription includes the following types of reports:

The Basic Four

History and Physical Report (H&P)

Consultation Report

Operative Report

Discharge Summary

Specializations

Medical Imaging Report

Pathology Report

Radiology Report

Electroencephalograms (EEG)

Electrocardiograms (EKG or ECG)

Autopsy Report

Labor and Delivery Notes (L&D)

Death Summary

Rehabilitation Notes

Emergency Room Notes (ER)

Psychological Report

Social Services Report

Transcriptionists must learn the format for each of these types of reports. The four basic reports generally adhere to a certain format with specific headings, subheadings, and styles for body text. The standardization of medical reports is actually fairly recent and is partially due to an agreement among several industry organizations, including the Joint Commission for Accreditation of Healthcare Organizations (JCAHO), to require physicians to include specific content in each type of report. Transcriptionists must therefore be familiar with these formats and be able to recognize them when heard on a dictation. Note that even with standardization, there are still variances in reporting formats from hospital to hospital, as each health information manager (formerly called medical records director) has his or her own preferences.

Medical office transcription formatting is different from hospital formatting. Medical offices more commonly follow one format for "chart notes" and another for consultations and referral letters. Chart notes usually appear in paragraph form, with the patient's name and date at the top. The most common chart note style is called SOAP:

- **S**—Subjective—the patient's complaint
- **O**—Objective—the physician's findings
- **A**—Assessment—the diagnosis
- **P**—Plan—the goals and direction of the treatment

Another common chart style is called HPIP.

- **H**—History
- **P**—Physical exam
- **I**—Impression
- **P**—Plan

Some physicians merge the two formats and dictate chart notes in the following form: Subject, History, Impression, Plan. Similarly, letters often follow a specific organization and content. Chart notes may be typed in standard block form or modified block form just as business letters. Whichever format is used, each physician usually has a preference that he or she wants a transcriptionist to follow.

Figures 4-1 and 4-2 illustrate two types of reports. Figure 4-1 shows an operative report; note the headings on the sides that have become standard in this type of report. Figure 4-2 shows a letter format from a specialist physician to a patient's primary care physician.

Figure 4-1

Transcription of an Operative Report. (Courtesy of Joan Walston, Words Times 3 Medical Transcription, Santa Monica, CA)

XXXXXXXXX AMBULATORY SURGERY CENTER
XXXXXXXXXXXXXXXXXXXXXXXXXXXXXX SUITE XXXX
XXXXXXXXXXXXX, CA. 90034

PATIENT NAME: xxxxxxxx xxxxxxx   **MEDICAL RECORD: #xxxx**

DATE Of SURGERY: xx-xx-9x   **SURGEON: xxxxxxx xxxxx, M.D.**

ANESTHESIOLOGIST: xxxxxxxxxxx, M.D.

OPERATIVE REPORT

PREOPERATIVE DIAGNOSIS: Stenosing tenosynovitis, right thumb.

POSTOPERATIVE DIAGNOSIS: Same.

PROCEDURE: Release of flexor tendon sheath, right thumb.

PROCEDURE IN DETAIL: Under 2% Nescacaine, a local infiltration anethesia, augmented by intravenous sedation, the right upper extremity was prepped and draped in the usual fashion. The operation was done under tourniquet control and using 3.5 power loupe magnification. A V-shaped incision was made at the volar base of the right thumb. Dissection was carried down to the underlying flexor tendon sheath. Bilateral digital nerves were carefully identified and preserved. The A1 pulley appeared stenotic and thickened. The patient had reproducible clicking on active flexion. The A1 pulley was then incised longitudinally and this allowed free and unencumbered excursion of the flexor tendon. The wound was irrigated and closed with nylon sutures.

Dictated: xx/cms
Date Dictated: xx-xx-9x
Transcribed: xx-xx-9x

_____

xxxxxxxxxxxxxxx, M.D.

The Technology of Transcription

We discussed earlier that transcriptionists may work in any of three styles: picking up tapes, having doctors call their home or office directly, or calling a central server from which they listen to the dictations or download them to their own units at home. The way in which you work thus depends extensively on the technology you have.

There are currently two technologies behind medical dictation and transcription—analog cassette tapes and digital computer-based technology. As you might imagine, digital technology is quickly gaining ground and will likely change the profession entirely over the next few years. Let's examine each one.

■ ■ ■ ■
Figure 4-2
Transcription of a
physician to
physician letter.
(Courtesy of Rochelle
Wexler, Medical
Transcription Service,
New York, NY)

xxxxxx, 199x

xxxxxx xxxxxxx M.D.
xxxxxxx Street
xxxxxxx, NY xxxxxxx

Re: xxxxxx   xxxxxxxx

Dear Dr. xxxxxxx:

Thank you for allowing me to once again see your patient, Ms. xxxxxx xxxxxx.

xxxxxx is a 55-year old woman with stage 0 CLL. I initially saw Ms. xxxx in 199x. Since that juncture, you have been following her. She has remained well with no evidence of infection, bleeding, pulmonary or skin manifestations nor adenopathy. On history, her review of systems is negative.

Physical examination reveals a blood pressure 140/88 mm Hg. There are no palpable nodes. Her chest is clear, her cardiac exam is normal. There is no palpable hepatosplenomegaly. Similarly, there is no skin infiltration nor neurological disease. On repeat CBC, her hemoglobin is 13.6 with a hemocrit of 40. Her white count is 73,000 of which 80% are lymphocytes which are mature in appearance. Her platelet count is 217,000. Her immunoelectrophoresis reveals a decreased IgM at 49, but otherwise is normal. Her LDH is not elevated, and her SMA-20 is normal except for a cholesterol of 291.

I believe that Ms. xxxxxxx is still "stage 0." Although the white count has increased over the three-year period, I do not at this point feel it indicates the need for therapy. I would ask that her hemotologic parameters be repeated when you see her. Hopefully, this would be in periods of roughly four months. I would be interested in discussing with you your hemotological findings.

Thank you once again for allowing me to participate in her care.

Sincerely,

xxxxxxxx xxxxxx, M.D., P.C.

THE OLD WORLD: ANALOG TAPES Cassette tapes are the basic technology that has dominated the medical transcription profession for decades. In general, cassette tapes are used as follows: doctors dictate into handheld cassette recorders or into desktop recording units that look like specialized telephones with microphones rather than a handset. Either of these dictation devices may use standard size or microcassettes. A transcriptionist then picks up the tapes—or perhaps a messenger service delivers them. The transcriptionist uses a machine called a transcriber that allows him or her to play the tape using a foot pedal that controls the speed of the play and the direction. The transcriptionist can advance the tape and type or rewind it if he or she needs to review a passage. When the transcriptionist is done, he or she must then return the hard copy of the dictation along with the original tapes to the physician.

In the 1970s and early 1980s, advances in communications equipment and tape technology led to further options. Both in hospital settings and medical offices, better phone systems and dictating units came on the market that allowed physicians to forgo a dictating unit in his or her office. Instead, the doctor could call an offsite transcriptionist from any phone. Using the phone keypad, he or she could control the tape for rewinding, reviewing, and re-recording the dictation as needed. These improvements in equipment greatly boosted offsite transcription services, but they also increased opportunities for telecommuting and home-based transcriptionists who likewise could now receive dictations called in directly to their offices without having to run around picking up cassettes.

Tape technology still largely dominates the medical transcription field, and new tape-based products continue to improve the equipment to this day. Companies such as Dictaphone and Lanier still produce tape-based dictation and transcribing equipment for use in hospital settings and offsite locations such as offsite transcription services and small- and home-based businesses. Today's best tape machines have multiple input ports and cassette trays that allow several physicians to call in and dictate simultaneously—while a transcriptionist can be playing another cassette and transcribing. The newest tape-based machines also include many sophisticated features, such as the ability to remove tapes without losing one's place and inserting another tape that contains priority work; voice-activated motion so that there is less wasted tape (the tape will stop moving when the physician is thinking rather than dictating); and LCD displays that show the amount of work contained on a cassette.

One reason that tape technology continues to lead is the sheer number of tape-based machines already in the field. Another reason is that many physicians still prefer to dictate into their own handheld dictation recorders or desktop units. The price range for sophisticated multiport tape systems is also within the budget of most small and home-based businesses that encourage physicians to call them directly.

However, tape technology has certain drawbacks. Despite the improvements, it is awkward and time-consuming to find a specific location on a tape. When the doctor or transcriber is searching for a specific text, the tape must be physically advanced or rewound. Second, tapes have a limited recording capacity (usually 60 or 90 minutes), so they must be watched and changed just before they run out of recording space. Finally, tapes can suffer from deterioration in voice quality, or become damaged, or worse, get lost.

THE NEW WORLD OF DIGITAL TECHNOLOGY   Beginning in the early 1980s, the birth of digital technology began to revolutionize the transcription business. Digital technology allows dictation to be done directly onto a magnetic disk (just like the hard disk of your computer). As the physician dictates, special voice software samples the sound at rapid intervals and stores the data as series of 0s and 1s (bytes) just as your software stores your word-processed documents or spreadsheet data.

The advantages of digital technology are especially applicable to medical transcription, since there are no tapes to change and no unreasonable limits on length of time recordings can go on, and a passage of text can be found very quickly (called random access). This makes dictating easier, because the doctor can quickly go back and revise a dictation, or insert new text, or jump ahead to another passage.

Digital technology also makes the transcriptionist's job easier. First, the displays on digital transcribers are like telephone LCD displays that automatically capture the "demographic" data on a recording, such as patient's name, date, priority rating, and so on. This makes identifying the passage much easier for transcriptionists. Second, the transcriptionist can use the random access feature to move through a dictation, quickly advancing or going back to passages as necessary. Finally, the quality of digitized voice is generally better than the analog recording found on tapes. Digital technology also allows passages to be speeded up without distortion, so that fast typists can plow through a dictation faster than it was recorded.

Digital technology was very expensive when it first came out, so it was mostly purchased by large hospitals and services that had thousands of reports to transcribe each day. Physicians were able to call a central server and dictate their reports over the phone right from their offices or from workstations on the hospital floors, assured that their voices were accurately recorded digitally. When their dictations were finished, either an *onsite* transcriptionist would then log onto the server with a transcribing unit to do the work, or an *offsite* transcriptionist would call the central server and transcribe the dictations while listening over the phone lines. In general, the offsite transcriptionist also needed special equipment to control the playback—fast/slow, advance/rewind—so that the transcription could be properly done. This equipment was often a proprietary desktop unit specifically coordinated with the digital machine at the hospital or a special phone with a foot pedal.

New technology, however, never seems to solve all problems at once. Despite the significant improvements digital technology offered, some glitches and drawbacks remained. The principal one was the cost of communications to get the digital documents. Offsite transcriptionists who called in to retrieve dictations needed to spend hours on the phone listening to the dictations and transcribing them. Because it can take up to four times as long to transcribe a dictation than to record it, offsite transcriptionists who lived far away either could not be used or would incur huge phone bills!

One way to avoid the high cost of phone charges for dial-up transcription was to "re-record" the digital dictations all at once to the offsite service or home-based transcriptionist rather than having the work done while the transcriptionist remained on the phone. Ironically, much re-recording was being done from a sophisticated digital server in a hospital to old-fashioned tape-based transcribers still in use at independent transcription services and home-based businesses.

The glitches do not end there, however. One problem still existed: re-recording took a great deal of time. In fact, re-recording took the same amount of time it took to record the original dictation, practically defeating the purpose. If 10 doctors called a central server and dictated 10 hours of material that eventually had to be re-recorded to home-based transcriptionists, the re-recording would then take 10 more hours to accomplish. This was a time-consuming drain on hospitals, services, and independent transcriptionists.

As a result, the newest technology today in the digital arena is special compression software that reduces re-recording time to a fraction of the original recording time. Some products can download 10 hours of dictation in 30 minutes. This new phase of digital re-recording technology allows telecommuters and home-based transcriptionists to dial up the server in a hospital, clinic, or service at any time of day or night, download their assigned dictations, and transcribe them at a later time without tying up phone lines or incurring large communications costs. Downloads can even be programmed to occur automatically in the middle of the night, so that the transcriptionist will have a body of dictations all ready to start on in the morning.

One major company in this field, Dictaphone, describes how this technology has helped its customers. A mid-size independent transcription service in North Carolina that used Dictaphone products was serving dozens of hospitals in several southern states and even had some physicians calling from as far away as Hawaii and California. The service had a staff of 25 transcriptionists, but many of them were offsite and needed to obtain the dictations by calling in and transcribing while on the phone. The service was thus chalking up huge phone bills from the offsite workers. For instance, one of its best offsite transcriptionists was a woman based in Louisiana; when she called in to do two hours of dictation, she would log about eight hours of phone time.

With the new re-record technology, this service now has a Dictaphone server unit, called a Dictaphone Digital Express 7000®, which automatically dials the offsite transcriptionist in the middle of the night to download her work. At her end, she has a corresponding Dictaphone unit called the Dictaphone Straight Talk®, which features the company's proprietary ExpressNet™ re-record technology that transfers the voice data in a fraction of the real time. As Dictaphone points out, "When the home-based transcriptionist is ready to start work at 8 A.M., her desktop system is full of high-quality, re-recorded digital dictation that is ready to be transcribed, eliminating the need for lengthy long distance calls." See Figure 4-3 for an illustration depicting how Dictaphone's ExpressNet™ technology works for this type of arrangement. (Note: several other companies produce similar equipment. Dictaphone is used only for example here.)

As good as this sounds, a problem with such re-record technology is that it requires the transcriptionist working with a large facility such as a hospital or service to invest in the proprietary equipment needed to coordinate with the server at the host site. For example, in the case just described, the service ended up buying every one of its transcriptionists a Dictaphone Straight Talk® unit. This can become expensive for a small business that subcontracts out to independents but cannot afford to buy each of them a unit. On the other hand, a home-based transcriptionist who wants to work with hospitals or services can voluntarily invest in the equipment but needs to know which brand to buy, based on which brand is used by potential clients. Most of the companies selling dictation/transcription equipment lease the units to make them more affordable.

However, an interesting development has occurred recently to eliminate the proprietary equipment dilemma. Several PC-oriented companies have entered the market with specialized hardware and software that allows ordinary personal computers to become dictation/transcription units. For example, one company called Narratek produces software called *VoiceWare*™ that gives an ordinary PC (assuming it has a sound card) the capability to record digital dictation. If the PC is located in a physician's office or hospital, physicians can thus record the dictation right into it (or if the physician prefers, he or she can use a standard handheld tape recorder and then have the secretary replay the tape into the microphone on the PC). Once the dictations are stored on the sound card in the PC, they can be sent by modem to an offsite transcriptionist who has installed Narratek's corresponding *VoiceScribe*™ software, which decompresses the voice data. The transcriptionist then has a foot pedal attached

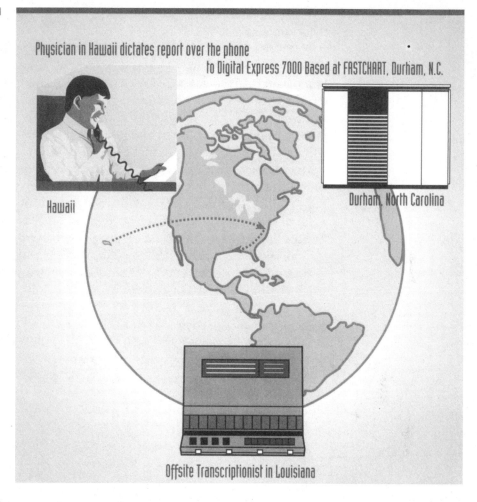

Figure 4-3
Brochure from
Dictaphone shows how
to go from dictation to
documentation in
minutes! "A physician in
Hawaii picks up a
phone, calls the Digital
Express® located at a
transcription service in
Durham, NC, then
dictates the report
The Digital Express,
equipped with
ExpressNet™
technology, transfers
voice file data at an
accelerated speed to
Straight Talk® in
Louisiana. The
transcriptionist plays
back the report,
transcribes it, then
transmits the completed
report back to the
service via modem or
fax. The service then
sends the finished
report either back to the
dictating physician or to
a referring physician.
The entire process, start
to finish, can be done
within 30 minutes with
ExpressNet. (Illustration
and text courtesy of
Dictaphone,
Stratford, CT.)

to the PC sound card to control the playback. Once the work is done, the transcriptionist can send the word-processed file back to the physician or hospital via modem, or, if preferred, he or she can fax, mail, or messenger the actual hard copies.

Narratek's software also works with DVI digital dictation systems (DVI is another of the leading companies in this arena). Just as with the re-recording scenario discussed earlier with the Dictaphone products, doctors call into a central DVI system and dictate their reports. However, rather than having the telecommuting or independent transcriptionist owning an expensive proprietary system, an ordinary PC can call up the DVI server and download the dictations to the PC's soundcard. The transcriptionist can then transcribe the reports using a foot pedal attached to the soundcard.

Narratek's systems are very cost-effective compared to traditional proprietary systems and may begin to attract an audience among small and home-based independent transcriptionists. However, some industry sources criticize PC-based software products such as Narratek's, claiming that these systems are not yet sophisticated enough and lack the security mechanisms that must be in place to protect patient confidentiality. You will need to judge this equipment for yourself.

One problem that transcription industry officials admit is that, at this time, there is still no standard data file format for compressing and storing voice data. Whatever file format is selected, it must take into account medical transcription's special requirements, such as the need to have digitized voice data capable of being played back at any speed without distortion, the need to have flexibility in the system so that physicians can insert and delete at will, and the need to have demographic data accompany the voice data. All of this means there will likely be many competing systems for quite a while, and that transcriptionists will need to choose from among them.

See Figures 4-4 and 4-5 for illustrations of some of the products offered by two of the leading companies in the transcription business, Lanier and Dictaphone.

Figure 4-4
Dictaphone transcription products. The ExpressWriter Plus™ uses microcassette technology. The Straight Talk® Plus unit uses digital technology and can link to Dictaphone dictation products used in hospitals and independent services, such as shown in Figure 4-3. (Photos courtesy of Dictaphone, Stratford, CT.)

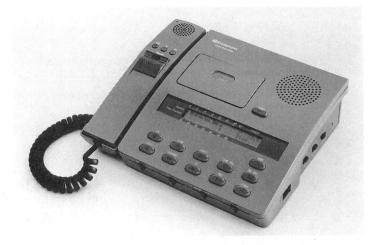

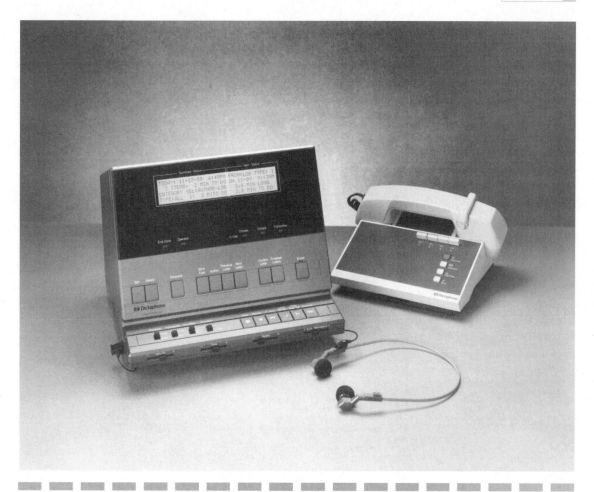

Figure 4-4 Transcription equipment from Dictaphone (Continued)

THE FUTURE WORLD: ONLINE TRANSCRIPTION As you can see, there are many exciting developments occurring in medical transcription. Digital technology is opening many new vistas for telecommuters and home-based independent transcriptionists. Furthermore, the future portends even more exciting developments, especially because of the Internet. Many industry insiders see the Internet as the eventual delivery vehicle for dictation and transcription.

Attaché IV

The Attaché IV combines the convenience of handheld dictation with standard cassette compatibility. Handy features, like one-button control and instructional queuing, help you stay productive anywhere your business takes you. Its superb sound quality ensures that your recorded voice is crisp and clear every time. And when you're ready to relax, use it to play back instructional tapes or listen to prerecorded music.

VoiceWriter 110/210

VoiceWriter 110 and 210 desktop dictation units offer crisp, clear sound and a host of features, like a pistol-grip microphone, one-button control, document queuing, telephone recording and half-speed recording. Additional features include an automatic recall, digital transcriptionist display and an optional foot control and headset. If your office uses standard cassettes for dictation, choose VoiceWriter 110. If you use microcassettes, choose VoiceWriter 210.

VoiceWriter 160/260

The VoiceWriter 160 and 260 offer all the features of the VoiceWriter 110 and 210, plus other capabilities. Digital Voice Operated Recording (VOR) automatically starts and stops the tape when you start and stop talking, automatically guarding against wasted tape and missed words. An expanded display panel features a voice level indicator for instant confirmation that you're recording. And the "store recall" feature lets you switch tapes for priority dictation without losing the display information for the original tape. VoiceWriter 160 uses standard cassettes, VoiceWriter 260 uses microcassettes.

VoiceWriter 650

The VoiceWriter 650 lets you multiply the productivity of your dictation and transcription operations. Featuring a rotating carrousel with four tapes, it lets you assign each tape to a different individual, or separate routine work from priority work. It allows call-in dictation using remote dictate stations or ordinary telephones, and can even function as an answering machine. The VoiceWriter 650 also functions as a transcribe station, with time-saving features like special instruction queuing, automatic recall and a work indicator light that lets you know when dictation is ready to be transcribed.

VoiceWriter Executive

The VoiceWriter Executive brings the power of digital technology to you by converting voice to digital information for storage on a computer hard drive. Digital dictation offers capabilities not available on analog systems, like automatic priority assignment, instantaneous random access and interactive verbal prompts. And because the voice signal is digital, it can be speeded up or slowed down without affecting the pitch, for easier transcription.

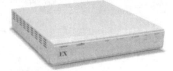

Lanier dictation products

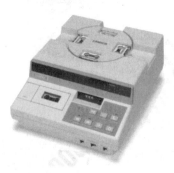

Figure 4-5 Lanier transcription products. The VoiceWriter 650, for example, allows for simultaneous dictation and transcription with its four cassettes. The VoiceWriter Executive uses digital technology to improve the quality of the sound and to provide more flexibility for the transcriptionist. Photos courtesy of Lanier, Atlanta, GA.

Imagine this scenario: the physician dictates into a recorder on her desk or at the station at the hospital. The recorder has a small credit-card size insert to store the dictation in digital form. When the doctor is finished, she removes the card and gives it to a clerk who inserts it into a PC. For each dictation, the PC automatically shows a screen containing the patient's name, age, and other identifying information. Meanwhile, the dictation is automatically digitized. The physician or secretary then presses one button and the PC connects to the Internet, locates the remote

Voice Recognition Software

Many transcription professionals have worried for years that voice recognition software would eliminate their jobs. Such software theoretically could take a dictated document and transform it into a printed one, using the ability of the computer to recognize sounds and identify them with an appropriate dictionary word that could be spelled out on the screen.

It now seems clear that voice recognition software is still a long way off from taking over medical transcription for many reasons. First, the software is simply not sophisticated enough to recognize the difference between many sound-alike words, such as ileum and ilium or perineal and peroneal. Second, the vocabulary of the medical profession changes rapidly with a steady stream of new drugs, procedures, and names for diseases. This means that the software would need constant updating. Finally, the most significant issue is that the current generation of voice recognition software requires physicians to speak in slow, monotone speech, at about 70 words per minute. The problem is, doctors tend to dictate at more like 200 words per minute, and they often do so while on the go, or eating lunch, or from a noisy room.

It may be that advances in chip speed and voice software algorithms will improve the software to the point that it can become a tool for transcriptionists. One potential use might be for a good voice recognition software product to create a first draft of a transcription, leaving holes or guesses at what the software thinks the word is. The transcriptionist could then work on the final draft by reviewing and editing the text with the correct words. If that were so, transcriptionists would probably welcome the technology because it would truly elevate them from the feeling of being rote typists to being medical language specialists.

site for the transcription company, and delivers the voice data and demographics within a few seconds. The transcriptionist—who may be located anywhere in the country—is notified of incoming mail and downloads it to his PC while working on another document. For the next few minutes, the PC decompresses the file in the background. When ready, the transcriptionist opens the file, and with an earphone connected to the PC, transcribes the report. The demographic data are automatically appended to the top of the file. Finally, the transcriptionist saves the file, logs onto the Internet, and e-mails the completed document back to the physician. All of this has taken about 30 minutes and has transpired with complete security and privacy for the information because of special keys used over the Internet to ensure data are delivered only to the appropriate destination.

If this future appeals to you, see the sidebar on page 222 for some interesting comments on technology from two industry leaders.

Comments from Two Industry Leaders

Scott Faulkner, Vice President, Healthcare, Western Region, Dictaphone

- In my view, the growth of the transcription industry cannot be underestimated. For example, new legislation requires that acute care facilities transcribe progress notes. This ties into the massive trend in healthcare for computerized medical records. There will likely be more and more work for people with less formal backgrounds and training (i.e., many medical reports of this nature, such as progress reports, are usually less technical). This means many excellent opportunities for people interested in medical transcription.
- One of the key developments in the medical transcription field is its expansion into the world of client/server architecture. A transcriptionist can dial into a central server (such as at a hospital) and download dictations and patient records from home. This erases the geographical boundaries that inhibit people from being able to work out of the home. Of course, we have had to overcome some limitations, such as the problems of telecommunications (the dilemma of local calls vs. long distance if the transcriptionist is calling in from far away). However, our view is that the next generation technology will utilize the Internet as the solution. The benefit of the Internet is that it makes a completely level geographic playing field. Anyone can download dictations from anywhere, do the work, and ship it back.
- Many people wonder about whether speech recognition technology will make a dent in medical transcription. In my view, it is unlikely, at least at present. Medical vocabulary is much too specialized, and there is a constant stream of new terms, such as for new drugs and pharmaceuticals. There will likely always be a need for human intervention.

Bernie Magoon, Marketing Manager, Voice Systems, Lanier

- The problem today is not having an appropriate technology to help the voice files go from point *a* to point *b*; the problem today is having enough transcriptionists to handle the workload.
- Technology is changing the profession today. It used to be that if physicians were calling your house to dictate, you were limited to your own geographic area for your customers. The market is now opening up and we will soon have a completely geographically free market. What we are trying to do today is take away the barriers so that you are not limited to your geographic location.
- What we will eventually have is real-time voice file movement and the ability to download quickly. It may very well be that transcriptionists of the future will work on ISDN lines.
- Ironically, technology today is helping home-based people get into the business at low cost; but it may eventually hinder them as the big players are able to lower their costs too. This remains to be determined.

The Transcriptionist's Lifestyle

Your lifestyle of a transcriptionist depends entirely on whether you are an employee, a telecommuter, or an independent.

An employed hospital transcriptionist usually has a hectic, pressure-filled, and demanding job. Transcribing many kinds of reports requires exceptional experience and knowledge, and many hospitals don't hire new entrants to the field; there is simply too much pressure to produce, and they cannot afford to have inexperienced people working on their reports. The advantage of a hospital boiler-room atmosphere is that it provides transcriptionists with a collegial atmosphere—friends to whom they can turn for help and support. Many transcriptionists report that they often get into a jam when they simply don't understand what the physician has said, but by checking with another transcriptionist who can offer a "fresh ear," they can finally figure it out.

On the other hand, the life of the telecommuter or independent transcriptionist is usually much more enjoyable—and less pressured. These transcriptionists have more time to spend with their families while having more flexible hours that allow them to work in the early morning, evening, or while a child is napping in the afternoon. Home-based transcriptionists also report that they are usually more productive because they can get to work without wasting time commuting. However, some independents say that they miss the company of colleagues and that maintaining self-discipline to work can be a challenge.

Many independent, self-employed transcriptionists cite that having their own business is what attracted them to the profession, and they would rather be independent than employed telecommuters. They like being able to choose their clients and schedules. Some of the home-based services work for only a few local physicians, while others do regular work for hospitals as well as handling physicians in private practice.

The sidebar on Terri Ford of Monarch Transcription and Joan Walston of Words Times 3 describes two successful transcription businesses. As you'll see, Terri is a good model of the home-based independent lifestyle, while Joan has a small agency working out of an office.

Knowledge and Skills Needed

Unlike medical billing services or even medical claims assistance, the preparation needed to become a transcriptionist is extensive and arduous. This is not to suggest that only the most gifted of individuals need apply,

Business Profiles: Terri Ford and Joan Walston

Terri Ford

Terri Ford owned a home-based daycare center in rural Maryland for nine years while her three children were growing up. When they entered school full time and she was left with only other people's kids, Terri decided it was time for a change. She already had a computer background, having been a bookkeeper for 10 years before her children appeared, and she now felt strongly that working with computers was the future.

A number of coincidences then followed. First, Terri read about medical transcription in an issue of *Money Magazine*, and learning that it was predicted to be a good business, she ordered the book *The Independent Medical Transcriptionist* by Donna Avila-Weil. From that book, she learned about the home-study program called the SUM Program for Medical Transcription Training. She contacted one of the vendors, Jennifer Martin, and purchased it. She was so ambitious to get her new career off the ground that she flew through the program in just five months. She loved the work and passed the exam with flying colors.

As coincidence would have it, Terri then saw an advertisement in her local newspaper from a service looking for home-based transcriptionists. The firm was looking to subcontract out some of its work. Although it did not pay her very much, Terri took the work to build her experience, especially since the owner would proof her work for mistakes. That was the start for Terri's company, Monarch Transcription.

Terri stayed with the service for four months, and then one day, she got a call from a family practice asking her to take over the transcription for their two doctors and part-time nurse practitioner. She accepted the job and began getting about two tapes per day, which amounted to nearly five hours of transcription plus another few hours for proofing and printing. (Terri notes that a typical family practice report is 10 to 20 lines long, and a report for a physical is about three pages.) Terri tries to provide 24-hour turnaround, and she picks up and delivers the tapes because the practice is only five miles away.

For her equipment, Terri uses a mini Pearlcorder and a standard transcriber made by Panasonic. She bought a Pentium IBM Aptiva P-100 with a 16 Mb hard drive, a 4-speed CD-ROM, and she uses *Microsoft Word*. She told me that she expected her family practice client to convert to digital soon, so she will be able to call in rather than driving each day to drop off her work and pick up new tapes.

Terri has found her new transcriptionist lifestyle perfect for her family. She achieved her exact goal: to work from home during the hours when her children were in school, without having to go out into the working world and be away from her children. The only downside is the loneliness of working solo (as many people who work from home experience). Terri would therefore love to have a partner so she could have some adult company during the day. To fill part of this need, she occasionally logs onto America Online's forum and chats with other transcriptionists (there's one on CompuServe too).

Joan Walston

Joan Walston is the antithesis of Terri Ford when it comes to the transcriptionist's lifestyle. When I first called Joan to interview her about her business, she told me she was so busy that I needed to schedule an appointment with her—two weeks later! Rather than working in a beautiful rural area for a small family practice,

(Continued)

Joan's business is located in a bustling medical area of Santa Monica, California. She leases an office amidst several hospitals and dozens of buildings containing thousands of private physician practices.

Joan Walston got into medical transcription 20 years ago, when the requirements for entry into the business were much less rigorous. She was an English major in college, and believing that she had excellent language skills, she decided to try medical transcription. Her first jobs were doing overflow work for hospitals. Today, Joan handles work for many physicians affiliated with one of the hospitals nearby, and she also works for several private practices. Over the years, Joan has developed expertise in nearly every area of medicine, so she can handle almost every type of medical dictation, from operative reports and patient visits to medical research papers and grant proposals. One doctor even has Joan keep his resume on file and regularly update it each time he adds a new paper or grant award to his credentials.

Joan's business has generally grown although it goes through ups and downs. Her company, Words Times 3 Medical Transcribers, generates enough work that Joan subcontracts some of it out, using anywhere from two or three independents at a time. She encourages phone-in dictations from her clients, so she has two four-line systems with multiport transcribers that allow both dictations and transcriptions to occur simultaneously. Because her office is in such a densely packed medical area, she also picks up tapes and delivers transcribed documents for some clients within the two to three block radius.

Joan believes strongly in providing a quality service. She says that "quality work is a distinguishing factor in my business." She notes that many doctors are very articulate but some of her clients depend on her to fix up their dictations into proper English. On that note, she advises that anyone interested in transcription needs to understand that there is only room for people who are really good if they want to have their own business. She feels that there is a greater possibility for lower standards in a big operation, so her goal is to continue growing but only large enough for her to maintain control on the quality her company produces.

but simply to help you understand that if you are planning a career in medical transcription, you should consider the training as a long-term endeavor and not become discouraged or disappointed with the path in front of you. You may need to devote 6 to 18 months to study, and then another few years in an apprenticeship position. In the long run though, a good education and training program will help you build a solid business or enable you to have your pick of employers.

The starting point for a career in medical transcription is not difficult for anyone with a high school diploma. In general, if you have a fairly good command of English, know how to spell and the rules of spelling, and can type from 50 to 80 words per minute on a computer, you are ready to begin a program for learning medical transcription. Following are the areas of knowledge you will need to develop:

- Medical terminology (word origins, spellings, meanings) and transcription styles

- Medical sciences—the basics, including anatomy, physiology, pathology, pharmacology, disease processes, as well as some areas of specialization such as radiology, neuroscience, cardiology, or psychology/psychiatry
- English grammar and punctuation as well as spelling
- Skills with PC computers and general word-processing software
- Business skills—marketing and sales

The section later in the chapter on "Resources and Training" explains in more detail the type of programs you can find to take such courses, but note for now that many community and junior colleges offer medical transcription training. You will also find several home-study programs such as the one mentioned in the profile of Terri Ford, the SUM program.

Medical Terminology and Transcription Styles

Medical dictations do not reflect the average daily speech of mortals. Although we can ask insurance companies and lawyers to write their documents in plain English rather than formal legalese, medical reports cannot be simplified to a level below the technical vocabulary used in medicine. There is no other way to express what happens in a surgical operation except to use the highly technical terms for body parts, chemicals and drugs, units of measurement, and medical equipment involved. Medicine is a field that, by its very nature, requires specialized terms for the thousands of body parts, diseases, processes, diagnoses, chemicals, and technical terms that physicians must describe and use.

How does a student learn all this terminology? One major aid to mastering medical terminology comes from the field of *etymology,* which focuses on the origins of words. Since most medical words are based on Greek or Latin roots, plus a prefix and/or suffix, a large part of your medical education focuses on learning a few hundred roots, prefixes, and suffixes. For example, the words neurology, neuritis, neuropathy, neurosurgery, and neurologist all use the root *neur-,* meaning *nerve.* You can learn to recognize many root words from related English words, but you may need to study extensively the hundreds of prefixes and suffixes used in medicine. For instance, consider the suffixes *-itis* (inflammation of), *-oma* (tumor), *-ology* (study of), and *-ectomy* (removal of).

Another medical language area you will need to study are homophones (words that sound the same) and antonyms (opposites), because these are critical to getting it right when you type a medical transcription. For example, you must be able to distinguish clearly between "The patient's hypertension" and "the patient's hypotension," since the first means high blood pressure and the second means low blood pressure. This can be difficult when listening to a doctor who speaks quickly or with an accent, unless you know and understand the context. Many medical words sound very similar, but you must be able to decipher them based on context.

You will also need to study how to punctuate, abbreviate, and capitalize medical terminology. For instance, you must know where to put periods when you type a series of blood tests, or where to put a comma when you list a group of statements. You must know how to type many proper nouns such as Bells palsy (capitalize the B and don't use an apostrophe on eponyms). An important standard is knowing to capitalize and underline any statements relating to allergies (THE PATIENT IS ALLERGIC TO IODINE) because it could save someone's life.

As indicated earlier in the chapter, you also need to learn the various styles and formats used in transcription. In short, you need to learn a multitude of conventions and terminology (and this book cannot do justice to teaching you even a few).

Furthermore, your learning does not stop once you complete your initial education. Each year, new medical equipment and surgical instruments are invented whose names you will need to learn. One of the major areas of change is pharmaceuticals. Each year, hundreds of new drugs are added to the list of prescriptions doctors may offer, and you need to learn to spell them. (Ironically, most doctors have no idea how to spell many of these new drugs, so you are often the keeper of such knowledge.)

Medical Science Training

A medical transcriptionist must have a solid understanding of the medical sciences: anatomy, physiology, pathology, pharmacology, and so on. This usually means taking an overview course in each area to become familiar with the terminology and procedures, though you do not need to go into the same depth as a pre-med student or nurse. Your goal is not to learn enough to identify and analyze a disease, but you must have at least an aural knowledge of this "foreign" language, that is, the ability to identify and understand the significance of the word when you hear it.

A transcriptionist cannot work in a vacuum, typing up reports as if the words were nonsense terms that simply need to be spelled correctly. The mark of high-quality medical transcription is that the documents make sense. While transcriptionists are not technically responsible for fixing errors dictated by a doctor, they should be able to recognize the meaning of a report and monitor it for sense and context. If a doctor starts a transcription discussing a procedure performed on the right side of the body and then accidentally uses terminology related to the left side, the transcriptionist needs to recognize that an inconsistency has occurred. He or she can then point out the problem to the physician or to the supervisor if the transcriptionist is working for a hospital or service.

English Language Skills

Transcriptionists still use English to connect the hard words. In other words, you still need to know how to write proper English, how to punctuate correctly, and how to maintain a consistent style. As Joan Walston and others I interviewed were all eager to say, physicians are not usually the best grammarians, often slipping into the passive voice or using misplaced modifiers (e.g., "The patient was examined by me on the table" instead of, "I examined the patient on the table"), or rambling when a single sentence would have done it. Although many transcriptionists, particularly those who work in hospital settings, are told to transcribe verbatim without making any changes whatsoever, many independent transcriptionists report that doctors expect them to improve the grammar in their documents. This means that although transcriptionists cannot change any medical terminology or phrasing, they need to use judgment in making a physician's report read intelligently, with well-articulated sentences and proper punctuation.

Computer Literacy

Today, all medical transcription is typed using computers and word-processing software. For telecommuting and independent transcriptionists, *WordPerfect 5.0* or *Word Perfect 5.1* for DOS (formerly owned by Novell and now owned by Corel) has long been considered the software of choice, but *Microsoft Word for Windows* has captured a growing share of the market as has the new version of *WordPerfect for Windows*. Many transcriptionists still use the DOS-based software, but as in all professions, Windows-based programs are becoming the new standard. (In the hospital environment, many other software packages are in use; these are actually interfaces built on top of *WordPerfect* or *Word* by independent companies that add such features as management reporting, digital dictation, autofaxing, e-mail, and electronic signature.)

Most transcriptionists now use a variety of productivity-enhancing add-on software products, the most important of which are specialized medical spelling checkers. These include programs such as *Stedman's 25/Plus* medical spell checker and dictionary containing more than 200,000 words.

Another new type of software product hitting the market recently is "word-expanding software," programs that allow you to type just one or two characters and then select from a list of frequently used words that start with those characters. Obviously, such software is intended to improve productivity, because some medical terms and pharmaceutical drugs are as many as 15 to 30 characters long. For example, consider the word esophagogastroduodenoscopy, a mere 26 characters; rather than type each of those characters, you simply need to type "eso" and then point to the word you want that appears at the bottom of the screen.

See Appendix C for a list of companies offering spell-checking software and word-expanding software. for medical transcription.

Business and Professional Skills

Many people believe that medical transcription is the right profession for them, so they obtain training and set off to get a contract with a physician, only to discover that they must sell themselves. They then become flustered and find they cannot attract clients.

In short, transcription is a business just as any other. You cannot become an independent transcriptionist without having the skills to get clients and operate your business with a profit. You must know how to market yourself, compete with other services out there, set your fees, and develop a reputation. If you want to be an independent or telecommuting transcriptionist, you also need self-management skills, since you largely work alone even if you report to a supervisor in a hospital or service setting.

As part of your business skills, you must also develop a highly professional demeanor and be able to tolerate the day-in, day-out nature of your work, while feeling proud of what you do. You must be extremely detail oriented, organized, and compulsive about doing a good job and handing in quality work. A medical transcriptionist needs to be as precise as a neurosurgeon, as sensitive as an interior designer, and as attentive as an orchestra conductor. While a small level of error can perhaps go unnoticed and may even be within a level of statistical tolerance, the transcriptionist's charter is truly to avoid mistakes and to be vigilant in monitoring the work. In short, you must be a person of high standards.

You must also enjoy the challenge of figuring out a puzzle, because you will find yourself truly stumped and unable to recognize the words used. Nevertheless, you must be patient, curious, and open to finding out exactly what was said on the dictation without becoming frustrated and willing to abandon your task easily.

You must also maintain a high degree of ethics because of the extremely privileged and confidential information you are working on. You must respect both the rights of the patient and the sanctity of the healthcare provider. In fact, the matter of confidentiality is so important in this profession that there are federal and state laws that protect patient privacy that you need to know about.

You must also keep some emotional distance from your work, as you are often transcribing tapes about people who are seriously ill or dying. While none of the transcriptionists I interviewed said they suffered from depression or sadness when transcribing reports, I am sure that there is an emotional challenge to spending your days transcribing reports about seriously ill or dying people.

Finally, while many people think that the best personality for this job is an "introverted" one, it actually helps to be at least a bit outgoing and interested in having an active lifestyle. Two of the primary detrimental aspects of the job are burnout and stress-related physical illnesses, such as carpal tunnel syndrome, radial entrapment in the arms, eye and ear strain, lower back problems, and a host of other ailments that stem from keyboarding and sitting. For that reason, the wise person recognizes that hobbies and physical exercise are important aspects of the work. You need to regularly seek out things to do outside of work and establish a regular schedule of outdoor activities for amusement and life enhancement.

Income and Earning Potential

Medical transcription offers an excellent opportunity to make a good living in a consistently high-demand field. (I am sure you have never heard of medical transcriptionists who were laid off in the past few years! Or if they were, they probably went out and started their own business without any problems.) Other than the stability of the job, the important question is, how much can a transcriptionist actually earn?

Unfortunately, the answer to the income question varies considerably. For transcriptionists employed in hospitals, the starting pay ranges between $8 to $15 an hour, with an average salary for an experienced transcriptionist at $30,000 a year or slightly better. For independent transcriptionists, the earning potential can be much greater, going as high as $70,000 if you are highly qualified, type quickly, and work slightly more than full time.

The reason for these variances is that, as with the other professions in this book, there are many ways that independent transcriptionists price their services, and there is also a wide variation in the fees they can get depending on their location in the country. In the past, transcriptionists have charged according to any of the following three standards:

1. Hourly fees ($15 to $24 per hour)

2. Per page ($5 to $6 per page)

3. Per line ($0.08 to $0.19 per line)

In recent years, the per line method of charging has come to be the dominant method used by independent transcriptionists in many areas. One confusion that exists is what constitutes a line. In some areas, a typed line of any length counts as one line, regardless of length. You may set your margins to 60 characters or 80 characters, but regardless of how many words are on a line, each line counts. If a report you transcribe has 32 short lines (e.g., lines that have only 2 or 3 words on them) mixed in with 200 full-length lines (e.g., 70 characters), they all count the same, and you would charge for 232 lines.

The line-count method is easy to do and reasonable. Of course, you need to define with your client in advance what you call a line. Some transcriptionists like to set their margin to 65 characters, but some physicians like 70 or 80. You can end up battling over what constitutes a line.

Today, some transcriptionists are moving toward using 65 characters as the standard unit of measure to count lines. Regardless of what your margins are or how many words are on a line, you agree to call 65 characters one line. A good reason for this is that word-processing software easily and quickly counts characters. When a document is completed, you simply run the character count macro and divide the result by 65. For example, if you completed a transcript and the software counted 8,565 characters,

TABLE 4-2

Range of Line Rates for Medical Transcription (cents per line)

Region of the U.S.	Low Range	High Range
Northwest	10—12	17—19
Western	8—11	12—17
Middle	8—9.5	16—17
Eastern	10	12—15
Southern	10—12	13—16

Source: The Independent Medical Transcriptionist, by Donna Avila-Weil, CMT, and Mary Glaccum, CMT.

you divide 8,565/65. The result is 132 lines. You then multiply 132 × the line rate you have established. If you were charging 12 cents per line, you would earn $15.84 for that document.

Line rates vary greatly by location. In general, transcriptionists in major cities are able to charge much more than those in small towns and rural areas. What part of the country you live in also makes a big difference. According to a survey taken by Donna Avila-Weil and Mary Glaccum, authors of *The Independent Medical Transcriptionist*, most respondents charged by the line with rates as shown in Table 4-2.

Whatever the line rate, most transcriptionists charge a slightly higher fee for emergency work (called STAT work, "STAT" means immediately). They may also charge fees for special delivery, copies, faxing, or reprints of reports that have been lost. In all, the area of fees is open to negotiation for the independent transcriptionist. You can negotiate your best rate with each client based on the following:

- Determine if you want to charge by the "gross line count" regardless of how long a line is or how many words it contains, or by the measured line count (such as a 65-character line).

- Ask for samples of work done for the physician by other transcriptionists so you can measure the margins used to determine the line rate you might be able to get.

- Find out what the going rate is in your city or town and which method most people are using.

- Determine if you can charge your standard line rate for everything you put in a document, including headers and footers.

What then is the bottom line for income potential for an independent medical transcriptionist? The answer to this question depends entirely on your productivity and hours worked. For simplicity, let's make some assumptions: an experienced medical transcriptionist using the latest computer technology including macro abbreviations and word-extending software can type 300 lines per hour. A novice might be able to type from 100 to 200 lines per hour. Table 4-3 shows your income potential at various line rates per hour assuming you work an 8-hour day 250 days of the year.

As you can see, the potential for a decent income is high even for the novice. The table indicates that a novice who transcribes 100 to 150 lines per hour can gross between $20,000 and $50,000—a reasonable gross income range for either a single person or a spouse who wants to contribute to the family income. Note, however, that this table shows gross income and excludes business costs: equipment, supplies, faxes, delivery charges, marketing costs, utilities, phone bills, and so on. Expenses in this business average 20 percent to 30 percent of fees.

As the table also shows, if you are ambitious and seek more income, you can work harder to achieve a higher line production rate, moving far beyond the $50,000 bracket, especially if you can bill at a rate greater than 10 cents per line.

TABLE 4-3

Gross Income Projections for Medical Transcriptionists

	@ 10¢ per Line	@ 12¢ per Line	@ 14¢ per Line	@ 16¢ per Line	@ 18¢ per Line
100 Lines per Hour = 800 Lines per Day	$80/day × 250 = 20,000	96 per day × 250 = 24,000	112 per day × 250 = 28,000	128 per day × 250 = 32,000	144 per day × 250 = 36,000
150 Lines per Hour = 1,200 Lines per Day	120/day × 250 = 30,000	144/day × 250 = 36,000	168/day × 250 = 42,000	192/day × 250 = 48,000	216/day × 250 = 54,000
200 Lines per Hour = 1,600 Lines per Day	160/day × 250 = 40,000	192 per day × 250 = 48,000	224/day × 250 = 56,000	256/day × 250 = 64,000	288/day × 250 = 72,000
300 Lines per Hour = 2,400 Lines per Day	240/day × 250 = 60,000	288/day × 250 = 72,000	336/day × 250 = 84,000	384/day × 250 = 96,000	432/day × 250 = 108,000

Deciding If This Business Is for You

By now, you have read about the rigorous preparation medical transcriptionists must have, the lifestyle they lead, and the potential rewards. The following checklist can help with your decision. Take a moment now to do this 15-question checklist before reading the remainder of the chapter.

- Do I enjoy medical terminology and descriptions of cases?
- Do I enjoy working behind the scenes, without contact with the public?
- Do I like words, details, and working on documents?
- Do I like working on my own?
- Will I enjoy listening to voices of physicians, some of whom I haven't met?
- Do I like figuring out puzzles and trying to identify missing pieces?
- Do I enjoy constantly learning new words and vocabulary?
- Do I have a good ear for sounds, language, and voices and a good eye for spelling, punctuation, and grammar?
- Am I willing to listen to something over and over again until I get it right?
- Do I have good concentration skills and an ability to block out distractions that interfere with my ability to work?
- Am I accurate, organized, and fastidious?
- Do I like writing, typing, and working with computers?
- Can I read or write about serious illnesses without becoming upset or sensitive?
- Am I trustworthy and able to not disclose medical information about people whose names I know?
- Do I mind working in a profession that is sometimes given short shrift?

If you have answered yes to the majority of these questions, or if you have some doubts but want to proceed, the next section provides brief guidelines on how to get started. This material will be organized differently from the preceding chapters, since it is unlikely you will start your business immediately. The next section includes the location of resources for training and education, information on equipping and furnishing your office for medical transcription, and a discussion of how to build your career once you've finished an educational program.

Section II: Getting Started

Resources and Training

In general, if you have a good educational background, such as a college degree and general language aptitude, you can learn medical transcription using one of the high-quality home-study programs. However, if you are not linguistically oriented or do not have a good general educational background, you may wish to consider attending a community college program in medical transcription. These can take from two to four semesters to complete. Let's start by looking at home-study courses, since my assumption is that for most readers of this book, full- or part-time school is not an option.

HOME-STUDY PROGRAMS Perhaps the most noted home-study course that has received excellent marks is the SUM (Systems Unit Method) Program for Medical Transcription Training, available from Health Professions Institute in Modesto, California. As the SUM program literature explains:

> The SUM Program for Medical Transcription Training was developed to educate medical transcription students to the level where they are productive from their first day of employment. The SUM program is used mostly in schools and hospitals, but has also been made available to transcription companies and to individuals by popular demand. The program uses carefully selected authentic physician dictation, sequenced by medical specialty on standard-size cassette tapes, along with academic textbook reading assignments and exercises. As a self-directed student, you will transcribe the dictation to the best of your ability, using all references at your disposal, then check your work against the corresponding transcript answer keys.

This SUM program is modular. The Beginning Medical Training (BMT) course is the first segment. This module consists of 12 hours of authentic dictation, including:

- 1.5 hours of narration on relevant topics by well-known authors and educators in the field
- 1.5 hours of narrative instruction for transcribing pharmacology, lab procedures, and the medical history and physical examination
- 9 hours of authentic dictation, including chart notes, letters, initial office evaluations, history and physicals, consultations, emergency department reports, and discharge summaries in 11 specialties (cardiology, dermatology, endocrinology, gastroenterology, neurology, ophthalmology, orthopedics, otorhinolaryngology, pulmonary medicine, urology, and obstetrics and gynecology)

Students can take the beginning program and seek employment in a physician's office, group practice, or small clinic. It normally takes 480 hours to complete the basic program, including all the recommended readings (12 weeks if you study for 40 hours per week; or 24 weeks at 20 hours per week).

Students can then follow the basic program with any or all of five specialty modules that prepare them for more advanced work in hospital settings, including cardiology, gastroenterology, orthopedics, pathology, and radiology. Each advanced course contains four hours of authentic physician dictation (except for radiology, which has three). Students should plan on spending 80 hours for each advanced course.

The SUM program has received excellent marks from many people in the industry for its comprehensive and authentic training, and also for its ease of use among self-motivated people. As Linda Campbell, director of Product Development for Health Professions Institute (HPI) told me,

> We sell our program to hospitals and colleges but also to individuals. Before our program, there was very little quality among college programs, in part because there were no standards for training in this industry. There was no federal agency or anyone to mandate standards. We brought out our program in 1987, and since then, we have proven that given the right program, a motivated individual can learn medical transcription on his or her own. Is self-study an ideal situation? No, the ideal situation would be to have a trained medical transcriptionist teaching students in a facility. But that is not realistic for many adults today who are changing careers for one reason or another, and for whom self-study is their only option. We have done the best we can in this program, and we now have hundreds of people who have passed the certification (CMT) exam given by the American Association for Medical Transcription (AAMT).

The Basic Medical Transcription course costs $840, plus a few hundred dollars for various textbooks that are required reading. The course includes the tapes, the answer keys, and a student manual, which contains the suggested curriculum. According to Linda Campbell, if you are uncertain, you can purchase the first tape separately to see if you like the program; the cost is $85.

The advanced courses are $280 each, except for Radiology, which costs $210. Each advanced course comes with a student guide, answer key, and a word and phrase reference book.

HPI also offers a 10-hour video program called *Building a Successful Medical Transcription Business*. This video is directed at students who have completed the basic SUM program and/or advanced courses and are interested in starting their own business. The videos cost $495 and also include a binder of reference materials such as sample contracts.

Finally, HPI offers its students an opportunity to join a network, the Medical Transcription Student Network. The benefits of joining include a quarterly newsletter and a 10 percent discount on many reference and word books that HPI sells by catalogue.

Contact HPI at P.O. Box 801, Modesto, CA 95353 or call 209-551-2112 for information. HPI also sells a wide assortment of reference and word books for medical transcriptionists, and it publishes a quarterly magazine, *Perspectives on the Medical Transcription Profession*. See Figure 4-6 for samples showing various items available from HPI.

Note that the SUM program as offered by HPI is not an interactive course; students do not submit their practice transcriptions by mail to an instructor at HPI. It is completely self-study. No degree is awarded when you complete the program, because the Institute is not an accredited school, but rather a for-profit research and development facility providing educational materials. As its brochure states, however, "independent study students who have properly completed The Sum Program should not encounter difficulty finding employment."

If you prefer to have an instructor work with you as you complete the SUM program, and/or a degree, consider the following two options:

- **Review of Systems (ROS).** This educational training program is offered by Jennifer Martin and contains the same SUM program basic modules (BMT) along with interactive instruction. Ms. Martin is a former instructor at Maple Woods Community College in Kansas City, Missouri, and has been a home-based medical transcriptionist for more than nine years. Essentially, when you purchase Review of

Figure 4-6
Brochures and training materials from Health Professions Institute

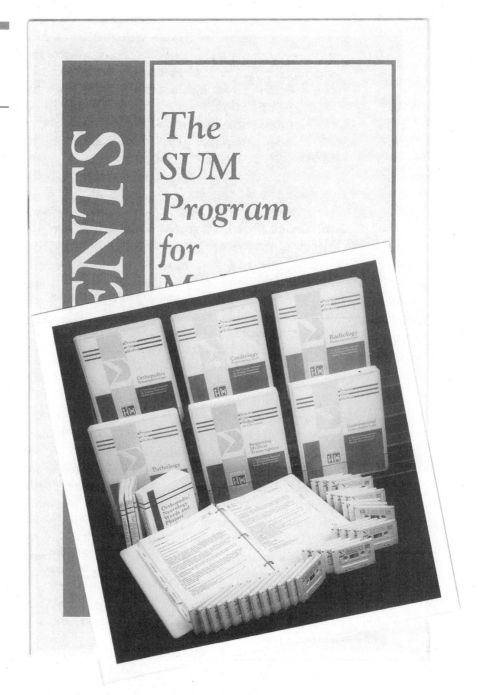

Systems, you get the very same beginning 12-hour SUM program offered by HPI, plus all necessary textbooks, a variety of reference and word books, and the expertise of Ms. Martin to correct assignments that you mail in as you complete them. ROS is sold in five modules, each costing $300, for a total of $1,500, slightly more than the fee charged by HPI for the basic program. You can contact Ms. Martin at 800-951-5559 or 816-468-4403. She is also available on e-mail at MTMonthly@AOL.com or at www.mtmonthly.com.

- **California College for Health Sciences (CCHS).** If you prefer to have an instructor plus earn a college degree, the entire SUM program is also offered as a home-study course through CCHS, an accredited degree-granting private postsecondary institution. CCHS offers the SUM program as part of an Associate of Science degree, which may entitle you to tuition assistance or reimbursement from an employer. You can contact the school at 222 West 24th Street, National City, CA 91950; phone 800-221-7374. See Appendix C for more information on CCHS.

Another home-study program is offered by a private company called At-Home Professions. This company began as a developer of home-study courses for court transcriptionists. The company realized that a related medical transcription course could also help many people who wanted to learn from home.

At-Home Professions' medical transcription course was developed under the guidance of Dr. Caroline Yeager, a UCLA physician who helped establish the Teaching Department at the UCLA School of Medicine, Martin Luther King Hospital. Caroline explained to me that in addition to being a radiologist, she had a long background in "instructional design" (the field of designing learning units for people, be it in banking or medicine), and so her interest in this area spurred her to write the course with At-Home Professions. In outlining the course, she pointed out that it follows "objective-based training" principles, meaning that you don't get an A, B, C, or D grade, which is a subjective view of your skills, but instead you move through the course by demonstrating that you have mastered one topic at a time. Caroline admitted quite modestly that the course won a prestigious award from a professional society of instructional designers of which she is a member.

The At-Home Professions program consists of five modules, with each module containing many lessons of written explanations, activities, and tapes that you do one at a time. According to company director Cole Thompson, At-Home Professions estimates that a student who studies an average of 20 hours per week can complete all five modules in about six months, although a few people have done it faster. "It's a completely self-paced program," he told me, "in which the students do the lessons at a pace they feel comfortable in. There are specific milestones in each module, and activities and assignments that students do that are self-correcting, followed by an activity that they mail in to us for correction." Cole added that in this program, students have regular one-on-one conversations with their instructors using At-Home's 800 phone number, so that it is not just a mail-order program with no contact between faculty and students.

Both Caroline and Cole were eager to reinforce that this program has tried to be as realistic as possible in teaching medical transcription. The course includes several hours of practice tapes using a broad range of voices similar to those of doctors—voices from Korea, India, Pakistan, Mexico, and many other locales, as well as voices eating lunch while dictating. The five modules teach all necessary medical transcription skills: specialty reports, hospital terminology, and operative reports, as well as essentials of anatomy and physiology. Cole also indicated that students are exposed to all the common specialties of medicine, such as orthopedics, chiropractic, internal medicine, and radiology.

The cost of the At-Home Professions program is $450 for each module, thus a total of $2,250. (Note: price is subject to change.) You can reach At-Home Professions at 800-528-7907, or by writing to 2001 Lowe Street, Fort Collins, CO 80525. The sidebar on Rochelle Wexler presents a profile of a transcriptionist who received her training using At-Home Professions' materials.

ACADEMIC STUDY   Home-study programs are often the only way that adults can learn a new profession, but if you have time or need the extra study, you might consider a broader based academic program offered through a college or community college. Academic programs differ in quality, so be sure to investigate the types of courses offered and the qualifications of the instructors.

The American Association for Medical Transcription (AAMT) recommends a model curriculum that it would like to see colleges adopt throughout the country. This curriculum includes two semesters of medical terminology and three to four semesters of practical experience in transcription, including one semester in a practicum. As you can see, this type of curriculum will take several years to complete. However, the advantages of attending a credentialed program are that you may get a more comprehensive education and that you may achieve a higher level of credibility in finding a job, especially in a hospital environment.

Business Profile: Rochelle Wexler

Rochelle came to medical transcription after a career in musical theater and a brief stint in publishing. She decided that she wanted to find a profession she could call her own, something that allowed her to work from home and to start up with a minimal investment in equipment and training. She had read the first edition of this book; and although she had no medical background, she realized that medical transcription fulfilled her needs.

Rochelle saw an advertisement for At-Home Professions in a magazine and called to receive its information. She double-checked the company's credentials and opted to purchase its training. Rochelle completely dedicated herself to completing the At-Home course quickly; she finished it within six months by working between 30 and 50 hours per week.

Rochelle says that the support staff at At-Home Professions gave her good advice about marketing her newfound career. Within two weeks, Rochelle obtained two clients using fliers that she created on her PC and samples of her work. Living in Manhattan, she was able to canvass a small area and give out 150 flyers in two days, which generated about six calls from various specialists.

Rochelle now has a variety of physicians for clients, including a urologist, cardiologist, oncologist, hematologist, endocrinologist, physical therapist, podiatrist, and pediatric pulmonologist. Some clients give her work sporadically, but she has several she "can count on." Rochelle points out that much of her work consists of referral letters and reports between primary care physicians and specialists. Her biggest client is a diabetes specialist who must heavily document patient visits.

Rochelle charges a line rate; she started at 13 cents per line and has been able to move most of her clients up to 16 cents per line. Her business philosophy is to do the best she can and to provide high-quality service. To this end, she does pick up and deliver tapes and documents. For her work, she used a plain vanilla 486 PC with *WordPerfect*. She has two transcribers, one for standard cassettes and one for micros.

Rochelle was kind enough to send in the photo in Figure 4-7 showing her workspace.

EVALUATING THE BEST PROGRAM FOR YOU Whichever method you prefer, academic or at-home study, degree or not, you should find out as much as you can about how the program works, how long it takes, how much it costs, who the instructors are, and what kind of instruction you will actually receive. In particular, ask if the program covers hospital transcription, physician transcription, or both (since hospital transcription tends to be more rigorous, with more technical vocabulary and more surgical procedures), and if it covers all of the major types of special reports. Then ask how many hours of listening you will receive, and if the audio component of the program includes a variety of accents and voices that increase the level of difficulty.

Following those questions, your next issue is to find out how well the graduates of the program have fared. Ask for a referral list so that you can speak to graduates to learn firsthand what they thought of the program

Figure 4-7
Rochelle Wexler,
medical
transcriptionist

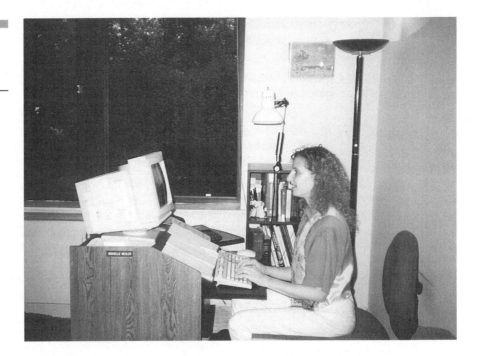

and how many of them got the jobs they were hoping to find. A good program will not hesitate to give you such a referral list as a good-faith demonstration that its graduates were qualified enough to have landed positions somewhere in the industry.

If you are considering a full-time A.A. or B.A. degree program, find out how many other general curriculum courses you will need to take; these will add time and expense to finishing your degree.

For comparison, many sources in the medical transcription industry prefer the SUM program to the At-Home Professions program. The SUM is generally considered to be more professionally oriented and more attentive to the rigorous demands of the profession. However, you should evaluate both of these programs and others you may find, as well as programs available at your local community college; find out which is the best option for you. Also, if you are investigating other home-study courses, be wary of any course that suggests that you can finish it in six weeks or three months, as any comprehensive program worth paying for will challenge you and take time to learn. It is simply a waste of your money if your program doesn't properly train you for the demands of real-life medical transcription.

ASSOCIATIONS The most noted association in the industry is the American Association for Medical Transcription (AAMT), with approximately 8500 members. Deeming themselves "medical language specialists," AAMT members lobby around the country, encouraging those in the medical community to better understand and reward more appropriately the high level of knowledge and professionalism that a duly-trained transcriptionist brings to the job. Through its own publication, the *Journal of the American Association for Medical Transcription* (JAAMT), the association informs its members about new technologies, new ways to get training and improve skills, and new ideas for making hospitals and physicians treat them more professionally.

AAMT is actively involved in nearly every aspect of the industry, from recommending a model curriculum to be used in college programs to working with many industry groups to establish new national standards for transcription formats. AAMT offers a certification exam that any transcriptionist can sit for, even if he or she is not a member. Upon successful completion of the exam, the individual receives the title CMT, or Certified Medical Transcriptionist. The exam actually consists of two parts: the first is a written portion and the second is a practical test. Each exam costs $150.

In recent years, AAMT has been mostly oriented toward full-time medical transcriptionists with professional or academic backgrounds. If you are a student working from a home-study program, you may find that the benefits of joining AAMT are not worth the membership expense. (AAMT has generally disapproved of home-study programs and does not produce one itself.) However, depending on your interests, you should obtain information about the organization and its potential benefits for you by writing to P.O. Box 576187, Modesto, CA 95357-6187 or by calling 800-982-2182 or 209-551-0883. Ask for the Director of Member Services.

Another organization that may be of growing importance to telecommuting transcriptionists is the Medical Transcription Industry Alliance (MTIA). Although this is a trade association for corporations such as large transcription services, it has formed an affiliate category for the transcriptionist employees. See Appendix C for more information about contacting MTIA.

NEWSLETTERS To fill a large gap in information available to the independent, former transcriptionist Jennifer Martin started a newsletter, *MTMonthly.* The newsletter contains a variety of articles, including updates on technology and medical terminology (especially new drugs that come onto the market regularly), as well as business tips and advice.

The annual fee for the *MTMonthly* is $48. To order, write *MTMonthly,* Suite 100, 1633 NE Rosewood Drive, Gladstone, MO 64118 or call 800-951-5559 or 816-468-4403.

ONLINE RESOURCES The world of online resources is growing in the medical transcription business. You can now find networks of people discussing medical transcription on CompuServe (in the Working from Home forum) and on America Online. The Internet is teeming with Web sites of interest to the new transcriptionist, including information from many of the companies that manufacture hardware and software for the industry, such as Dictaphone, Lanier, DVI, Narratek, and others. There is also a newsgroup dedicated to transcriptionists and other health professionals. See Appendix C for a list of sites to explore.

BOOKS There is one book that can especially enlighten the person interested in becoming an independent transcriptionist. Aptly titled *The Independent Medical Transcriptionist,* its authors Donna Avila-Weil and Mary Glaccum have a combined total of more than 50 years in the transcription business. The book includes extensive information on every topic touched on in this chapter, including education and training, setting up your business, legal issues, pricing, contracts, and more. You can order the book from its publisher Rayve Productions Inc., P.O. Box 726, Windsor, CA 95492; order phone is 800-852-4890.

Equipment and Furnishings

TRANSCRIPTION EQUIPMENT As described earlier in the sections of this chapter that discussed technology, the equipment you need to enter the business depends extensively on three factors:

1. Which type of business you are in (employee vs. telecommuter vs. independent)
2. What type of technology your customers use (digital vs. tape-based)
3. How you organize your service (physicians calling you vs. you calling into a server)

All these factors determine if you end up picking up cassettes from your clients and transcribing them at home using an inexpensive transcriber as Terri Ford does; or if you end up purchasing a multiport transcriber that allows for simultaneous call-in and transcription, such as the one Joan Walston uses; or if you invest in propriety digital technology equipment, such as the Straight Talk® unit from Dictaphone that coordinates with a large server at a hospital or service; or if you purchase PC-based software to turn your standard sound card into a dictation device or downloader device that allows you to decompress files that are sent to your machine via modem.

In general though, you may not need to worry about these decisions if you are just starting out. Most training programs, such as the SUM program and At-Home Professions and even college courses, simply require that you own an inexpensive standard cassette transcriber (not the micro-cassette size). This transcriber unit is made by many companies, including Lanier, Dictaphone, Sony, VDI, Phillips, and Panasonic, and the cost is usually less than $250. Some machines have adapters that allow you to use either standard cassettes or microcassettes. The more sophisticated of these transcriber units have many fancy buttons, such as ones that control the speed of the dictation, the volume, and the tone and know how many dictations are on the tape, and how long they are. It is generally recommended that you buy your transcriber unit from an authorized dealer or sales representative of a company rather than an office supply store, which tends to sell lower quality brands.

As you come closer to being ready to open your business, you can then decide if you want to invest in a multiport system and have doctors call you, or if you want digital equipment that coordinates with a large national service or a local one, or if you want PC-based software that enhances your PC. It is likely that the price of digital technology will come down by the time you are reading this book, and more facilities will adopt it. If so, you may still need to choose among various setups, such as purchasing proprietary hardware from Dictaphone, Lanier, or another major company versus the use of generic re-recording technology.

COMPUTER   Most medical transcription today requires a 386 or 486 PC using DOS-based word-processing software such as *WordPerfect*. However, it would not make sense to get into business—unless you absolutely had to—using this type of equipment. Prices on Pentiums are dropping dramatically, and a Windows-based environment will generally improve your productivity.

The common recommendation made today is to purchase a Pentium with 16 Mb of RAM, a 500 Mb hard drive, and a CD-ROM to use for the increasing amount of reference materials such as dictionaries and word books that are now available in that format. It also helps to have a backup tape unit or other backup equipment. You cannot risk losing completed reports to accidents, vandalism, or breach of security (such as a computer virus that destroys your hard disk).

PRINTER For your printer, a good dot matrix printer is acceptable, as long as it has "near-letter-quality" output. However, more and more people are moving to using laser printers, as their purchase cost and per page expense go down.

SHREDDER Because of the high level of patient confidentiality that you must maintain as an independent transcriptionist, it is also recommended that you own a paper shredder to destroy drafts of documents and transcriptions. Small shredding machines are now quite inexpensive and well within the budget for a home business.

OFFICE FURNISHINGS Because you will be spending so much time at a keyboard, be sure to find an ergonomic desk that allows your arms and wrists to rest on a pad to avoid muscle spasms, inflammation of the wrist, and nerve entrapment due to swelling of the wrist. Dr. Earl Brewer, M.D, a specialist in arthritis in Houston, Texas, and author of *The Arthritis Sourcebook* (Lowell House), cautions that overuse of the wrists and arms by people who heavily use computers is one of the primary causes of long-term injury to the muscles and joints of that area, and therefore a contributing factor in arthritic problems.

It has also long been known that poor ergonomics (the study of how fit and function interrelate) combined with repetitive motions can lead to cumulative trauma disorders (CTDs), which include tennis elbow and carpal tunnel syndrome, a debilitating disease of the wrists. As a result, it is usually recommended that you have a chair with arm rests that allow you to relax your forearms. It is also useful for the chair to have castors so that you can move around easily to change positions, and that its height be adjustable. Ideally, you should aim to not need to stretch your neck, arms, or wrists to reach your keyboard. You can also purchase a keyboard platform to raise or lower your keyboard to accomplish this. (I have had this problem and it led to a very debilitating three months of bursitis in both shoulders, due to poor positioning of my arms relative to my keyboard and mouse.)

You also want your monitor to be at about a 20-degree angle lower than your line of sight, and positioned between 13 and 18 inches away from your eyes to avoid eyestrain. You might consider an antiglare filter, which absorbs reflected light on your screen that can overload the eyes.

Call BackSaver Products at 800-251-2225 for more information on back support products, and BackCare Corporation in Chicago at 312-258-0888 for information on their products to help typists. Read computer magazines for regular reports on new furniture, lighting equipment, and ergonomic computer designs that can improve your office or study conditions. One new product, for example, is called the HandEZE AE Fingerless Glove. As its name suggests, it is a glove worn while typing, but it has been ergonomically designed to alleviate muscle fatigue and pain caused from carpal tunnel, tendonitis, arthritis, and numbness. It costs only $19.95 per pair. Call for a catalogue and brochure from Therapeutic Appliance Group at 800-457-5535.

REFERENCE BOOKS Today's medical transcriptionist has a great need for a number of reference books on his or her desk. There are literally scores of dictionaries, word books, style guides, and medical reference sources. Some are general, but many are reference materials that you need to specialize in one medical field or another, from new technological vocabulary to psychology to pharmacology. Because new names are continually invented for diseases, procedures, diagnoses, instruments, and drugs, these books are constantly updated and so you need to purchase new editions frequently.

You can order reference materials and word books from several organizations and publishers of medical books. See Appendix C for details.

Building Your Career

If you finish a training program in medical transcription, you will probably be eager to get your new business going. However, it is commonly said that there is a Catch 22 in this industry for new transcriptionists: you can't get a job until you have two to three years of experience but you can't get experience without a job.

Nevertheless, because of the demand for transcriptionists everywhere, predictions are that even the newest graduates will find work, just as Terri Ford and Rochelle Wexler did within a few weeks of completing their programs. You may wish to start by interviewing in a medical records department of a hospital where you can obtain continued support and training. Because hospital work is so varied, you will also expand your breadth of knowledge and experience.

Alternatively, you might discuss opportunities for employment with a local service, such as that run by Joan Walston, who seeks out distinctive individuals to train. There is now a growing number of extremely large national services that hire hundreds of transcriptionists, many of whom are offsite. It is likely that many such services will need people and be willing to hire new recruits who can demonstrate quality work and a commitment to learning. It is expected that the next century will open up even more professional training programs in this field to handle the growing demand for transcriptionists.

Many industries have similar future outlooks. As with insurance, banking, and publishing, you will need to put in a few years to pay your dues and learn the ropes before you can move out on your own. There is actually some value in this, because obtaining real-world experience and getting paid for it benefit you in many ways. If you must obtain a job rather than start your own company, this is the time to learn about dealing with doctors, with poor dictations, with voices you didn't encounter in school or in your home-study program, and with the myriad other details that no one taught you. This is the time to perfect your working style so that when you go off on your own, you are not surprised at your mistakes or the little idiosyncrasies that you thought you never had when you were under pressure.

Many people say that one to two years of experience in a hospital are sufficient as background to start your own business or to work for a small service that provides flexible hours and possible telecommuting opportunities. One key to assuring that you can control your own destiny is to pick an area in which to specialize. Learn the vocabulary of one field and develop your knowledge of its trends. With medicine itself becoming an industry of specialists, you would be wise to imitate the doctors in this way. As a matter of fact, it is probably better to specialize in a few areas, to be sure you do not become attached to a small clientele. If one doctor for whom you do most of your work moves or changes practice, you would be left without a source of income.

Related to this issue of having only one client, if you are a free-lance independent medical transcriptionist (or any other professional for that matter), you must be careful about working exclusively for one client since the IRS may then determine that you are not really an independent contractor but a statutory employee. If that happens, the financial penalties for you are severe. Charging on an hourly basis is one indication the IRS may use against you, so be sure to charge by the page or line, and to have many clients so you will be perceived as an independent contractor. Be sure to consult your accountant and attorney to review the IRS questions that are used to determine if a person is an independent contractor or an employee.

ESTIMATING START-UP EXPENSES   Like medical claims assistance, one advantage of this business is that, in general, start-up costs are very low for the home-based person. Your investment in office equipment (including a computer, printer, transcriber, and phone) and supplies such as books and reference materials can be as low as $2,000. If you can afford it, you may want to spend $2,500 to $6,000 for better computer and transcription equipment.

Your expenses might amount to

Office equipment (computer, printer)	$1,500—$3,000
Transcriber (if purchased new)	$300—$1,000
Business cards, letterhead, envelopes	$100—$200
Fliers	$100—$500
Office furniture	$400—$800
Phone	$100—$200
Books	$200—$300
TOTAL	$2,700—$6,000

Note: sophisticated tape-based or digital transcription equipment can be leased for as little as $150 to $250 per month.

MARKETING YOUR SERVICE   A home-based medical transcriptionist is as much a businessperson as the other two medical professionals in this book. You must therefore know how to market to prospective clients if you want to remain in business.

The first avenue open to a qualified transcriptionist is to obtain overflow work from permanently staffed locations. Nearly every transcriptionist reported that hospitals and services are continually overloaded or need to fill in for vacationing staff, forcing them to farm out work to independent contractors on a regular basis.

The second avenue to marketing your service is to pursue a field of specialization and create a niche for yourself. When you have such a specialization, you can write a letter of introduction to every doctor in your area who performs that specialty and announce your new business. You can easily tailor a direct marketing letter to a small number of doctors who might use your services. One transcriptionist I interviewed used her background in both medical and legal transcription to specialize in personal injury (PI) and worker's compensation cases, since doctors involved in these cases must extensively document the patient's injuries. She obtained a list of all doctors who do worker's comp from the state board in California and then sent a letter to each one. She got many responses, some of whom became clients when she followed up with a personal call and an interview.

Finally, the next most useful marketing strategy is word of mouth. Like accountants, lawyers, and consultants, doctors use recommendations and referrals for finding services they need. You should do the same. After working with a doctor for a few months, ask for a referral to one of his or her colleagues. It's easy to get referrals if you have been performing well and the physician knows what kind of person you are.

As with many professions, starting up your own business can be slow and painful, but a few months of lean times can pay off big in the end.

PRICING As discussed earlier in the chapter, your goal is to maximize your fees. At the same time, you are likely faced with a classic situation of needing to compete with a few others who lower their prices to get the business. This dilemma points to the fact that the transcription market is fairly price sensitive. For example, Joan Walston of Words Times 3 says that she can charge $24 per hour, but she has not been able to go above that figure for many years because of resistance in the market.

You therefore need to have a sense of what your competition charges and what your clients are willing to accept if they like your work. If you are a fast typist in an area in which per line rates are low, you may be better off charging by the page. On the other hand, if your product is high quality, but your work takes longer than another transcriptionist, you might do better charging by the hour to more fairly compensate you for the extra effort you put into making sure that your documents are perfect.

Ultimately, you need to watch out for what one medical transcriptionist called the "bad mental connection." She explained,

> What I mean is that your presence in the doctor's office signifies trouble to the physician, as in "Oh, no, here goes more of my money." You don't want the doctor to think like that. You want the physician to associate your presence with help, not with a drain on money. That's why you also learn to invoice physicians whenever they pay their other employees, so that they don't think that every time you walk in the door while there's a roomful of patients waiting for them, that they have to pull out their checkbook and pay you.

CONTRACTS Many independent transcriptionists have only an informal contract with their clients, but most seek to operate formally and so ask the physician to sign a contract for their services. Given the efforts you may have expended to sign a new client, it is certainly advisable that you try to work with a contract as often as possible. Contracts can spell out the turnaround times, schedules, fees and method of pricing, and all the variables you need to protect you from the whims of new office personnel who want to fire you and put in their friend. Remember that turnover is rampant in medical staffing, and it is easy for a new office manager to suddenly dislike your work and insist on hiring someone else. Consult a lawyer to create your contract, and make it for at least a three- or six-month period of time to start, so that both you and the physician can make sure the relationship is working.

Finally, while medical transcriptionists are not technically responsible for the correctness of the documents, it is often suggested that you carry errors and omissions (E&O) insurance to protect yourself. Or if you don't, Donna Avila-Weil and Mary Glaccum recommend that your contract clearly state that you do not carry E&O insurance and that you are not responsible for errors in your documents unless proofed by the dictating physician. One transcriptionist I interviewed places a footer at the bottom of every page that reads, "Dictated but not read unless signed." This more or less forces the physician to sign each document to verify the accuracy of the transcription.

Building Your Business

Medical transcription demands rigorous training and in-depth technical knowledge and is an extremely intense occupation, but the rewards can be worth the effort. The current shortage of transcriptionists is critical, and it bodes well for a properly trained individual to enter the profession and find steady work with a good salary. For this reason, it is a profession on the forefront of the home-based business movement, allowing thousands of people to establish their own work schedules and run their own businesses from the comfort of their home.

While some predict that new technologies such as voice recognition and computer-based patient records (CPR) may change the face of the profession over the next decade, it is actually far more likely that the evolution of such technology will not remove the need for human intervention in this highly demanding field. For this reason, you can truly count on a fertile environment for good transcriptionists who have the knowledge and skills required in this business. In short, this is a profession in which you can be proud to participate.

Ten Steps to Starting Your Business

The goal of this chapter is leave you with a way to think about a broad range of start-up business advice. Rather than throw out random suggestions and tips, I have developed a brief mnemonic scheme—a device that helps you remember—to assist you in recalling the steps you now need to take. The mnemonic is DREAM BIG for $, which stands for the following sequence of steps:

- Step 1: **D**ouble-check your decision
- Step 2: **R**esearch your business
- Step 3: **E**stablish goals and a business plan
- Step 4: **A**rrange your office
- Step 5: **M**otivate yourself
- Step 6: **B**e professional
- Step 7: **I**nvigorate your marketing
- Step 8: **G**row your business
- Step 9: $$—Make Money!—$$
- Step 10: —Enjoy Yourself!—

Notice that this mnemonic device is upbeat and bright; it even includes that trite little happy face that was popular years ago that most of us now hate. Nevertheless, it has come to represent a certain "Don't worry!" philosophy of life that even the most serious entrepreneurs need to recapture once in a while. The goal of this mnemonic is to remind you at all times of the 10 necessary functions that you must accomplish and keep in mind while undertaking your own business. A good mnemonic sticks in your head for years and years and thus becomes a permanent way to remember a great deal of data that would otherwise confound the mind. Like the mnemonics "Every Good Boy Deserves Fudge" (for the lines of the music staff: EGBDF) and "My Very Excellent Mother Just Sells Nuts Until Passover" (for the planets: Mercury Venus, Earth, etc.), I hope this mnemonic will come to be memorable and significant to you too.

Let's examine now the elements of the mnemonic, exploring what you need to remember at each step of the way.

Step 1: Double-Check Your Decision

It's truly amazing how many people want to be in business for themselves. Though there are no official figures, recent estimates indicate that nearly 36 million people are self-employed and work from home in either full-time or part-time businesses. Small businesses especially are growing, with hundreds of thousands of new incorporations each year, and hundreds of thousands more starting sole proprietorships and partnerships. Another statistic of note is that the fastest growing segment of these new businesses are those started by women.

However, statistics also show that many businesses fail each year, as many as two out of three (and usually within the first year) for a variety of reasons, including excessive spending, poor management, cash flow problems, inadequate marketing, and bad service/product. The point is: are you sure you are ready and able to launch your venture? While pessimism is not useful, and in fact can destroy a positive attitude that contributes to success, I simply suggest that you take time in this initial phase of your thinking to reflect upon your decision and explore its pros and cons in as much depth as you can. Although your choice of a business may arise from your previous background and experience, or from a strongly held desire to work in one of the medical fields, you need to ask yourself several critical questions about your plans:

- Do you have the personality traits that are needed to market a new business?
- Are you willing to learn what you don't know?
- How hard can you work to make your business a success?
- How much are you willing to sacrifice?
- Do you have the character to survive the challenges of start-up?

It can be difficult to force yourself to answer such questions objectively. We are all a product of our own minds and often cannot see our own faults. Some people have a higher opinion of their capabilities than is justified, and may answer such questions with the conviction that they can overcome any challenge. This is usually a good attitude to have, but overstating your qualifications can lead to serious business myopia. You can't afford to miss your own internal problems. This is why, in my opinion, so many people fail in new businesses: they just aren't willing to seek training when they need it, or they fail to ask the right questions because they think they know all the answers.

On the other hand, I also believe that many people discount their talents and shortchange their capabilities. They don't give themselves enough credit for their native intelligence and skills. Many people can prosper in their own business if they recognize that they truly have the talents, skills, and learning ability to succeed. The problem is, people often tend to glamorize entrepreneuring and exaggerate the personal talents and skills needed to do it. They end up fearing that they don't have these skills or abilities, or that their intelligence is insufficient to learn them.

The truth is, few people fit into the category of genius (and that kind of intelligence doesn't necessarily guarantee success anyway). Entrepreneurs are everywhere. Thousands of businesses are started by "ordinary people" every day, except these people believe in themselves and have a deep understanding of their strengths and weaknesses. Their self-knowledge gives them direction and reflection; they know where and how to focus their energy, when to say "I need to learn something new," and when to change course.

The secret to success is best expressed in the adage from Socrates, "Know Thyself." Knowing yourself well allows you to make more meaningful assessments of your skills, abilities, and interests. Don't jump to conclusions about your capability to start a business. Really think through your interests, motivations, strengths, and weaknesses to see if you are minimizing or overstating them.

Table 5-1 contains a list of questions you should consider in double-checking your decision to start a health service business. Rather than having you answer the questions with a simple yes or no, there's a column for your "qualifying thoughts" in which you can reflect deeply about why you said yes or no, and what additional factors you may need to consider to support your conclusion. Consider this column to be the "gray area" in which you are honest in admitting that you don't really know something, or that you actually do believe you could learn something in a relatively short period of time if you put your mind to it.

You might decide, for example, that although you said no to the question that asks about your mastery of accounting and bookkeeping, your qualifying thought might be that you have always enjoyed math. As a result, rather than letting your ignorance of the topic count as a simple *no* that could deter you from your entrepreneurial pursuit, your gray area points out that you recognize your potential to learn about accounting. This will help you see your *potential* energy, rather than your static energy.

Depending on your answers to these questions, you may be ready to get going—or to cancel your plans. If the latter is the case, this book may have saved you a lot of time, headaches, and money. You needn't feel bad about your decision or feel that you have failed. Not starting a health services business does not reflect a deficit in your abilities; it simply indicates that you have wisely chosen otherwise. Perhaps you can explore other entrepreneurial ventures that better match your personal interests and goals. With the growth of home-based work today, you can probably find a wide range of opportunities that might satisfy your personal and professional objectives.

For example, Daniel Lehmann and Patricia Bartello, of DAPA Support Services, the medical billing company mentioned in Chapter 2, spent more than a year evaluating career options. Both had a long-time interest in running their own business, but after a year of exploring franchises and business opportunities, they felt most comfortable choosing a business that matched Pat's previous background in the health field and Dan's background in business. Similarly, Nancie Cummins was coming from an insurance sales background when she decided she wanted to run her own business. She looked at many options, including accounting and medical transcription, but she finally chose medical billing after evaluating her skills and personal interests. In both situations, the individuals involved took their time exploring options and weighing the pros and cons of each.

If you haven't firmly decided to start your own business, you may wish to check the resources in Appendix D. These sources can assist you in eval-

TABLE 5-1

Questions to Ask to Double-Check Your Decision

QUESTIONS	Y	N	QUALIFYING THOUGHTS
Personal Questions			
▪ Have you had an interest in running your own business for a long time?			
▪ Have you worked in a related business area or had any experience relevant to medical billing, claims assistance, or transcription?			
▪ If you haven't worked in a related field before, are you sure that you want to abandon the work experience you already have to learn a new field?			
▪ Do you enjoy technical details, formal systems such as health insurance, and complex terminology?			
▪ Are you willing to learn new things and to work in a profession that requires continual learning?			
▪ Is income potential more important to you than enjoying your work and the people with whom you work?			
▪ Are you independent and a self-starter?			
▪ Are you persistent, organized, disciplined, trustworthy, creative, and not easily discouraged?			
▪ Are you confident about yourself and comfortable working with professionals such as doctors, nurses, and medical personnel?			
▪ Is your family supportive of your interest and effort to start your own business?			
▪ Are you willing to change your lifestyle so that you can work more hours and more intensely, at least at the beginning of your enterprise?			
▪ Do you enjoy working alone without feedback or praise from others?			
▪ Have you considered working with a partner?			
Business Questions			
▪ Have you had any business training in management, marketing, or sales?			
▪ Do you know how much money you will need to get started?			

(*Continued*)

TABLE 5-1

Questions to Ask to Double-Check Your Decision   (Continued)

QUESTIONS	Y	N	QUALIFYING THOUGHTS
Business Questions (Cont.)			
■ Have you determined your minimum income needs?			
■ Do you know how to do bookkeeping and accounting?			
■ Do you enjoy taking classes on business issues or reading about business in newspapers and magazines?			
■ Do you enjoy working with computers?			
■ Are you open to learning to use new software in desktop publishing, accounting, database management, and other areas?			
■ Do you enjoy negotiating?			
■ Are you willing to do cold calling and selling?			
■ Are you willing to seek business advice from others and accept suggestions and criticism?			

uating your career options and clarifying your true desires. (Even if you have decided to start a medical billing, claims assistance, or transcription business, many of these books will be valuable to you.)

Step 2: Research Your Business

Many people do not like the idea of doing research, preferring to follow their gut feeling, intuition, or perhaps the advice of others. They think research is not action, but rather busywork that does not influence how they act and cannot accomplish what they want to do.

However, given that many new businesses fail during their first year, and that bankruptcy and failure are destructive patterns of behavior, it would seem to be clearly in your best interest to research your new venture. Why risk your money and your goals for lack of a few days of information seeking and asking the right questions? Research not only helps you prevent failure, it also allows you to maximize your potential. If research can help you earn $45,000 in your first year rather than $30,000 because you uncovered a new clinic opening in your community and were the first one to get there, wouldn't that put your business interests in better shape?

The goals of your research should be to find out about the size of the market for your business in your community; to scope out and know your competition, if any; to determine as best you can the optimal way to target your market; to define your company in terms of how your business fits into the industry; to understand the patterns of pricing for your business in your geographic area; and to learn what kinds of mistakes people typically make in your business.

These issues are all vital to making sure you have the best advantage when you get underway. The data you find in researching such issues can influence what title you pick for your company name, how large a geographic area you decide to cover, whether to use direct mail, how many clients you might be able to get in your first year, how long it may take you to break even, and a host of other critical issues that determine whether you remain in business. As you know, most first-year businesses fail, so if you intend to stay in the business, research allows you to better plan your activities and goals, and to be better prepared than the next guy to outlast your competition.

Don't underestimate the power of research! Make some phone calls to doctors' offices and speak with the staff or to the doctor himself or herself. Call a hospital healthcare information department (formerly called medical records) and ask to speak to the supervisor for transcriptionists. Call a local clinic and ask if it has anyone it recommends to those patients who need help filling out claims. Open up the *Yellow Pages* in your city and those within 50 miles, and find out how many companies are listed under Medical Transcription, Billing Services, or Insurance Claims Assistance. Log onto the Internet and search Alta Vista or another search engine for medical transcription or medical billing and review the entries listed. Visit the Web sites of the many organizations and companies involved in the allied health fields, such as NACAP, NEBA, AAMT, HPI, Dictaphone, Lanier, and DVI to learn about trends in your industry.

Call competitors and tell them your plans. Paul and Sarah Edwards report that this method is actually quite useful. If you find that competitors are open about the business and willing to talk, it is a good sign that there is enough business to go around. (You might even get some overflow work simply by doing this.) If you find that people are close-mouthed, you may conclude that times are rough and so you may need to rethink your plans. I found, in researching this book, that all the people I called were open and willing to speak about their businesses. Not only did this indicate to me that they were doing well, but that all the businesses I am covering have ample opportunity for additional players.

Another overlooked avenue for information are your own physicians. Why not use them for information and feedback on your business plans? You will probably find that they are flattered to be asked and might accept an offer to take them to lunch.

Through this footwork and phone calling, you can learn, for example, that you would fare best if you planned to focus on one specialty, such as anesthesiology, because there may already be enough competition in other specialties.

Through your research, you may also find a person who is interested in becoming a partner with you. Some people recognize that they cannot handle all the work, or that they would benefit greatly by having a partner who has different skills, such as marketing experience or a nursing background. You may recall from Chapter 2 that Mary Vandegrift and Heidi Kollmorgen each started out on her own, but both realized shortly thereafter that they didn't enjoy the marketing aspect of medical billing. Each met another woman who had just the talent needed, and now both have successful partnerships. While this option isn't for everyone (many people simply insist on being on their own), collaborations and partnerships, often called strategic alliances, are becoming a more popular and useful paradigm for doing business. (In fact, I have just finished authoring a book with Paul and Sarah Edwards on this topic. Called *Teaming Up*, the book explains how to develop any of ten different types of collaborations and provides legal and financial advice for doing so.)

So, there are many benefits to research. Whether your research period lasts a few days or months, just do it! Although you can also do too much research, and procrastinate starting your venture out of fear, statistics generally indicate that most people don't do enough.

Step 3: Establish Goals and a Business Plan

There are many ways to establish goals, but writing a business plan is the best one. A business plan can range from a formalized document if you are applying for a business loan, to a more informal outline of your future plans and financial projections. Whichever method you choose, a well-conceived written business plan is a map to your destination. It plots the route showing how you will get from point A to point B and serves as a continual reminder of your course.

A business plan usually begins with what is called your company's "mission statement," a terse articulation that explains the heart of your business. This statement expresses what you want customers to think about you, so don't include such statements as "I will make $100,000 within two years." An example of a mission statement for a billing service might be: "To be a dedicated service-oriented company that guarantees the satisfaction of its clients through consistent attention to detail and timeliness on electronic claims and full practice management services."

Don't assume you can eliminate this step if you already have a background in the medical area, such as working for a physician. Despite your experience, writing a business plan will prevent you from falling into the trap of believing that you know how to run a business. Working for someone else is not the same as working for yourself.

An outline of the remainder of a typical business plan is shown in Table 5-2. Each subsection serves a purpose in defining and qualifying your goals, financial expectations, and principles. The more precisely you identify and verbalize your objectives and responses, the better you will fare. Business planning enables you to weed out faulty thinking; it forces you to examine your goals accurately and in detail. By writing down your ideas and thoughts, you can discover inconsistencies and gaps that you failed to notice before.

One important aspect of your business plan is your company name. Now is the time to select it. Your company name is a critical factor in many businesses. You can choose a name to reflect your location, your service, your motto, or your personal attention. Think, for example, of the businesses described in the profiles in this book and the names their owners chose:

- *Billing:* Business Medical Services (Dave Shipton); Medical Management Billing (Nancie Cummins); H/D Medical Receivables, Inc. (Heidi Kollmorgen); Linda's Billing Service (Linda Noel); DAPA Support Services (Daniel Lehmann and Patricia Bartello); AccuMed Solutions (Sheryl Telles and Kathy Allocco)

- *Claims Assistance:* Claims Security of America (Harvey Matoren); In Home Medical Claims (Tom and Nancy Koehler); Claim Relief Inc. (Barbara Melman); Medical Claims Management (Rikki Horne)

- *Transcription:* Words Times 3 (Joan Walston); Monarch Transcription (Terri Ford); Medical Transcription Service (Rochelle Wexler)

TABLE 5-2

Business Plan Outline

I. EXECUTIVE SUMMARY

1. General description of the business plan

2. Introduction to the company

3. Mission statement

4. Brief description of your business goals and financial requirements

II. COMPANY ANALYSIS

1. Strengths and weaknesses analysis

2. Company history

3. Product, program, and service offerings

4. Technology and resources

5. Major competitors and competitive positioning

6. Factors determining success

III. INDUSTRY ANALYSIS

1. Definition and description of industry

2. Growth rate and key factors

3. Financial characteristics of the industry

IV. MARKET ANALYSIS

1. Size of total market

2. Market segmentation and share

3. Market barriers

4. Market demand

5. Price structures and policies

6. Marketing mix (advertising, public relations, direct selling, and sales promotions)

V. STRATEGIC ANALYSIS

1. Goals and objectives

2. Key performance and indicators of success

3. Tactical plans and completion schedules

4. Operating assumptions

TABLE 5-2

Business Plan Outline   (Continued)

VI. MANAGEMENT ANALYSIS

    1. Identification of key personnel

    2. Organizational structure

    3. Management and customer service philosophy

VII. FINANCIAL ANALYSIS

    1. Budget projections and pro formas

    2. Financial schedules and statements

As you can see, some of these owners chose names to suggest their medical expertise, while others emphasized a function of their service or their own name. Spend some time considering your business name. Create several options, and then sound them out with friends and professional acquaintances. Choose one that is memorable and portrays a suitable image in your market. Avoid names that sound like other companies in your area.

For assistance in developing a business plan, consider the following sources:

Business planning software. If you are going into medical billing, the association NEBA has a partially formatted business plan on disk that you can use as a template for your own company. The plan comes with a copy of the well-known software program *Tim Berry's Business Plan Tool Kit,* which you can use to modify the template according to your needs. If you go into claims assistance or medical transcription, you can buy Tim Berry's software, as well as another program, *BizPlanBuilder* by JIAN Tools, in any software or office supply store. (A portion of the NEBA business plan for medical billing is included on the CD-ROM accompanying this book. See Appendix A for information about contacting NEBA and Tim Berry's company, Palo Alto Software.)

Books: There are literally several dozen books that teach how to write a business plan. Look in your local bookstore in the small business section.

Government assistance: Many states publish through their Department of Commerce pamphlets and publications that can help you organize yourself and learn about business planning. There are also various bureaus often affiliated with business schools that can assist you in developing your plans. You might also contact the Small Business Administration at 800-827-5722, from which you can obtain information on a host of topics ranging from business planning and financing to women's and minority business issues. There is also the SBA Office of Women's Business Ownership, which you can reach at 202-205-6673. Every state also has one or more branches of the Small Business Development Centers (SBDC) that are specifically intended to help new entrepreneurs create their business plans and objectives. Call your closest SBA office to find out the location of your nearest SBDC.

The National Association of Women Business Owners, founded in 1978 and now with over 10,000 members and scores of chapters across the country, can also be of service to women seeking information and mentoring when opening a new business. It can be reached at 1100 Wayne Avenue Suite 830, Silver Spring, MD 20910, 301-608-2590 phone, 301-608-2596 fax.

Step 4: Arrange Your Office

Now is the time to organize your home-based business. If you are not a neat, organized person by nature, you can benefit by taking a few days to plan your home office, organize your files, purchase supplies, and set up your computer system.

If you are purchasing new equipment, whether it is a new phone system, a computer, or new software, give yourself time to become comfortable operating it. Many software programs have a "quick start" lesson that teaches the basics in a few hours, but to take full advantage of the software's most powerful features, you need to spend time practicing and using it just as you would for your business.

One caution in setting up your home office according to Herman Holtz, author of several consulting books: don't spend excessive amounts of money equipping your business. A rule of thumb is to buy only when the equipment improves your productivity and pays for itself in your next job. For example, if you need to send out direct mail letters and by purchasing a laser printer, you can save $500 in typesetting and design, this purchase is worthwhile. Similarly, spending an additional $75 on a high-speed 28,800 modem rather than a 14,400 modem can pay off in faster transmissions and less wasted time on the Internet. In general, upgrading to better business equipment that significantly improves your productivity is worthwhile, even if you have to purchase it on credit (interest on business debt may be tax deductible for you; check with your accountant).

If you buy office equipment such as computers, furniture, chairs, or lamps, you can write off up to $18,000 (this amount will increase each year between 1997 and 2003 to $25,000) against your gross business income in that year (assuming you made a profit); you cannot write off expenses to create a loss as long as your earnings are at least $10,000 in that year! In other words, you can only write off against earnings; you cannot use business expenditures to create a loss.

Speaking of taxes, here's an important tip about setting up your home office. Be sure to do it so you can legally take a home office deduction for using part of your living quarters as office space. Even if you use part of a bedroom, you can deduct it as an expense (pro-rated according to its percentage of space compared to the total living space in your home) as long as you use it strictly for business purposes. If you make any improvements to your home office, you can also deduct those direct expenses. Of course, you can also deduct against business income standard business expenses, such as office supplies, stationery, business cards, software, shipping/ postage charges, professional publications and books, business insurance, and advertising. Be sure to check with your accountant for advice on your specific situation before taking any business or home office deductions. If you take such deductions, make sure you have kept records of all your purchases and office supplies to verify them.

To handle their business finances, many home-based business owners use one of the easy-to-learn accounting programs, such as *Quicken, Cash-Graf, DacEasy Accounting 95, Peachtree Accounting*, or *One Write Plus*. These programs have become very easy to use, even for people unfamiliar with accounting and bookkeeping principles. Because none of the businesses covered in this book carry inventory, your accounting will generally be straightforward, and you can most likely keep your books on a "cash" rather than "accrual" basis. If you need assistance in understanding accounting for a home business, go to a bookstore and choose from the many books available on basic accounting procedures.

Step 5: Motivate Yourself to Work and Win

The field of personal performance improvement is growing quickly in the 1990s, as many people have come to recognize that concepts such as creativity, positive thinking, and peak learning are not New Age babble but scientific areas that are researched every day by training and development specialists, instructional designers, and even military planners. In fact, many fascinating general audience books have been published in the past decade that extrapolate on this research.

Starting your own enterprise demands that you maximize your work flow and personal habits. You need to stay motivated and upbeat, learn how to tackle challenges and overcome defeats, and work to your best ability if you want to succeed—and stay healthy. Poor management, one of the leading reasons for business failure, does not only indicate that the entrepreneur did not understand accounting, cash flow, or marketing mix. Poor management can also indicate that the owner has a bad attitude, alienated customers, or became so discouraged that an opportunity to save the business passed right in front of his or her eyes. It is probably an understatement that 50 percent of small business failures happen because people did not have the right personal management skills to keep their business going through rough times.

To motivate yourself, read some of the books listed in Appendix D. These books have helped many people gain greater control of their time, their productivity, and their creativity in business.

Step 6: Be Professional

This step encompasses the many bureaucratic tasks you must take care of to establish your business legally in your community. It also includes the actions you can take to enhance your business image in the eyes of your clientele and the public.

Nearly all home businesses must obtain proper city or county licenses to operate as businesses. You need to make sure that your neighborhood is zoned for home-based businesses, even if you don't have clients coming to your home. If you are doing medical claims assistance, and you have people coming to your home office, be sure that you don't incur the wrath of your neighbors and that you have the proper licenses to run the business from home. You can never tell what might upset a neighbor. One CAP who lived in a condominium complex related to me how her neighbors complained to her association because she had one or two clients per day coming during normal business hours.

In most locales, you need to pay your city or county a few hundred dollars in business license fees. To find out what you owe, check with your city hall or county clerk's office.

If your company uses a name other than your own, you should file a fictitious-name statement, which requires advertising your business name in a local newspaper for a few days and filing paperwork with your city or county. This ensures that you are not accidentally usurping another name already in use.

If you sell any type of product (and some types of services), you may need to register with your state's sales tax board and pay quarterly or monthly sales tax to the state. Check with your accountant about your specific city and state laws.

As mentioned in Chapter 3, if you become a CAP, you may need to be licensed by your state as an insurance broker or public adjuster.

Because you are self-employed and do not have federal taxes and Social Security withheld from a pay check, you will need to file and pay federal and possibly state estimated quarterly taxes on your income. These are due each year on April 15, June 15, September 15, and January 15 for income that was earned in each preceding three-month quarter. One component of what you pay is the "self-employment tax" for your share of Social Security and Medicare taxes. When you work for a company, one-half of this is paid by the employer and the other half is deducted from your paycheck. When you work for yourself, you pay both halves, according to a schedule tied to your net income. Consult your accountant for details about these payments, as there are methods to reduce your liability for the Social Security portion of the tax. Note that you need to keep good records of your income to file these estimates.

Last, you may wish to consider increasing your home insurance to include your home-based business equipment and liabilities. Such extra insurance can usually be done as a rider to your policy for a small additional premium. Whether or not you should buy "errors and omissions insurance" for protection in the event of mistakes you make in your business is difficult to judge. Consult your accountant and lawyer for advice on this issue, as it depends on what assets you need to protect and what risks you take in your business.

Regarding your business image, you can easily enhance the impression you make on your clients by having well-designed and neatly printed stationery and business cards. Try not to settle for the $29.95 special at the local office supply store, as standard business typefaces and logos are not distinctive enough if you want to give the impression of a professional business. Use a desktop publishing software to devise your own logo, or hire a designer to create a specialized logo for your company.

Invest in a high-quality answering machine or voice mail system that allows you to have separate messages for different purposes. A good phone system would have at least two message options (A and B) so that you can record one message for when you are in the office but busy and another message for when you are out. The message you leave on your answering machine or voice mail is important. Don't record an informal or unprofessional message. Call your own machine and listen to your message once in a while to make sure it is working properly and sounds professional. You'd be surprised at how fast, or long, or boring your message may sound to a caller. Many machines allow people to press the star (*) key to bypass the message if they are a frequent caller, so be sure to tell people that.

You should maintain a professional appearance in any of the professions in this book. If you are a male in the medical billing or transcription business, wear a jacket but no tie to meetings with your clients—and don't carry a briefcase. Several people told me that this will prevent receptionists from pegging you as a pharmaceutical salesman and blocking your access to the doctor. You'll have to try this out for yourself.

For many of these issues, it is best to consult a lawyer and an accountant to review your specific situation. For additional assistance in some of the areas of this step, consider joining the newly formed home-based business organization, Small Office Home Office Association (SOHOA). Members of this organization get a variety of benefits, including group health, life, and business insurance; access to a legal service plan that provides with legal advice; the capability to do credit checks on your customers using Dun & Bradstreet services; and the ability to take credit cards (which is difficult to obtain for most home-based businesses). You can reach SOHOA at 1765 Business Center Drive, Reston, VA 22090; phone: 1-888-SOHOA11. Another home-business association is the American Association of Home-Based Businesses, P.O. Box 10023, Rockville, MD 20849, phone 202-310-3130 or 800-447-9710.

Step 7: Invigorate Your Marketing

Each of the chapters in this book has focused on some of the most important marketing concepts for that business. Every home-based business must squarely face the marketing issue, because without customers, you aren't in business. There is no escaping the fact that you should constantly do marketing *all* the time, even when you have a few clients.

This step uses the term "invigorate" quite intentionally. As a home-based business, you don't have the wherewithal to compete with large companies in direct mail volume or in advertising dollars. You need to be creative, originating marketing ideas that make your potential client base take notice of you—and then take action to hire you. Appendix D contains a list of many useful books on marketing, sales, and publicity. Here are some important concepts to keep in mind:

1. Be classic in the design of your marketing materials; don't overdo glitz. This approach provides the professional appearance cherished in the medical market.

2. Have people come to you instead of going to them. Focus your marketing efforts on publicity, networking, and special promotions that make people want your service. Save presentations for someone who has already expressed a strong interest in your service.

3. Obtain personal meetings with your clients, so that they can see who you are and what you can offer. Be pleasant and professional. It's hard to turn down a request for business from a person with whom they've spent some time and have begun to develop a relationship.

4. Referrals are your very best source of business. Use networking to obtain as many leads as you can.

5. Don't lose sight of your cold prospects; call them occasionally to see if their situation has changed.

6. Test your marketing materials. Prepare several different versions of direct mail cards or letters of introduction so that you can test out which one seems to draw the most clientele.

7. Present your information in a simple way that concentrates on what value the customer will get from your service.

8. Devote at least 10 percent to 20 percent of your time on continuous marketing efforts, regardless of how many clients you have. If for some unforeseen reason, a client leaves you and you must replace that business, you will have a much shorter way to go if you have a few warm prospects waiting in the wings.

Step 8: Grow Your Business

When people start their own business, they often don't think they will achieve their target, and so are surprised when they become successful. However, it is important to grow your business slowly while paying attention to the quality of your service. For example, if you find yourself with too many clients to handle alone, your service may suffer and your customers will be disappointed.

Remember to do continuous planning to keep in step with your situation. Revise your plans every few months. Don't let old projections of business growth get stale. If you are to grow your business, you need to keep track of all the details that influence your rate of growth, such as cash flow, hours worked, number of clients, new clients each month, and productivity levels. Accurate record keeping and review will inform you when you might need to put in extra hours to get new clients, or when you might need to hire a temporary assistant.

You also need to grow at a pace that is right for your personality and work habits. You may have dropped out of a corporate job because you were tired of 12-hour days and coming home stressed. If your new home-based business causes you to feel the same stress, you have not gained much. By looking into your heart and taking stock of your true goals, you can reformulate your business direction and reduce the problems that detract from being your own boss. For example, the medical transcriptionist Terri Ford, mentioned in Chapter 4, knew that she wanted to run a home-based business that still gave her time to spend with her children, so she structured her day around that goal and did not force herself to take on more clients than she could readily handle.

Spend one day a month charting your progress. Although you may have started your business because you enjoy the specific work in that field, you still need to be like the president and CEO who stands vigil at the control tower to be sure there are no accidents.

Step 9: $$—Make Money—$$

How do you know if you are making money? Most people look in their checkbook to see if the balance is greater today than yesterday. But this does not mean that you are making money; balances can be deceptive. If you have invoices to get out or collections to make, you are missing money and your checkbook balance does not tell you that. That is why it is better to use an accounting program.

Don't be fooled by your mental or temporary picture of your financial status. Again, use your computer and an accounting package to keep track of your money. Know when you need to get clients to pay, or when you might delay paying a bill yourself to improve your financial picture.

Consider any hesitations you have about making money and refute them. Some people say that they are in business because they like the work, but this is often foolhardy if they are not making enough money to support their business or their families. Why should you settle for $25,000 when you could be making $35,000 or more if you worked more efficiently or priced your service more aggressively? Don't underestimate your potential. If you think you can charge an extra $65 registration fee, do so. If you think you can get the physician to pay $500 for you to do the setup of patients in your medical billing software, by all means ask for it. If the physician disputes your fees, say, "I am just not able to work for free. It will take me two days to enter all your patients, and just as you get paid for your work, I have to get paid for mine." You can always back down and settle for a compromise figure. You need to speak from a position of strength although you needn't hesitate to compromise when necessary. But it isn't worth going into a situation with a compromised position!

Step 10: —Enjoy Yourself!—

If you are going into business for yourself, you probably had a dream that included greater control of your life and more self-respect. On this basis, I highly recommend that you periodically take stock of your business and make sure that you enjoy your work.

One important element are your clients. Do you enjoy working with them and are they worth the financial rewards you gain? Entrepreneurs often feel desperate to accept business even though some customers bring in more problems than profits. We all know that the medical field has its share of egotistical doctors who can be bad businesspeople. There are also front office staff people who, when faced with tremendous pressure to do more than one job, may take their anger out on you. If you are experiencing personality problems with a client, or what appears to you to be an unusual number of snafus, you need to do something about the situation. Either speak up or get out. You do not need to increase your anxiety or financial distress with customers who blockade your success and happiness. This is not to suggest that you abandon clients at the drop of a dime if they are troublesome, but that you look for patterns of behavior that indicate to you that the client is disreputable, egotistical, sexist, or simply not worth your time. Conversely, situations like these may give you an opportunity to test out your personal communication skills. Can you make the situation better by trying to find a way to clear the air?

In short, run your business according to your pleasure and taste. If you are to succeed, you might as well do it your way! I wish you the best of luck in your venture, whatever that might be.

Appendix A

Medical Billing Business Opportunity Vendors

The companies listed on page 274 are all business opportunity vendors. They sell billing and practice management software *plus* some type of training to prepare you to enter the medical billing field. Some people may benefit from purchasing a business opportunity, especially if they do not have a background in health insurance, medical practice management, or sales/marketing. The training and support that a business opportunity vendor provides can improve the chances of success.

There are many medical billing business opportunity vendors in the country. However, it is important to be sure that you buy from a reputable business opportunity dealer. There are reports about vendors who use high-pressure sales techniques to entice you to buy their package, but then do not provide adequate training to help you understand how to use the software or develop a high-quality marketing program to get clients. To protect yourself, please see the suggestions in Chapter 2 for finding a good medical billing business opportunity vendor and some caveats to help you identify unscrupulous vendors.

To simplify your search, the following list includes vendors that, in my view, are among the most reliable and knowledgeable in this business. These vendors offer medical and dental software along with either live training onsite at their offices with professional trainers, or offsite training via phone conference calls and reference materials. Please be aware that purchasing from one of the vendors on this list is not a guarantee that you will succeed in medical billing, nor does it ensure that you will never encounter any problems.

Note that all vendors change their packages and prices, so specific information on prices is not included here. You are encouraged to call each vendor and obtain a brochure showing what is currently included in its package in terms of software (DOS or Windows-based), the extent of study materials provided in its package, the type and location of its training, the cost of ongoing technical and marketing support, and the amount of marketing assistance provided. Which vendor you finally select will be based on your own criteria. Be sure to get a firm understanding with each vendor about how much marketing support you will receive, because marketing your business is the key to success.

ClaimTek
President: Kyle M. Farhat
222 SE 16th Avenue
Portland, OR 97214
800-224-7450 phone
503-239-8316 phone
800-503-9461 fax

Electronic Filing Associates (EFA)
President: Ed Epstein
6900 East Camelback Road
Suite 800
Scottsdale, AZ 85251
800-596-9962 phone
602-481-0464 phone
602-994-9826 fax

Medical Management Software
President: Merry Schiff
1730 South Amphlett Blvd., Suite 217
San Mateo, CA 94402
800-759-8419 phone
415-341-9759 fax

Santiago Data Systems
President: Tom Banks
Director of Sales: Mary Lee Hyatt
1801 Dove Street
Newport Beach, CA 92660-2403
800-652-3500 phone
714-852-6600 phone
714-852-6626 fax

Medical Billing Software Companies

The following companies sell medical and dental billing software only. They do not sell support or training on how to market to healthcare providers. They supply only technical support on using their software.

You may wish to buy directly from one of the following software companies if you believe you have the skills and background to make it on your own. As an alternative to buying from a medical billing business opportunity vendor, you could supplement a direct purchase of software with a home-study course listed in a later section. However, note that this method of studying still requires that you have a good background in health insurance, medical practice management, and marketing. Home study for medical billing without the support of a trained professional is not recommended for those who have a minimal background in the field.

The Computer Place—Medisoft
Contact: Jeff Ward, Marketing Director
Darlene Pickron, Marketing
916 E. Baseline Road
Mesa, AZ 85204
800-333-4747 phone
602-333-4747 phone
602-892-4804 fax
Web site: www.azmedisoft.com

Lytec Software
Lytec Systems
7050 Union Park Center, Suite 390
Midvale, UT 84047
800-735-1991 phone
801-562-0111 phone
801-562-0256 fax
Web site: www.lytec.com

Oxford Medical Systems
President: Gary Boehm
230 Northland Blvd., Suite 223
Cincinnati, OH 45246
800-825-2524 phone
513-772-5102 phone

Associations

The following two organizations are important to join for anyone interested in medical billing:

National Electronic Biller's Alliance (NEBA)
2226 A Westborough Blvd., Suite 504
S. San Francisco, CA 94080
415-577-1190 phone
415-577-1290 fax
Web site: www.nebazone.com

NEBA is a new organization for people in medical billing. The association offers an extensive array of marketing support materials, a home-study course, a newsletter, a template business plan, and certification. Through the association, you can meet many other people who are in the profession and share information and assistance.

New Organization of Claims Assistance Professionals
c/o Lori A. Donnelly
Donnelly Benefit Consultants
2475 Willow Park Road
Bethlehem, PA 18017
610-974-8271 fax
E-mail: dbclad@aol.com

Based on the old NACAP organization, this emerging association, under the leadership of Lori Donnelly, has many members who perform both medical billing and CAP functions. NACAP went out of business just as this new edition of this book was going to press. You can contact Ms. Donnelly for more information about medical billing and claims assistance.

Online Resources

You can find excellent information and an opportunity to chat with colleagues and other people interested in medical billing by going online. The two largest online services in this field are CompuServe and America Online.

- *CompuServe.* First, use the Go command and type "Work." When you enter the Working from Home forum, go to the Library menu and select "Medical Transcription and Billing." This library contains dozens of files with information, reports, and transcripts of conversations or e-mail that are useful to anyone interested in medical billing.

- *America Online.* Enter the key word "Business Strategies," then go to the "Home Business Message Board." Then enter "New" and "Medical Claims Processing."

If you are not a member of either CompuServe or America Online, you can easily subscribe. Both services offer free sign-up disks, which can be found in computer magazines on newsstands everywhere. Otherwise call CompuServe at 800-487-0453 or America Online at 800-827-3338.

Newsletters and Directories

AQC Resource Newsletter
175 N. Buena Vista Avenue, Suite B
San Jose, CA 95126
408-295-4102 phone

Noted medical billing industry watcher Gary Knox publishes this excellent newsletter bi-monthly. The newsletter contains reviews of software, business opportunity companies, notes on healthcare trends.

AQC Resources also publishes **The Directory of Medical Management Software.** This is an excellent compilation of the many companies involved in the medical billing field, including software publishers, business opportunity vendors, clearinghouses, and associations. The directory includes reviews of most of the leading software products and business opportunity vendors.

NOTE: *Readers of this book can purchase the AQC Directory of Medical Management Software at a 10% discount off the usual AQC price. The discounted price is $40.00 including first class shipping and handling. (California residents: add 8.25% state tax, totaling $43.00.) Please make your check out to Rick Benzel and send it to: Benzel/AQC Order, 11670 National Blvd., Suite 104, Los Angeles, CA 90064. Allow 10-14 days for processing and first class delivery.*

Code Facts Newsletter
Published by Medicode
5225 Wiley Post Way, Suite 500
Salt Lake City, UT 84116
800-678-TEXT (8398) phone

This twice-monthly publication includes articles on coding tips, questions and answers, office management strategies, and Medicare policy changes.

Magazines and Professional Journals

Before subscribing to the following magazines and journals, look at a copy at a library or call to ask for a sample copy to determine your level of interest.

Journal of Medical Practice Management
  800-638-6423 or 410-528-4100
  $134 per year

Medical Economics
  800-223-0581
  $94/year

Clearinghouses

There are literally dozens of clearinghouses you can work with. Your software may require you to go through one specific clearinghouse. However, you can likely work with any clearinghouse you want. Contact the following clearinghouse for a competitive rate:

Electronic Translations and Transmittals Corporation (ET&T)
Frank Haraksin, President and Founder
Victorville, CA
619-955-1788 phone
800-950-3868 for information

The following clearinghouse is developing the capability to handle insurance eligibility requests electronically:

EDI Pathways Corporation
Kathy Allocco, Sheryl Telles, and Noreen Sachs
7898 East Acoma Drive, Suite 101
Scottsdale, AZ 85260-3480
888-EDI-CORP phone
602-368-9200 phone

Supplier of Medical Coding and Reference Books

Medicode
5225 Wiley Post Way, Suite 500
Salt Lake City, UT 84116
800-678-TEXT (8398)
Web site: www.medicode.com

Medicode publishes and distributes medical information books, such as ICD-9 and CPT coding books, as well as many others. Ann Jacobsen, Account Specialist, will help you with your reference book needs. For readers of this book, she offers a 15 percent discount on Medicode publications, and 10 percent on other publications. To receive your discount, identify yourself as a reader of this book.

Recommended titles from Medicode:

Understanding Medical Insurance: A Step-by-Step Guide, 3d Edition by Jo Ann C. Rowell

Coders' Desk Reference, published by Medicode

Reimbursement Manual for the Medical Office: A Comprehensive Guide to Coding, Billing, and Fee Management, published by PMIC.

PMIC

4727 Wilshire Blvd., Suite 300
Los Angeles, CA 90010
800-MED-SHOP

PMIC publishes a variety of medical reference books, including books on coding, billing, and practice management. Call for a catalogue. See especially the books on practice management, which can help you understand the physician's point of view.

Home-Study Courses

National Electronic Biller's Alliance (NEBA)

2226 A Westborough Blvd., Suite 504
S. San Francisco, CA 94080
415-577-1190 phone
415-577-1290 fax
Web site: www.nebazone.com

NEBA offers a detailed home-study course in medical billing. The course contains in-depth information on what you need to know to get into medical billing and how to market your services.

At-Home Professions

2001 Lowe Street
Ft. Collins, CO 80525-9949
800-528-7907

At-Home Professions offers a multivolume home-study course in medical billing and also one in medical transcription.

Marketing Support Materials

National Electronic Biller's Alliance (NEBA)
2226 A Westborough Blvd., Suite 504
S. San Francisco, CA 94080
415-577-1190 phone
415-577-1290 fax
Web site: www.nebazone.com

NEBA offers a wide variety of marketing support materials, including an excellent tape program, templates you can use for your brochures and fliers, phone consultations, and software you can use during your presentations.

Communications Plus
Brenda Borneman
28 Coy Park Drive
Newark, IL 60541
815-695-5223 phone

This company supplies mailing lists of medical providers who do not file electronically—exactly what you need for your business. You can order from Brenda directly.

General Business Books

See Appendix D for a list of books on entrepreneuring and marketing your business.

In addition, if you are interested in software to help write your business plan or to assist with your marketing planning, contact the following company about their software products: *Tim Berry's Business Plan Pro* and *Tim Berry's Marketing Plus.* These are two of the best software products available for entrepreneurs.

Palo Alto Software
144 East 14th Avenue
Eugene, OR 97401
800-229-7526 phone
541-683-6162 phone
E-mail: info@palo-alto.com
Web site: www.palo-alto.com

Contact NEBA at the address and phone number on page 280 for a special version of *Tim Berry's Plan Pro* that contains a business plan template for a medical billing business. A sample of this template is included on the CD-Rom accompanying this book.

General Health Information

Health Care Financing Administration (HCFA)
U.S. Department of Health and Human Services
7500 Security Boulevard
Baltimore, MD 21244
Web site: www.hcfa.gov

HCFA is the federal government agency that operates Medicare and Medicaid. You must understand Medicare and Medicaid billing rules and regulations. You can download from HCFA's Web site the most current edition of the *Medicare Handbook,* which will give you a general overview of how Medicare works and what benefits it pays to enrollees. [Note: to view the document just as it is printed, you will need to first download the Adobe Acrobat Reader, which is available free at http://www.adobe.com/acrobat/readstep.html. Then when you go to the hcfa.gov Web site to download the *Medicare Handbook* as a "pdf" file, it will automatically appear on your screen exactly as printed in booklet form. Alternatively, you can visit the hcfa.gov Web site and download the handbook as a straight text (.txt) file, but it will not be formatted in columns and with photos as you would find in the printed document.]

However, this document is intended for the general public, so it is not specific enough to teach you about billing issues you may encounter as a professional medical billing service. To learn more about Medicare, check with the insurance carrier in your state or region that is responsible for handling Medicare claims. Enroll in the billing seminars it offers.

Health Insurance Association of America (HIAA)
1025 Connecticut Avenue NW
Washington, DC 20036-3998
800-828-0111 to order the *Source Book*

HIAA offers an excellent annual publication containing information and statistics about the healthcare industry, particularly relating to health insurance. If you enjoy facts and statistics or want to use such data in your presentations to potential clients, order a copy of the *Source Book of Health Insurance Data,* usually published in a new edition in March of each year.

Appendix B

Associations

New Organization of Claims Assistance Professionals
c/o Lori A. Donnelly
Donnelly Benefit Consultants
2475 Willow Park Road
Bethlehem, PA 18017
610-974-8271 fax
E-mail: dbclad@aol.com

As indicated in the text, the old NACAP organization went out of business just as this new edition of this book was going to press. A new organization is evolving, under the guidance of several active members of NACAP, spearheaded by Lori Donnelly. You can contact her about the status of the new organization and its membership. As the new organization develops, there will be many opportunities for leadership roles and networking.

Training Programs

Institute of Consulting Careers (ICC)
222 SE 16th Avenue
Portland, OR 97214-1488
800-829-9473 phone

ICC is a publisher of professional business training materials. ICC produces a home-study course coauthored by CAP Lori Donnelly and Rick Benzel. The course includes two manuals, two videos, and a diskette containing sample letters, forms, and agreements. The course sells for $495, but ICC will provide a 10 percent discount to readers of this book.

Claims Security of America
Harvey Matoren
3926 San Jose Park
P.O. Box 23863
Jacksonville, FL 32241-3863
904-733-2525 phone
800-400-4066 phone

Harvey Matoren offers workshops and seminars in CAP work. He also has a software program developed for use in his own business. Harvey is an extremely knowledgeable and experienced practitioner of CAP work.

Donnelly Benefit Consultants
Lori Donnelly
2457 Willow Park Road, Suite 219
Bethlehem, PA 18017
610-974-8447 phone
610-974-8271 fax

Lori Donnelly offers workshops and seminars to teach CAP work as well as medical billing. She will also come to your location for a fee to train you in either business.

Information on Medicare

Health Care Financing Administration (HCFA)
U.S. Department of Health and Human Services
7500 Security Boulevard
Baltimore, MD 21244
Web site: www.hcfa.gov

HCFA is the federal government agency that operates Medicare and Medicaid. You must understand Medicare if you work as a CAP. You can download from HCFA's Web site the current yearly edition of the *Medicare Handbook* to get a general overview of Medicare benefits. This publication is updated annually and contains a description of Part A and Part B benefits, deductibles, and copayments. The document is intended for the general public, but it is a good start if you have little knowledge of Medicare. [Note: to view the document just as it is printed, you will need to first download the Adobe Acrobat Reader, which is available free at http://www.adobe.com/acrobat/readstep.html. Then when you go to the hcfa.gov Web site to download the Medicare Handbook as a "pdf" file, it will automatically appear on your screen exactly as printed in booklet form. Alternatively, you can visit the hcfa.gov Web site and download the handbook just as a straight text (.txt) file, but it will not be formatted in columns and with photos as you would find in the printed document.]

General Books on Medicare and Health Insurance

Check your local bookstore for a variety of books that are continually published intended to help consumers understand Medicare and Medigap, such as *Medicare and Medigaps: A Guide to Retirement Health Insurance* by Susan and Leonard Hellman, and *Medicare Made Easy* by Charles Inlander and Charles MacKay. You can also benefit by reading *Understanding Medical Insurance* by Jo Ann C. Rowell, available from NACAP or Medicode (see Appendix A). These resources can add to your general knowledge, although you will need a more in-depth understanding developed through experience and networking with other CAPs.

Hospital Bill Auditing Business Opportunity

Healthcare Data Management, Inc.
President: Bill Conlan
60 Chestnut Avenue, Suite 103
Devon, PA 19333
800-859-5119 phone
610-341-8608 phone
610-989-0658 fax

HDM offers a business opportunity in "hospital and doctor bill auditing." This field is related to CAP work but focuses more specifically on auditing hospital bills. The business opportunity includes software, manuals about the hospital billing business, general business manuals, contact management software, sample marketing materials, and two days of training in the Philadelphia area (airfare not included).

Appendix C

Home-Study Programs

Many community colleges and vocational schools offer training for medical transcription. However, if you are not inclined to attend an academic program, consider the following home-study programs:

SUM (Systems Unit Method) Program for Medical Transcription Training
Health Professions Institute (HPI)
P.O. Box 801
Modesto, CA 95353
209-551-2112 phone
Website: www.hpisum.com

The SUM program is considered to be the top-ranked program for learning medical transcription. The basic program, called the Beginning Medical Training (BMT), consists of a specific syllabus of readings plus 12 tapes that utilize authentic dictations. It normally takes 480 hours to complete the basic program, including all the recommended readings. (That amounts to 12 weeks if you study for 40 hours per week; or 24 weeks at 20 hours per week.) The advanced program consists of five additional modules in various specialties: cardiology, gastroenterology, orthopedics, pathology, and radiology.

HPI also sells a wide assortment of reference and word books for medical transcriptionists, and it publishes a quarterly magazine, *Perspectives on the Medical Transcription Profession*.

Review of Systems (ROS)
Jennifer Martin
1633 NE Rosewood Drive
Gladstone, MO 64118
800-951-5559 phone
816-468-4403 phone
E-mail: MTMonthly@AOL.com
Web site: www.tyrell.net/~mtmonth

ROS uses the same materials from SUM program, but in an interactive format. Ms. Martin provides personal feedback on your assignments, grades

287

your tests, and generally helps you with your progress in accomplishing the SUM program. ROS is useful for people who want to study independently but would like a watchful eye helping them along the way.

California College for Health Sciences
222 West 24th Street
National City, CA 91950
800-221-7374 phone
Web site: http://cchs.edu

CCHS offers an Associate of Science degree program specializing in medical transcription. CCHS is a recognized degree-granting institution for distance education. The program in medical transcription utilizes the SUM program materials.

Medical Management Software
President: Merry Schiff
1730 South Amphlett Blvd., Suite 217
San Mateo, CA 94402
800-759-8419 phone
415-341-9759 fax

Medical Management Software is a reseller of the SUM program. Contact Merry Schiff to learn about the discount offered for the beginning SUM program for readers of this book.

At-Home Professions
2001 Lowe Street
Fort Collins, CO 80525
800-528-7907 phone

At-Home Professions offers its own independent study course in medical transcription, consisting of five modules. Each module contains a study manual/workbook and tapes.

Newsletter

MT Monthly
Suite 100
1633 NE Rosewood Drive
Gladstone, MO 64118
800-951-5559 or 816-468-4403 phone
Published by Jennifer Martin
$48 per year or $90 for two years

The newsletter contains articles of interest to the home-based transcriptionist, including business issues, product reviews, updates on new terminology and technology, new drug information, and humor. You can download a copy from CompuServe, on the Working from Home forum, in the library section for medical transcription. You can also see a recent copy on the Internet at www.Tyrell.net/~mtmonth.

Business Training

For an in-depth examination of becoming an independent medical transcriptionist, see

The Independent Medical Transcriptionist
Donna Avila-Weil and Mary Glaccum
Rayve Productions, Inc.
Box 726
Windsor, CA 95492
800-852-4890 phone

This book contains a detailed presentation of the issues involved in becoming an independent transcriptionist. Recommended reading if you are serious about this profession.

Medical Terminology, Word, and Reference Books

Medical transcriptionists need an assortment of reference and words books to check spelling of terms and definitions. You can order a wide variety of reference and terminology books from Health Professions Institute and AAMT. See their listings for ordering information. You can also order reference materials from the American Medical Association; to obtain its catalog, call 800-621-8335 and ask for customer service.

In addition, there are many major publishers of medical reference and word books, including

- F.A. Davis Company, 1915 Arch St., Philadelphia, PA 19103, 800-523-4049
- J.B. Lippincott, East Washington Square, Philadelphia, PA 19105, 800-638-3030

- South-Western Publishing, 4770 Duke Drive, Suite 200, Mason, OH 45040, 800-242-7972

- Springhouse Publishing Company, 1111 Bethlehem Pike, Springhouse, PA 19477, 800-346-7844

- W.B. Saunders Company, 6277 Sea Harbor Drive, Orlando, FL 32887, 800-545-2522

- Williams & Wilkins, 428 East Preston Street, Baltimore, MD 21202, 800-638-0672

Spell Checking Software

The following companies produce specialized spell checking databases in the medical field that work either with a standard word processor such as *WordPerfect* or with a proprietary word processor:

- Spellex Development (medical spell check for DOS and Windows) 800-442-9673

- Sylvan Software (medical spell check for DOS and Windows) 800-235-9455

- W.B Saunders Company (medical spell check for DOS and Windows) 800-545-2522

- Williams & Wilkins (medical spell check for DOS, Windows, and Mac) 800-527-5597

Word-Expanding Software

Word-expanding software allows you to type just the first few characters of long medical words and have the entire word appear, saving keystrokes and time. The following companies provide such word-expanding software:

- Hawk Technologies, Inc.—Product: *ShortCut*—770-640-1151

- Narratek—Product: *Smartype*—617-566-1066

- Productive Performance—Product: *Medical Macro Expanders*—206-788-8300

- Productivity Software International—Product: *PRD + MedEasy*—212-818-1144

- Summit Software—Product: *FlashForward*—800-577-6665

- Textware Solutions—Product: *InstantText*—800-355-5251

- Twenty-First Century Research—Product: *Explode-It!*—800-563-5418

Associations

Health Professions Institute (HPI)
P.O. Box 801
Modesto, CA 95353
209-551-2112 phone
209-551-0404 fax

HPI is not actually an association, but if you are a student of medical transcription, you can join its network MTSN (Medical Transcription Student Network). Benefits include a free subscription to HPI's magazine *Perspectives* and to a special newsletter for students *MTSN Gazette*. You also receive a 10 percent discount on reference books purchased from HPI and Williams and Wilkins.

Medical Transcription Industry Alliance (MTIA)
Executive Director: Catherine Baxter
Houston, TX
713-313-6050 phone
713-313-6051 fax
e-mail: csbmtia@icsi.net
Web site: www.wwma.com/a2/mtia

Begun as an association for owners of large medical transcription services, MTIA has branched into representing transcription businesses of any size, including one- and two-person small-office and home-based independents. Today, MTIA is geared to meet the educational and networking needs of many transcription businesses and interested students who are planning a career in medical transcription. Among the goals of MTIA are to promote uniform performance standards, to educate transcriptionists about new technologies and industry changes, and to provide business information for committed entrepreneurs. MTIA has several membership categories, including an associate membership for those who are just getting under way in an independent business. The CD-ROM accompanying this book contains a document about the history of MTIA.

American Association for Medical Transcription
Pat Forbis—Associate Executive Director
P.O. Box 576187
Modesto, CA 95357-6187
800-982-2182 phone (Ask for Director of Member Services)
209-551-0883 phone
Web site: www.sna.com/aamt

AAMT is oriented toward promoting the continuing education and high-level ethical and professional standards for transcriptionists. In general, it is not oriented toward teaching you the entrepreneurial skills of starting and running a small or independent medical transcription business, although it now has a business issues subgroup. If you are a student in a full-time college program or a working transcriptionist, you may wish to join AAMT to obtain its benefits: an excellent quarterly journal, *JAAMT*, which contains many articles to help you continue your medical transcription education. AAMT has local subchapters in many areas as well. AAMT also offers a certification exam that may add credibility to your business. The exam is in two parts—written and practical; you must pass the first portion before you can take the second. You do not need to be a member of AAMT to take the certification exam.

Online Services

- *CompuServe.* To find the forum for medical transcriptionists, use the GO command and type WORK. This will take you to the Working from Home forum; then choose LIBRARY, and select "Medical Billing and Transcription." This library contains files of interest to medical transcriptionists, including transcripts of past conversations among transcriptionists and reviews of hardware and software.

- *America Online.* You will find the transcriptionists under EXCHANGE, Home/Health Careers, on the Careers Bulletin Board.

- *Prodigy.* You will find medical transcriptionists on the Careers Bulletin Board under the Medical Transcription Topic.

- *Genie.* Genie has its own software (Aladdin), which can be downloaded once you have registered and are online. You will find the MTs on the Medical Bulletin Board.

In addition, the Internet has become a burgeoning resource for transcriptionists. There is a medical transcription newsgroup called sci.med.transcription, where you can chat with many others and read previous conversations between transcriptionists who debate the fine points of which associations to join and which technology to use. There are also many home pages belonging to transcriptionists on the Net. For example, see the Web site, www.angelfire.com.

Appendix D

Resources for Double-Checking Your Decision

- *To Build the Life You Want, Create the Work You Love,* by Marsha Sinetar, St. Martin's Press
- *Finding Your Perfect Work,* by Paul and Sarah Edwards, Jeremy P. Tarcher/Putnam
- *Growing a Business,* by Paul Hawken, Fireside/Simon & Schuster
- *Honey, I Want to Start My Own Business: A Planning Guide for Couples,* by Azriella Jaffe, HarperBusiness
- *How to Find Your Mission in Life,* by Richard Bolles, Ten Speed Press
- *On Your Own: A Guide to Working Happily, Productively and Successfully at Home,* by Lionel Fischer, Prentice Hall

In addition to these books, contact the various associations listed in Appendices A to C, including NEBA, NACAP, AAMT, HPI, and MTIA, to obtain general information about the professions they represent. Speaking to people in these associations can often be useful in helping you decide if you want to enter the career they represent.

Resources for Motivation

- *Aha: Ten Ways to Free Your Creative Spirit and Find Your Great Ideas,* by Jordan Ayan, Random House
- *The Greatest Salesman in the World,* by Og Mandino, Warner
- *How to Succeed on Your Own: Overcoming the Emotional Roadblocks,* by Karin Abarbanel, Holt
- *How to Think Like an Entrepreneur,* by Michael B. Shane, Bret Publishing
- *The Secrets of Successful Self-Employment,* by Paul and Sarah Edwards, Jeremy P. Tarcher/Putnam

- *Seven Habits of Highly Effective People,* by Steven Covey, Fireside/Simon & Schuster
- *Seven Laws of Spiritual Success,* by Deepak Chopra, Amber Allen Publishing

Resources to Invigorate Your Marketing

- *Do It Yourself Marketing,* by David Ramacitti, Amacom
- *Grow Your Own Business with Desktop Marketing,* by Steven Morgenstern, Random House
- *How to Get Big Results from a Small Advertising Budget,* by Cynthia Smith, Carol Publishing
- *How to Get Clients,* by Jeff Slutsky, Warner
- *Secrets of Savvy Networking,* by Susan RoAne, Warner
- *Successful Presentations for Dummies,* by Malcolm Kushner
- *The Ultimate Sales Letter,* by Daniel Kennedy, Bob Adams Publishing
- *Street Smart Marketing,* by Jeff Slutsky, Wiley
- *The World's Best Known Marketing Secret,* by Ivan R. Misner, Bard & Stephen

SPECIALTY ITEMS

- *The Business Generator,* by Paul and Sarah Edwards, includes a copy of *Getting Business to Come to You* plus a special program created by the Edwardses to help you understand your preferred marketing methods and develop an effective marketing strategy. Call 800-561-8990 for orders.

Business Planning Books

- *Business Planning Guide,* by David Bangs Jr., Upstart
- *How to Write a Business Plan,* by Mike McKeever, Nolo Press
- *Preparing a Successful Business Plan,* by Rodger Touchie, Self-Counsel Press
- *Successful Business Plans: Secrets and Strategies,* by Rhonda M. Abrams, Oasis Press

SOFTWARE

- *BizPlanBuilder,* Jian Tools for Sales, Inc.

- *The Medical Billing Business Plan Template,* available from NEBA (see listing in Appendix A), includes a copy of Tim Berry's *Business Planning Software*

General Business Books

- *The E-Myth: Why Most Small Businesses Don't Work and What to Do About It,* by Michael Gerber

- *The Home Office and Small Business Answer Book,* by Janet Attard, Henry Holt

- *The Idiot's Guide to Starting Your Own Business,* by Edward Paulson with Marcia Layton, Alpha Books

- *Running a One Person Business,* by Claude Whitmeyer, Salli Rasberry, and Michael Philips, Ten Speed Press

- *Teaming Up,* by Paul and Sarah Edwards and Rick Benzel, Putnam/Jeremy P. Tarcher

- *Streetwise Guide to Small Business Startup,* Bob Adams, Bob Adams Publishing

- *Working from Home,* by Paul and Sarah Edwards, Jeremy P. Tarcher/Putnam

In addition to these books, visit the web site for Paul and Sarah Edwards at www.workingfromhome.com. Here you will find a wealth of information about home-based professions. The Edwards are also the hosts of a weekly radio show which you can hear in many cities on the Business Radio Network, or you can hear it live at the web site www.cfra.com (assuming you have installed audio plug-in software that allows you to download broadcasts and sounds off the Internet using Netscape or Microsoft Explorer). You can also order an interactive CD-ROM version of their noted book on marketing, *Getting Business to Come to You,* by calling 800-756-0339.

General Business Associations

National Association of Women Business Owners (NAWBO)
1100 Wayne Avenue, Suite 830
Silver Spring, MD 20910
301-608-2590 phone
301-608-2596 fax

NAWBO is the premier organization for women entrepreneurs. There are hundreds of local chapters that provide business information, support, and opportunities for networking.

Small Office Home Office Association (SOHOA)
1765 Business Center Drive
Reston, VA 22090
1-888-SOHOA11 phone
1-703-438-3049 fax

SOHOA provides networking and educational opportunities for self-employed individuals. Through the power of the association, you can purchase automobile, home, health, and life insurance at group rates. It also has a special program with a bank that allows you to accept credit cards for payment.

Appendix E

CONTENTS OF THE CD-ROM

The CD-ROM accompanying this book contains "demos" of seven medical billing software programs and a demonstration copy of the medical billing business plan template available from NEBA. In some cases, the demonstration versions are live working software, although they have been disabled or limited in some fashion, such as the number of patients they can store or actions they can perform. In other cases, the demonstration is a self-running presentation of the software.

Note: All of the software publishers included here may have put out newer versions of their software since this CD-ROM was compiled. Please call the vendors directly to obtain information about any new releases they have; their direct phone numbers are provided below.

The following information explains how to use the CD-ROM.

Installation Procedures

To install the software programs on your computer from the CD-ROM, follow these instructions:

For Windows 95 systems:

Save and close all programs and documents currently running. (One of the demos requires you to restart your computer after its installation, so you don't want to lose any data you may be in the middle of working on when this occurs. It is therefore important to save your data first and close all running applications before starting this installation procedure.)

Insert the CD-ROM into the drive. Select the [Start] button.

From the Start menu, select the "Run" option.

At the "Run" prompt, type the following: E:\SETUP.EXE (or use whatever drive letter is associated with your CD-ROM drive)

Follow the prompts on the screen to complete the installation. You will

299

be prompted to select the programs you want to install, and you may "uncheck" any programs you don't want.

All the programs (except OneClaim Plus) will automatically be installed to your hard drive. These will be grouped together and listed as "Benzel Demos" on the Programs submenu of your "Start" menu.

The last program, OneClaim Plus, has its own installation program. After the first seven programs have been automatically installed, a separate installation wizard will automatically take over and install OneClaim Plus. It will then prompt you to restart Windows before continuing. **Note:** OneClaim Plus will not be listed as part of Benzel Demos; it has its own listing in your Programs submenu.

After the installation, look at the "Copyright and Contacts Readme" file before using any of the software. This file contains information about your warranty from McGraw-Hill, as well as listing all the addresses and phone numbers of the software companies included on this CD-ROM. You may wish to print out this file.

To run any program (except for OneClaim Plus), go to "Benzel Demos" and select it. Further details are provided below. To run OneClaim Plus, it is listed as a separate title on your Program menu. Some of the software programs also contain Readme files that explain the specifics of how to use them. Read these files for assistance in how to use each software product.

For Windows 3.1x systems

Save and close all running applications first to be sure you do not lose any data.

Insert the CD-ROM into the drive. From the "File" menu, select "Run."

At the Run prompt, type the following (use the drive letter associated with your CD-ROM drive): D:\SETUP.EXE.

Follow the prompts on the screen to complete the installation.

The presentation will be installed in a group folder named "Benzel Demos" which will appear on your desktop.

To run any software, click on its icon or on a Readme file associated with that software. Further details are provided below.

There is also a "Copyright and Contacts Readme" file which you should read first. This contains a listing of all the software companies and warranty information.

NOTE: *Santiago's OneClaim Plus operates only with Windows 95. When you are installing the other 7 programs, you will receive a prompt reminding you that this software will not install on your system if you are working under Windows 3.x. Be sure to "uncheck" this software from the install box if you are running Windows 3.x.*

Uninstall Procedures

For Windows 95 systems

For all Benzel Demo Applications:

Select the "Uninstall Readme" icon from the Benzel Demo Applications program group. This contains specific information about how to uninstall the programs, including OneClaim Plus.

For Windows 3.x systems

To uninstall the software, refer to the "Uninstall Readme" file under "Benzel Demos."

Detailed Guidance to Use Each Program

1. InfoHealth Demonstration Software: The Claims Manager
InfoHealth (a division of Synaps Corporation) has provided a demonstration of its medical billing software, The Claims Manager. The demonstration includes a working but limited version of the company's software with complete instructions for a walk-through.

To run the software:

Select "InfoHealth Presentation" from the program group Benzel Demos. A main menu screen will appear, containing 3 categories.

Opportunity—under this category, two buttons appear: The Industry and Synaps Corporation. Clicking on each button will reveal a document you can read.

The Solution—under this category, the Features and How to Order buttons also contain documents to read.

Software Showcase—under this category, there are 3 buttons:

Overview—this button provides a self-running tour. (Use the right arrow key to advance through the tour; hit the escape key if you want to exit it.)

Instructions—this button provides important information for using the demo.

Demonstration—this button launches you into a demo of the Info-Health software.

Important note: Before trying the demo, click on the "Instructions" button and print them out; you will need them to operate the software and get a feel for how to use it.

NOTE: *When trying the actual software, try printing out sample patient statements and monthly reports. If you want to do so, be sure to change the parameter for "Print Device" from "Output1.opt" by pressing the F1 key and selecting "Printer1."*

Additional note: Do not uninstall this demo from the main menu. Use the uninstall Wizard that comes with the Benzel Demos and uninstalls all the software programs at once (except for OneClaim Plus).

For more information, contact Synaps Corporation/InfoHealth at 800-455-2544.

2. Lytec Systems Demonstration Software: Lytec Medical for Windows Lytec has provided a working but limited copy of its medical billing software, Lytec Medical for Windows.

To run the software:

Open the instructions found in the file called Lytec Readme. Print out the file, as this contains a tutorial to help you walk through the software using sample data.

Select the software Lytec Medical from Benzel Demos. Follow the instructions for using the software in the Readme file. The demo includes hypothetical sample data that is automatically loaded, allowing you to practice with the software.

There is also a Lytec Help file in Benzel Demos that contains general Help screens about the software.

For more information, contact Lytec Systems at 800-735-1991.
Lytec is also sold by the following two business opportunity vendors:

Medical Management Software (800-759-8419)

Claim-Tek (800-224-7450).

3. Santiago SDS, Inc. Demonstration Software: OneClaim Plus
Santiago SDS, Inc. has provided a demonstration copy of its software, OneClaim Plus. This is a working but limited version of the software.

NOTE: *This software requires Windows 95, a Pentium processor, and 20MB of free space on your hard drive. Remember, this software does not appear under Benzel Demos on your Programs menu; it is listed separately. However, the Readme and Help files for this software are located in Benzel Demos.*

To run the software:

Open the "OneClaim Plus Readme" file located in Benzel Demos that provides complete instructions for using the demo. You may wish to print out this file before using the software.

Select "OneClaim Plus for Windows" located on your Programs menu of your Start Button. (Remember, this program is not located under Benzel Demos. It insisted on having its location on the Programs menu of your Start menu.)

There is also a Santiago Help file located under Benzel Demos. This file contains general help screens about the software.

For more information, contact Santiago SDS, Inc. at 800-652-3500.

4. ClaimTek Systems Demonstration Software: Data-Link
ClaimTek has provided a demonstration copy of its medical practice management software for Windows, Data-Link. This software is not a medical billing program; it is intended to be used in a physician's office, to which your independent medical billing service would be linked. The staff in a

physician's office uses Data-Link to record patient visits and perform practice management for the physician. The independent billing service links up with Data-Link over the modem to download the data that the office staff has keyboarded, with which it can perform the billing and electronic claims submission. The medical billing service then uploads updated account information back to the physician's office. Data-Link interfaces with Lytec Medical for Windows, which ClaimTek sells you with Data-Link.

To run the software:

NOTE: *There are no specific instructions with this demo program. Begin by clicking on the "Locate Patient" button and then type in "Smith." This will bring up a patient into the main field, and you can then click on any of the other buttons to peruse the screens.*

For more information, contact Claim-Tek at 800-224-7450.

5. *Medisoft Demonstration Software á Medisoft Advanced Patient Accounting*   Medisoft has provided a demonstration copy of its software, Medisoft Advanced Patient Accounting (DOS-based). The software includes a self-running screen show demo that walks you through the software. Medisoft is developing a Windows-based version of this product.

To run the software:

Select "Medisoft Patient Accounting" from Benzel Demos. The program will load and begin. The main menu screen gives you the option of choosing a self-running demo or using an actual version of the software. It is recommended that you select the self-running demo first. Hit any key to walk through the self-running demo. Hit Escape to exit the demo and go to the actual software.

When you are working in the actual software, use your down arrow key on the main menu to select the option "Exit" when you want to quit. The escape key does not exit the software and return you to Windows.

For more information, contact Medisoft at 800-333-4747.

6. *Oxford Medical Systems Demonstration Software: WinClaim IV for DOS*   Oxford Medical Systems has provided a demonstration version of its software WinClaim. (Note: the program is DOS-based.) The demo contains both a self-running presentation and a working but limited copy of the software that you can actually use to run a medical billing business. (The live software is limited to 500 patients, but it will keep records and print HCFA 1500 forms. However, it will not send electronic claims.)

To run the software:

Select "WinClaim Demonstration" from Benzel Demos to see a self-running demo of the software. Hitting any key will advance you through the demo.

Go to Benzel Demos and select "WinClaim Readme." This provides information on how to use the actual software. After you have printed out this Readme file, go to next step.

Select WinClaim Introduction" from Benzel Demos. The WinClaim software will start. Follow the directions in the Readme file.

For more information, contact Oxford Medical Systems at 513-772-5102.

7. Healthcare Data Management, Inc. Demonstration Software: Medical Bill Auditing   This company has provided a self-running presentation of its medical bill auditing business opportunity. The demo does not include the software HDM sells for hospital bill auditing. Be sure to ask the company for a demo of its complete software before investing.

To run the demo:

Select "Healthcare Readme" from Benzel demos. Read the file for information on using the demo.

Select "Healthcare Presentation" from Benzel Demos to start the software.

Anytime you want to advance to the next slide, press the enter key.

When you see a blue box, click the left button of your mouse on this box and it will display additional information about the topic.

When you want to exit the program, press the escape key.

For more information, contact Healthcare Data Management, Inc. at 800-859-5119.

8. *Business Plan Pro—Medical Billing Business Planning Software Demo* The National Electronic Biller's Alliance has produced a business plan template for people starting a medical billing business. This template operates by using the well-known software program, Tim Berry's Business Plan Pro_, produced by Palo Alto Software. This demo version allows you to read the entire business plan and see the graphics that accompany it. However, you cannot print the business plan or edit it. (You need to purchase a copy to customize it for your business.)

To run the software:

Select "Business Plan Pro" from Benzel Demos.

When the main menu appears, click on the button for "Open a business plan." Choose the existing plan called "Ezclaim1.bps."

The medical billing business plan template will load and your screen will divide in half. The top half explains what section of the business plan you are in. This half of the screen provides directions on what to write if you were actually writing a business plan yourself. The bottom half of the screen shows you what is already written in the medical billing template. When you first open up the template, you are automatically placed into the first section of the business plan, Executive Summary.

You can read the existing business plan template, going from section to section to see what someone starting a medical billing business might have written. To see other parts of the business plan, click on the buttons on the bottom of the screen "Next Topic" or to go back to what you have already read, click on "Previous Topic." You can also see a list of the entire contents of the business plan by clicking on the "Select Topic" button. This will reveal a full listing of all business plan sections, and you can jump to any one of them.

As you read each section of the business plan, the top of the screen will occasionally reveal a "table" icon or a "graph" icon. This indicates that this section of the business plan has an accompanying table or graph. Click on the icon to view the table or graph.

You cannot print the business plan in this demo version, but you read the entire document in print preview mode. Go to "File" menu, select "Print," then "Print Preview." This allows you to read it more quickly. If you want, you can go back to each section of the business plan and read it in detail, as well as see the type of instructions the business planning software provides to people who are writing their own plans.

The "save" and "print" function of this software have been disabled out of consideration for the publisher and NEBA who sell them. Obviously, you must purchase a copy of the software and business plan template if you want to edit, rewrite, and customize it for your own business. To purchase a full working copy of the business planning software with the medical billing business plan template that you can customize for your business, contact NEBA at 415-577-1190. You can also contact Palo Alto Software at 144 E. 14th Ave., Eugene, OR 97401 (phone: 800-229-7526) to purchase just the business planning software. Note: only NEBA sells the combined software plus medical billing business plan template. Palo Alto Software sells only their business planning software.

For further information, contact NEBA for questions about the content of the business plan template, or for technical questions, contact Palo Alto Software at the phone numbers above.

NOTICE: *All software names are either Copyrighted, Trademarked, or Registered by their respective owners.*

Books Available from Rick Benzel
Ordering Information

Directory of Medical Management Software published by AQC Resource Books $36.00

Making Money in a Health Service Business on Your Home-Based PC $29.95

Working from Home, by Paul and Sarah Edwards $15.95

Finding Your Perfect Work, by Paul and Sarah Edwards $16.95

Teaming Up: The Small Business Guide to Collaborating with Others to Boost Your Earnings and $13.95
Expand Your Horizons, by Paul and Sarah Edwards and Rick Benzel

Aha! Ten Ways to Free Your Creative Spirit and Find Your Great Ideas, by Jordan Ayan, edited $15.00
by Rick Benzel

Note: California residents must add 8.25% sales tax to their total.

*Add $4.00 for the first book ordered and $2.00 for **each** book thereafter to cover shipping and handling fees.*

Send your check to
Rick Benzel
11670 National Boulevard, Suite 104
Los Angeles, CA 90064

Indicate which title(s) you want, and clearly print your name, shipping address, and phone number.
Allow 10-14 days for delivery. Remember to add shipping and handling fees as indicated.

Discounts are available for quantity purchases. Please write to the address indicated.

INDEX

About the Author

Rick Benzel is a freelance writer specializing in entrepreneurial opportunities and home-based business. He works closely with Paul and Sarah Edwards, and is the coauthor with them of *Teaming Up: The Small Business Guide to Collaborating with Others to Boost Your Earnings and Expand Your Horizons.*

SOFTWARE AND INFORMATION LICENSE